BTEC NATIONAL

Health and Social Care

Book 1

Eleanor Langridge

With:
Lisa Bossons
Deborah Boys
Val Michie
Jacky Roe

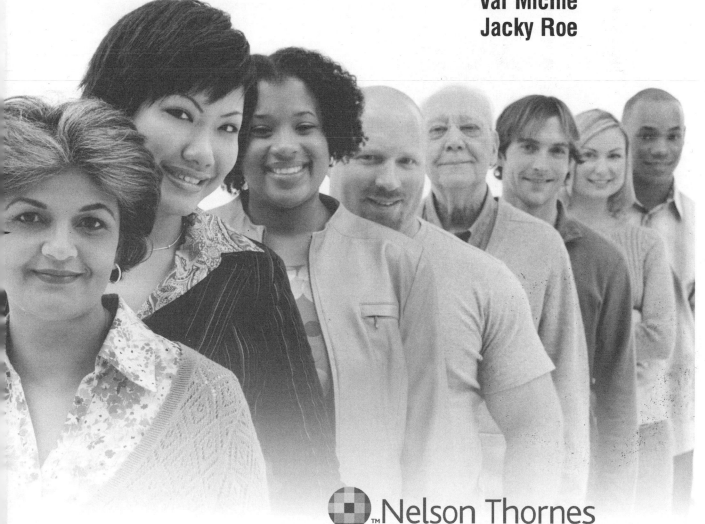

™ Nelson Thornes
a Wolters Kluwer business

Text © Eleanor Langridge, Lisa Bossons, Deborah Boys, Val Michie and Jackie Roe 2007
Original illustrations © Nelson Thornes Ltd 2007

Published in 2007 by:
Nelson Thornes Ltd
Delta Place
27 Bath Road
CHELTENHAM
GL53 7TH
United Kingdom

07 08 09 10 11 / 10 9 8 7 6 5 4 3 2 1

A catalogue record for this book is available from the British Library

ISBN 978 0 7487 8404 2

Cover photograph/illustration by Digital Vision
Illustrations by Angela Lumley
Page make-up by Pantek Arts Ltd, Maidstone, Kent

Printed and bound in Slovenia by Korotan

Contents

Introduction

Health and social care workers work with diverse groups of vulnerable people including children, young adults, elderly people and people with mental health problems and learning difficulties. They work in a variety of settings such as hospitals, care homes and people's own homes. Now is an exciting time to be a care worker because reforms are creating new jobs and flexible ways of working, and there is a huge amount of opportunity for career progression. If you are committed to working in care and enthusiastic about training and development, you can be assured of a challenging and rewarding career. The BTEC National Diploma in Health and Social Care will get you off to a flying start by preparing you both for work in health and social care and for further study.

How do you use this book?

Covering all 8 core units of the new 2007 specification and 2 specialist units, this book has everything you need if you are studying BTEC National Certificate or Diploma in Health and Social Care. Simple to use and understand, it is designed to provide you with the skills and knowledge you need to gain your qualification. We guide you step by step toward your qualification, through a range of features that are fully explained over the page.

Which units do you need to complete?

BTEC National Health and Social Care Book 1 provides coverage of 10 units for the BTEC National Diploma in Health and Social Care. To achieve the Diploma, you are required to complete 8 core units plus specialist units that provide for a combined total of 1080 guided learning hours (GLH). *BTEC National Health and Social Care Book 1* provides you with the following:

Core Units	Specialist Units
Unit 1 Developing Effective Communication in Health and Social Care	Unit 10 Caring for children and Young People
Unit 2 Equality, Diversity and Rights in Health and Social Care	Unit 11 Supporting and Protecting Adults
Unit 3 Health, Safety and Security in Health and Social Care	
Unit 4 Development Through the Life Stages	
Unit 5 Fundamentals of Anatomy and Physiology for Health and Social Care	
Unit 6 Personal and Professional Development in Health and Social Care	
Unit 7 Sociological Perspectives for Health and Social Care	
Unit 8 Psychological Perspectives for Health and Social Care	

BTEC National Health and Social Care Book 2 offers coverage of a further 8 specialist units (plus additional free online resources), providing the 1080 Guided Learning Hours required for the Diploma.

Is there anything else you need to do?

1   Talk to people who use health and social care services. Find out how they want to be cared for and what sort of qualities they would like to see in their care workers.

2   Talk to people who work in the health and social care industry. Find out what qualifications, skills and experience they needed to get their job and what their work involves.

3   Get as much experience as you can in the care industry and be aware of what your experiences teach you.

4   Take responsibility for learning about service users and the health and social care industry. In addition to completing all the work your teacher or tutor sets, ask questions and watch, read and listen to anything that will improve your knowledge and understanding.

5   Never be afraid to ask for help when you need it.

We hope you enjoy your BTEC course - Good Luck!

Features of this book

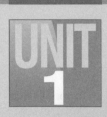

UNIT 1

Developing effective communication in health and social care

This unit covers:

- Effective communication and interpersonal interaction
- Factors that influence communication and interpersonal interactions in health and social care settings
- Knowing how patients and service users may be assisted by effective communication
- Demonstrating own communication skills in a caring role

People who work in health and social care require good communication skills in order to carry out their roles effectively. This chapter explores what communication skills are and how they are used to help clients and service users in health and social care settings. Factors that enhance and inhibit communication will also be examined in detail so that interpersonal skills can be reviewed and developed.

Learning Objectives

At the beginning of each Unit there will be a bulleted list letting you know what material is going to be covered. They specifically relate to the learning objectives within the specification.

Grading Criteria

The table of Grading Criteria at the beginning of each unit identifies achievement levels of pass, merit and distinction, as stated in the specification.

To achieve a **pass**, you must be able to match each of the 'P' criteria in turn.

To achieve **merit** or **distinction**, you must increase the level of evidence that you use in your work, using the 'M' and 'D' columns as reference. For example, to achieve a distinction you must fulfil all the criteria in the pass, merit and distinction columns. Each of the criteria provides a specific page number for easy reference.

grading criteria

To achieve a **Pass** grade the evidence must show that the learner is able to:	To achieve a **Merit** grade the evidence must show that, in addition to the pass criteria, the learner is able to:	To achieve a **Distinction** grade the evidence must show that, in addition to the pass and merit criteria, the learner is able to:
P1 describe different types of communication and interpersonal interaction, using examples relevant to health and social care settings Pg 6	**M1** explain how the communication cycle may be used to communicate difficult, complex and sensitive issues Pg 19	**D1** analyse how communication in health and social care settings assists patients/ service users and other key people Pg 43
P2 describe the stages of the **communication cycle** Pg 19	**M2** explain the specific communication needs patients/service users may have that require support, including the use of technology Pg 42	**D2** analyse the factors that influenced the interactions undertaken Pg 45
P3 describe factors that may influence communication and interpersonal interactions with particular reference to health and social care settings Pg 31	**M3** explain how own communication skills could have been used to make the interactions more effective Pg 45	
P4 identify how the communication needs of patients/service users may be assisted, including **non-verbal communication** Pg 42		
P5 describe two interactions that they have participated in, in the role of a carer, using communication skills to assist patients/service users Pg 45		

Activities
are designed to help you understand the topics through answering questions or undertaking research, and are either *Group* or *Individual* work. They are linked to the Grading Criteria by application of the D, P, and M categories.

---

activity
INDIVIDUAL WORK
1.1

P1

Write a placement log or diary that describes examples of communication and interpersonal actions that are relevant in a health and social care setting. Remember that you will need to obtain permission from the people concerned and that confidentiality must be maintained.

---

case study
1.1

Misheard information

Antonio Roberts is a marathon runner aged 26 who sustained an injury to his right foot which requires rest and an adjustable shoe. The plaster nurse, Joe Germodo, has measured his feet accordingly and has ordered a size 8 shoe for the left foot and a size 10 shoe for the right foot. The plaster department were short-staffed that day and instead of writing the message down before he went off duty, Joe made a verbal request to the department via a new student nurse.

When the shoes arrived for Antonio to try on several errors had occurred. The right shoe was size 8 and the left shoe was size 10 and they were both pink! Antonio's name had been turned into Antonia and the shoe sizes had been mixed up. The student nurse spotted this straight away, filled out the correct order form and the correct pair arrived.

Case Studies
provide real life examples that relate to what is being discussed within the text. It provides an opportunity to demonstrate theory in practice.

An **Activity** that is linked to a Case Study helps you to apply your knowledge of the subject to real life situations.

---

activity
GROUP WORK

Make up your own message and pass this on around the group, for example Antonio Roberts aged 26 requires a size 8 shoe for his left foot and a size 10 shoe for his right foot due to swelling.

1　What do you think happens:
- as information is passed on over time
- with information given to a large number of people
- to information that is complex?

2　What are the implications or effects to people if this information is confidential or is particularly important?

Keywords
of specific importance are highlighted within the text and then defined in a glossary at the end of the book.

One-to-one communication in a **health care setting** occurs, for example, when a doctor gives medical information to a patient. An example in a social care setting is when a councillor assists a client in therapy.

Professional Practice
boxes highlight any professional practice points relevant to the topic being covered.

Professional Practice

The following are different types of communication you may need in a professional setting:
- one-to-one situations
- verbal communication methods
- visual communications.

Remember boxes
contain helpful hints, tips or advice.

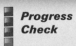

The nature versus nurture debate is concerned with two key questions.

 Link　See page 130 in Unit 4 for more information about the nature-nurture debate.

Links
direct you to other parts of the book that relate to the subject currently being covered.

 Find more slang on www.urbandictionary.com

Information bars
point you towards resources for further reading and research (e.g. websites).

Progress Check

1　List the different types of communication.
2　Describe what is meant by non-verbal communication.
3　Give an example of communication using visual technology.
4　What is a *phoneme*?
5　Describe the language development of a 3-month old child.
6　Describe the stages in the communication cycle.
7　What is a *communication passport* and how does it help the individual?
8　Name five environmental factors that can affect communication.
9　List barriers to effective communication.
10　Describe how these barriers can be overcome.

Progress Checks
provide a list of quick questions at the end of each Unit, designed to ensure that you have understood the most important aspects of each subject area.

Acknowledgements

Extract from 'A system for the natation of proxemic behaviour, American Anthropologist, No 5 65 1003-1026 october 1963 © 1963 by American Anthropological Association. Reproduced with permission of American Anthropological Association via Copyright Clearance Center

Communications pie chart figure 1.12 from Mehrabian, A. (1981) Silent Messages: Implicit communication of emotions and attitudes. Belmont, CA: Wadsworth, currently being distributed by Albert Mehrabian (am@kaaj.com) Reprinted with permission of the author

Table 1.9 First Languages spoken in the UK, from Ethnologue: Languages of the World, Fifteen Edition, by Raymond G. Gordon, 2005. Reprinted with permission of SIL International

Two Handed Fingerspelling Alphabet' from www.british-sign.co.uk. Reprinted with permission

Use of short quote by Dr. Rob Hicks BBC Health online. Reprinted with kind permission of the author. Check out Dr. Rob at www.drrobhicks.co.uk

Crown copyright material is reproduced with the permission of the Controller of HMSO

Quote from Royal Association for Deaf People reprinted with permission

Extract re Melcombe Day Hospital. Reprinted with permission

National Statistics Website www.statistics.gov.uk Crown copyright material is reproduced with the permission of the Controller of HMSO

Punch cartoon of Miss Triggs. Reprinted with permission of Punch Limited

Extract from 'General Social Care Council - Codes of Practice - for Social Care Workers and Employers' © General Social Care Council

Mindless discrimination' by Graham Thornicroft, The Guardian, July 26th, 2006. Copyright © Graham Thornicroft. Reprinted with kind permission of the author

Reprinted with the permission of Scribner, an imprint of Simon & Schuster Adult Publishing Group, from ON DEATH AND DYING by Dr. Elisabeth Kubler-Ross. Copyright © 1969 by Elisabeth Kubler-Ross; copyright renewed © 1997 by Elisabeth Kubler-Ross. All right reserved

Use of Phil Race's (2005) Experimental Learning Cycle. Copyright © Phil Race 2005. . Reprinted with the kind permission of the author

Extract - case study 6.2 from www.vso.org.uk. Reprinted with permission

Use of Professor Graham Gibb's Reflective Cycle (1988) © Graham Gibbs 1988. Reprinted with permission of the author

Front cover of leaflet 'Who regulates health and social care professionals'. Reprinted with permission of the Health Professions Council

Use of the Career Framework Table Copyright © East Midlands Healthcare Workforce Deanery. Reprinted with permission

The Mental Health Foundation's definition of Mental Health. Reprinted with permission of The Mental Health Foundation www.mhf.org.uk

Extract from 1986 Ottawa charter, © World Health Organization. Reprinted with permission

Investing in mental health - WHO definition of Mental Health. © World Health Organization. Reprinted with permission

Chapter list from 'Who International Statistical Classification of Diseases and Related Health Problems 10th Rev, 2007. © World Health Organization. Reprinted with permission

Short quote from The United Nations Children's Fund (UNICEF) study published in February 2007

Freud's Eight Defence Mechanisms from THE EGO AND THE MECHANISMS OF DEFENCE by Anna Freud, published by International Universities Press Inc,

Madison. Copyright © IUP 1936. Reprinted with permission

Extract from CHILDHOOD AND SOCIETY by Erik H. Erikson, published by Chatto & Windus. Reprinted by permission of The Random House Group Ltd

Maslow's hierarchy of needs from 'A Theory of Human Motivation' by Abraham Maslow, Psychological Review, 50, pp 370-396 1943 published by American Psychological Association (APA)

Poster 'SOS - the sun safety tips to SAVE OUR SKIN' Copyright © British Association of Dermatologists. www.bad.org.uk. Reprinted with permission

Use of RETHINK poster. Website www.rethink.org. Reprinted with permission

Use of 'Laura's Story' from www.in-control.org.uk

Table 8.4 Mary Sheridan's child development scales, from Early Years Level 2 pg 29-32, published by Nelson Thornes Ltd

Turning things around' by Charlotte Ashton, first published in The Guardian, 9th March 2006. Copyright © Charlotte Ashton 2007. Reprinted with the kind permission of the author

3 quotes from C. Henry Kempe, Sexual Abuse, Another Hidden Pediatric Problem: The 1977 C. Anderson Aldrich Lecture Pediatrics, Sept 1978: 62: 282-289. Reprinted with permission of American Academy of Pediatrics

Short extract from 'BTEC National Early Years' by Penny Tassoni, published by Heinemann, Reprinted with permission of Harcourt Education

Extract adapted from Good Practice in Child Protection by C Hobart and J Frankel, Stanley Thornes

Keepsafe Code, from www.kidscape.org.uk. © Kidscape. Reprinted with permission

Extract from BTEC National in Early Years by S. Green, published by Nelson Thornes

Lyrics to *Reggae Music* by UB40. Reproduced by kind permission of Sanctuary Kobalt (UB40) Ltd.

Photograph credits:

Alamy/ Bubbles Photolibrary: 120; Almay/ ImageState Royalty Free: 141; Almay/ By Ian Miles-Flashpoint PIctures: 142;Alamy/ Adrian Muttitt: 50; Alamy/ Angela Hampton: 5; Alamy/ Avatra Images: 9 (left); Alamy/ Bill Wymar: 239 (right); Alamy/ Bubbles Photo Library: 352; Alamy/ David Pearson: 246 (left); Alamy/ David Young Wolff: 350 (right); Alamy/ Frances M. Roberts: 184; Alamy/ Jeff Greenberg: 246 (bottom right); Alamy/ Juliet Brauner: 351; Alamy/ Libby Welch: 93; Alamy/ Marco Secchi: 98; Alamy/ Nick Kirk: 9 (right); Alamy/ Photofusion Picture Library: 239 (top), 350 (middle) Bernafon 2006: 38; Chubb Fire Ltd, reprinted by kind permission of Chubb Fire Ltd: 95; Corbis/ Artiga Photo: 49; Corbis/ Helen King: 4 Corbis/ Peter M. Fisher: 350 (left); Corbis/ Peter Macdiarmid: 246 (right top); Digital Stock 5 (NT): 142; Digital Stock 12 (NT): 141, 241 (left & right); Digital Vision Parents & Babies (NT): 237 (right); General Social Care Council: 74; Getty Images/ John Foxx: 186; Image 100 (NT): 10; Instant Art Signs (NT): 15, 22; John Birdsall Photography: 7, 86, 239 (left); PA/ Empics: 291; Photodisc 2 (NT): 152 (bottom); Photodisc 40 (NT): 229 (left), 241 (middle); Photodisc 63 (NT): 237 (middle); Photodisc 66 (NT): 9 (middle); Photodisc 79 (NT): 237 (left); Photodic 83 (NT): 168 (fig 5.21); Photofusion Picture Library: 8, 16, 75, 229 (right), 284; Report Digital/ Duncan Phillips: 107; Science Photo Library/ CNRI: 168 (fig 5.25); Science Photo Library/ Dr Klaus Boller: 168 (fig 5.26); Science Photo Library/ Eye of Science: 100; Science Photo Library/ John Cole: 87; Science Photo Library/ Kenneth Edward/ Biografx: 152 (top); Science Photo Library/ NIBSC: 169 (fig 5.27); Science Photo Library/ Steve Gschmeissner: 168 (fig 5.22, 5.23 & 5.24); Wellcome Images: 105

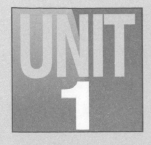

UNIT 1

Developing effective communication in health and social care

This unit covers:

- Effective communication and interpersonal interaction
- Factors that influence communication and interpersonal interactions in health and social care settings
- Knowing how patients and service users may be assisted by effective communication
- Demonstrating own communication skills in a caring role

People who work in health and social care require good communication skills in order to carry out their roles effectively. This chapter explores what communication skills are and how they are used to help clients and service users in health and social care settings. Factors that enhance and inhibit communication will also be examined in detail so that interpersonal skills can be reviewed and developed.

Communication underpins all aspects of care work and used effectively it can enhance people's lives considerably. Developing communication skills in a caring role requires awareness of your own communication style, awareness of individual needs and potential barriers. Knowledge is also required in terms of listening, observation, reporting and recording.

grading criteria	To achieve a **Pass** grade the evidence must show that the learner is able to:	To achieve a **Merit** grade the evidence must show that, in addition to the pass criteria, the learner is able to:	To achieve a **Distinction** grade the evidence must show that, in addition to the pass and merit criteria, the learner is able to:
	P1 describe different types of communication and interpersonal interaction, using examples relevant to health and social care settings Pg 6		
	P2 describe the stages of the **communication cycle** Pg 19	**M1** explain how the communication cycle may be used to communicate difficult, complex and sensitive issues Pg 19	

grading criteria

To achieve a **Pass** grade the evidence must show that the learner is able to:	To achieve a **Merit** grade the evidence must show that, in addition to the pass criteria, the learner is able to:	To achieve a **Distinction** grade the evidence must show that, in addition to the pass and merit criteria, the learner is able to:
P3 describe factors that may influence communication and interpersonal interactions with particular reference to health and social care settings Pg 31		
P4 identify how the communication needs of patients/service users may be assisted, including **non-verbal communication** Pg 42	**M2** explain the specific communication needs patients/service users may have that require support, including the use of technology Pg 42	**D1** analyse how communication in health and social care settings assists patients/service users and other **key people** Pg 43
P5 describe two interactions that they have participated in, in the role of a carer, using communication skills to assist patients/service users Pg 45		
P6 review the effectiveness of own communication skills in the two interactions undertaken Pg 45	**M3** explain how own communication skills could have been used to make the interactions more effective Pg 45	**D2** analyse the factors that influenced the interactions undertaken Pg 45

Effective communication and interpersonal interaction

Communication means the act of sharing or exchanging information, particularly new information. In this section we will look at types of communication, types of interpersonal **interactions** and the communication cycle. There are many ways of communicating information and these can be verbal or non-verbal. Methods may include sharing information between people which is known as interpersonal communication. This would occur in **one-to-one** interactions or in group work. Communication can be formal, informal or both. People may correspond with each other by text, such as in a note or letter or by the written word, such as in books, through oral communication as in speech, or through visual information as in signs, sign language, symbols, pictures or diagrams. Listening forms a large part of sharing information and is just as important as talking! Communication may occur through our other senses, for example, via touch; through music and drama, arts and crafts and communication methods that use technology. It is said that effective communication utilises most, if not all of our five senses.

In health and **social care settings**, it is important to be aware of the different methods of communicating. **Clients** will have different communication needs: some may speak a different language, some have hearing problems, some have problems interpreting written language.

Effective communication in health and social care settings is therefore vital. If instructions are misunderstood or information is not shared appropriately, clients may suffer. Staff need to be aware and understand what care is required. Staff 'handover', when new staff arrive on duty ready for the next shift, is a good example of the importance of sharing information. The care staff who are going off duty 'hand-over' information regarding clients gathered during the shift. Initially this will be a verbal account read from a written report. An equally important example of the need for effective communication is in enabling clients to share information concerning their needs so that staff can carry out their roles in supporting them effectively. This is usually shared verbally but may occur in the form of written information given during admission to the health and care setting such as in a care plan.

Written information from a report

Sunny Dale Elderly Care Centre			
Date	Note:	Action by:	Completed
12.5.06 9.00 a.m.	Could an appointment be made for Mrs. Allen to see the chiropodist please? Her toenails need trimming and are causing her some discomfort.	Staff Nurse Coleman	

Types of communication

Sometimes it is better to speak to someone about what you are intending to do and at other times it is better to write instructions about what you need to share. How do we know which is the most appropriate method? We are now going to look specifically at the different ways that communication occurs and its relevance and appropriateness in care settings. If you have the opportunity to gain work experience you will be able to witness first hand how these methods are applied.

One-to-one

This method of communication occurs between one person and another. No one else is involved. It ensures that each person communicating has each other's attention in a given moment. This may be while giving and receiving personal care or it may be a letter from the sender to the recipient. It is one-to-one if someone is receiving a phone call or text message. Given appropriately, one-to-one attention can make a person feel special and cared for as it is a means of saying to an individual that you are making time for them and they have your undivided attention. One-to-one communication is important to help aid self-esteem and feelings of general well being. For some people, however, this might be overwhelming if they have not had one to one attention very regularly or if they have been in some way isolated through lack of opportunity to communicate, for example, because of disease, disability, bereavement or other age- or life-related events.

One-to-one information sharing is important between professionals as well. Usually this will only occur where strict confidentiality needs to be maintained, for example, if a member of staff has a personal issue that the manager may need to know but that will not affect other members of staff or clients.

One-to-one communication in a **health care setting** occurs, for example, when a doctor gives medical information to a patient. An example in a social care setting is when a councillor assists a client in therapy.

Advantages and disadvantages of one-to-one communication

Advantages	Disdadvantges
It enables attention to be given to an individual person.	Quality of interaction is dependent on the skills of the person giving one-to-one.
The person may feel more comfortable communicating personal information.	The person may feel uncomfortable with specific attention.
It enables feedback to specific questions or concerns.	Preparation may be required to give accurate and informative answers to questions.
Interaction may take place over a series of formal or informal sessions.	It may be difficult to arrange several consecutive meetings.
Confidentiality is more likely to be guaranteed and maintained.	Interactions may be misinterpreted by individuals unless checked for understanding.

Group

Group communication is usually used as a way of sharing views, ideas, urgent or important information to a few or many people on one or on many occasions at a given time or over a period of time. Group information sharing is useful for presenting or sharing ideas from individuals or other groups. Solutions, new policies, new practice and procedures can be imparted in this way. An example of group communication in a health and social care setting is a meeting to ensure that staff and clients are aware of the fire evacuation procedures or an impending social event. Group communication can also be used to bring people together who share common aims or who require information from a person with specialist knowledge, for example, in a teaching session.

Group work is effective when clear aims and objectives are identified and people receive the information in a format that is clear and easily understood. In a large group situation, however, it is not always possible to know if everyone has understood or received the information in the same way. This can occur especially when assumptions are made about people's ability or understanding of the subject matter.

Group communication in a health care setting occurs, for example, at a meeting when hospital management communicate information and procedures to staff. An example of group communication in a social care setting is a communal therapy session when a councillor assists several clients together.

Advantages and disadvantages of group communication

Advantages	Disdadvantges
Same message can be delivered to a large group, saving time.	The message may not have been understood by everyone present.
The individual hearing the message may remain anonymous within group.	Some people may not have heard the message clearly.
The person hearing the message may not have to give an opinion or answer as the information is simply given.	Some people may not be able to interpret the information.
Information is given objectively and should be factual and informative.	Questions may not be invited.
Lively debate may open up more questions and answers.	Group information may not be repeated on another occasion or in same way.

Fig 1.1 Group presentation: Can everybody hear? Can everybody see?

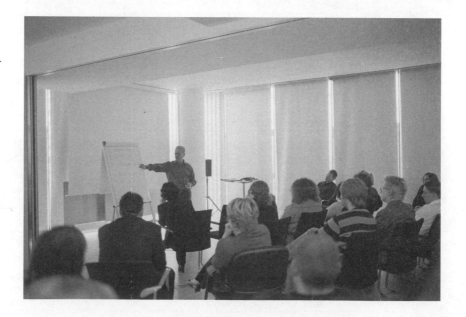

Formal

Formal communication usually follows a convention or set of rules and uses formal language. Information sharing using this method occurs in workplace settings between employers and employees and between professionals and clients. This may take the form of written letters, directions on how to take medication, fact sheets or posters that convey important messages or care plans. When formal language is used, the tone is respectful, there are usually no slang words and are written or spoken in a tone that conveys that the message should be listened to so that appropriate actions can be taken.

Formal communication in a health care setting occurs, for example, when a specialist examines a patient during a ward round and gives direct instruction as to how care should be carried out. In a social care setting, formal communication occurs, for example, during a case conference between two members of a care group to discuss how to support a customer care family.

Advantages and disadvantages of formal communication

Advantages	Disdadvantges
Information is structured and relayed in professional terms so that it can be acted upon.	Technical or specialist language may be used which could create anxiety for the individual.
Information given follows codes and conventions and is usually factual and to the point.	Information shared can seem intimidating to the receiver as it may use formal terms and references.
Information is shared for a reason and is usually given within a set time frame	The timing of the information may not be convenient to be heard by the receiver.
Information is given as guidance to be followed.	Communication may be one-way only, i.e. to be listened to rather than discussed.
Formal information may confirm what has been discussed and agreed.	Information may be misinterpreted.

Fig 1.2 Formal information sharing

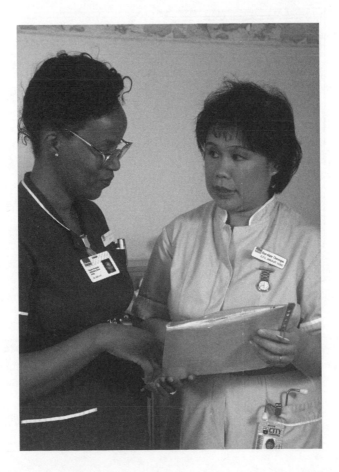

Informal

Informal communication is given without ceremony or fuss. This is used mainly between people who know each other and where a relationship may have been built up. Language tends to be spoken or written by using words that are familiar to the client. For example, a client might be greeted by saying 'Hi Mavis' instead of 'Good morning Mrs. Smith'. Notes written on pieces of paper that would not necessarily be filed are also forms of informal communication.

Fig 1.3 Informal
communication

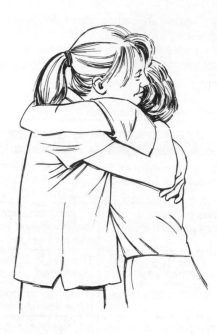

Fig 1.4 Formal
communication

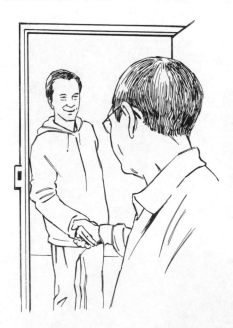

activity
INDIVIDUAL WORK
1.1

P1

Write a placement log or diary that describes examples of communication and interpersonal actions that are relevant in a health and social care setting. Remember that you will need to obtain permission from the people concerned and that confidentiality must be maintained.

The following are different types of communication you may need in a professional setting:

- one-to-one situations
- communicating to groups of people
- verbal communication methods
- written communication methods
- visual communications.

Music and drama

Music and drama are sometimes used as an alternative communication method. These activities have great value in opening up communication between friends and strangers. Music and drama therapy is valuable especially in helping clients to express feelings or to indicate needs that may be difficult to express verbally. Role play is a good example of this, where people benefit from the opportunity to act or re-enact situations that maybe painful to cope with. Music can stimulate and relax and so is excellent for promoting conversation, working in groups and for helping people to unwind. Music therapy and drama therapy are effective methods for helping people to communicate but tend to be used only when health and social workers have experience or are confident in using these forms of communication. Further training and development of staff can also help group dynamics as it can break down barriers.

Arts and crafts

Arts and crafts, such as painting, drawing, clay modelling, and other creative activities using a range of materials, are an important means of helping people to communicate through making something to share with others or for their own personal pleasure. These activities can provide a topic of conversation or talking point which can be a useful means of asking people's opinions and helping them feel valued. In some cases a renewed sense of self worth is achieved by creating an outlet for expressing themselves that does not necessarily rely on the written or spoken word. Independence can be gained especially where there is choice of what, when and how to use materials. Work produced can also be sold which could then provide an extra source of income.

Art can also serve as a useful **therapeutic** tool and may be used to unlock the memories in the subconscious mind. This is achieved, for example, through drawing or making things. The art therapist may suggest a theme or suggest the client chooses their own theme. The skilled art therapist will be able to guide the process and help clients to understand how to unlock barriers to the subconscious mind.

Fig 1.5 Role play activity at Melcombe Day Hospital

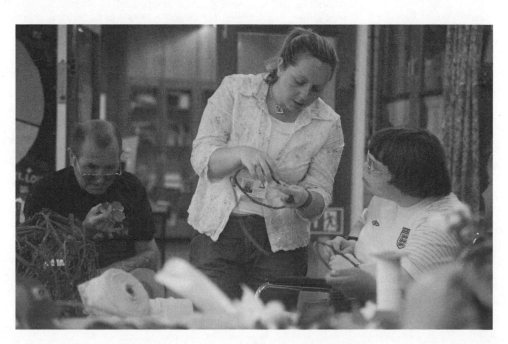

In a similar way, a drama therapist will be able to help clients replay aspects of their life in a safe and supportive environment. Unlocking memories and helping clients to deal with situations by assisting them through guided therapy to view things from a different perspective aids this communication process.

Reminiscence

In **reminiscence** therapy, people are brought together to remember how life used to be and to help people think about memories from the past. This can help people to connect with the present and future. Reminiscence therapy using everyday objects to stimulate discussion about when the articles, clothes, newspapers or objects were used and what impressions they create helps in stimulating discussions and opening up communication through interaction. This activity can also be used for teaching life skills to young adults about to move into 'supported housing'.

Fig 1.6 Kitchen activity for young adults with special needs

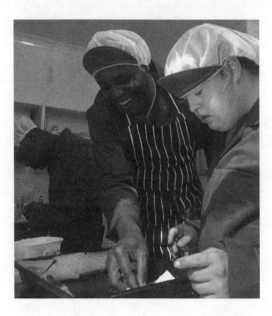

Communication using technology

The society in which we live is considered to be 'information rich' in terms of the variety of ways information is communicated and shared and the number of people it reaches. Huge amounts of money are spent on advertising and producing messages that may be conveyed to people. Different languages, different forms of media such as TV, radio, DVDs, films, magazines, newspapers, books which may also be written in large typeface, Braille or taped.

Fig 1.7 Using technology to communicate

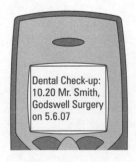

Dental Check-up:
10.20 Mr. Smith,
Godswell Surgery
on 5.6.07

The wide extent and growth of communication is evident also in technology used to communicate between people and peoples. The telephone that used to be fixed and could only be used where it was plugged in, is now portable and can be used anywhere. This has had a huge impact in many areas of our lives in terms of the wealth of information that is available to us at the tips of our fingers or push of a button. People are able to keep in touch and to help people much more easily. In spite of this, do we communicate with each other any better or more effectively?

Fig 1.8 Communication using different technologies

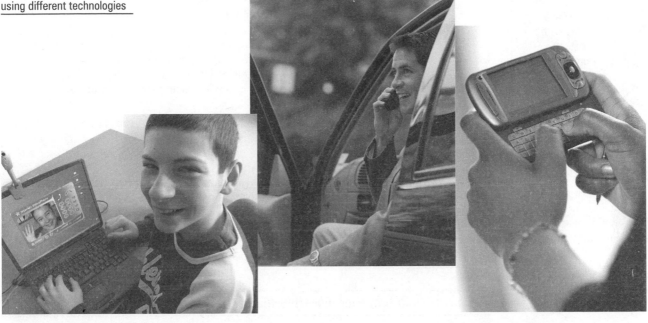

case study 1.1 — Misheard information

Antonio Roberts is a marathon runner aged 26 who sustained an injury to his right foot which requires rest and an adjustable shoe. The plaster nurse, Joe Germodo, has measured his feet accordingly and has ordered a size 8 shoe for the left foot and a size 10 shoe for the right foot. The plaster department were short-staffed that day and instead of writing the message down before he went off duty, Joe made a verbal request to the department via a new student nurse.

When the shoes arrived for Antonio to try on several errors had occurred. The right shoe was size 8 and the left shoe was size 10 and they were both pink! Antonio's name had been turned into Antonia and the shoe sizes had been mixed up. The student nurse spotted this straight away, filled out the correct order form and the correct pair arrived.

activity
GROUP WORK

Make up your own message and pass this on around the group, for example Antonio Roberts aged 26 requires a size 8 shoe for his left foot and a size 10 shoe for his right foot due to swelling.

1   What do you think happens:

■   as information is passed on over time

■   with information given to a large number of people

■   to information that is complex?

2   What are the implications or effects to people if this information is confidential or is particularly important?

Types of interpersonal interaction

Language is the way we convey information. This can be verbal, as in the spoken or written word, or it can be non-verbal, as in body language or pictures. Some researchers argue that verbal and non-verbal information should not be considered separately but just simply as communication.

See page 210 in Unit 6 for more information about communication.

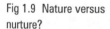

remember

The nature versus nurture debate is concerned with two key questions:
Are human beings a product of what we have inherited through our genetic make-up and are born with? (nature)
or
Are human beings a product of the experiences and influences that surround us as we develop throughout life? (nurture)

Speaking and writing are the two main forms of language production. Speech is the use of spoken symbols and the study of language is known as linguistics. Psycholinguists study how language is acquired.

Language plays a central part in our lives and there are many theories that describe how language develops. The rules that are used to construct language are called grammar. This can be divided into three separate areas: phonology, which is a language's sound system, syntax, which is the rules for combining words into phrases and sentences, and semantics, which is the meaning of words and phrases.

The nature versus nurture debate is still very much evident when it comes to explaining how language develops. What is known is that we seemed to be able to learn language from birth. A nativist theorist would say that we are born being able to carry out a task such as speaking. It is an ability that we have innate within us; Noam Chomsky (1928–) a nativist, believes that we have a Language Acquisition Device (LAD) in the speech area of our brains known as Broca's area that enables humans to transmit, translate and understand these symbols. Nurture theorists, on the other hand, believe that we learn language as a result of feedback and stimulation, as in operant conditioning for example, where information is reinforced due to positive stimulation. For example, a baby smiles, the parent returns the smile; the baby is receiving attention from the parent and repeats the smile; the baby's behaviour is reinforced.

See page 130 in Unit 4 for more information about the nature-nurture debate.

There are strong arguments that support both nature and nurture theories. Common sense may tell us that we are influenced and affected by both what we are born with and the experiences within our environment that shape our overall development.

Fig 1.9 Nature versus nurture?

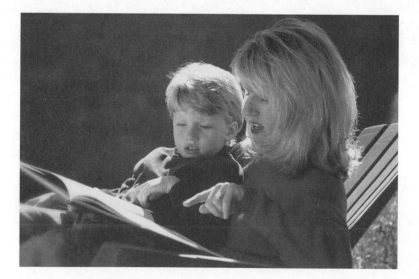

Speech

The expressive sounds (**phonemes**) we utter to convey what we are thinking is known as speech. We can vary the way we speak through tone and pitch. Organs of speech are our mouths, teeth, tongue and voice box (larynx). As children, we learn to speak in stages with increasing complexity.

- The pre-linguistic stage: from 0 to 12 months
- Linguistic stage 1: holographic speech (one-word speech with gestures)
- Linguistic stage 2: **telegraphic speech** (two-word phrases and then three-word phrases, and so on)
- Mastery of all the sounds (phonemes) necessary to produce speech: by about seven years of age

In the pre-linguistic stage of language development, babbling is said to occur at roughly the same time all over the world. Deaf babies or those born to deaf-mute parents, who therefore hear very little speech, babble too. However by 9 to 10 months, phonemes become restricted to those used in the baby's native tongue. It is therefore possible to say that babies from different countries no longer sound alike. Significantly, deaf babies normally stop babbling at around 9 to 10 months. This is thought to be due to lack of feedback from their own voice. Environment plays an important part in speech in terms of accent and intonation. It is fair to say that the more opportunities there are to practise speech, the more fluent we become at it.

Knowledge of how speech develops helps us to see the complex mechanisms involved in learning how to communicate using language. These components are formed through listening to others, interpreting language and meaning, remembering language, using gestures and facial expressions and using body language. Writing, visual and audio stimuli, such as books, pictures and sounds, also aid this process because these can be used on more than one occasion and so help with practising how to communicate.

In a health and social care environment, we can see how speech is crucial to aid interpersonal interaction. It is how we convey and express our thoughts and feelings. Speech may be difficult to understand if the organs of speech are affected by illness, disease or simply old age. Note how teeth help form sounds, so not having teeth or dentures in place affects this ability. As we grow older, our memories and ability to recall details may also become impaired. In people who have Alzheimer's disease or senile dementia, communication can be severely affected because the thought processes that help to decipher language and meaning are blocked or difficult to access. This leads people to become confused and disorientated because they are not able to express what they are thinking.

See page 31 for more information about barriers to communication.

Language

Different countries and regions have different languages, and within each country or region variations of the central language occur which may be dependent on factors such as cultural variation, dialect or local and regional terms for objects, places and people. Because language is central to human communication, it is constantly evolving, with new words coming into our vocabulary on a regular basis. Some new words describe new technology, such as 'WiFi' for the wireless internet or 'blog' for news and opinions posted on a web page. Some words deal with new or different situations or events, such as the term 'carbon footprint' as a measurement of a person's effect on the environment. Some words are familiar to particular groups of people, such as those used in this reggae song by UB40, describing how the band met as friends first and then formed to make music for people like themselves:

> 'I said we friendship come first, the band did come second
> And that's why I decided to put it in a song
> So listen crowd of people and throw up unnu hands
> If you love dem their style and you love dem pattern
>
> Reggae music can't refuse it
> So give us what we want and mek we gwan'

Reggae music written by UB40.

Stages in language development

Please remember that whilst language is seen as a developmental process, not all children will develop at the same rate. This chart is a general guide to language development.

Age	Language development
Pre-linguistic stage	
0–3 months	■ cries to show hunger, tiredness and distress ■ recognises different tones of voices ■ coos and gurgles when content ■ smiles
3–6 months	■ cries to show distress but can be soothed ■ babbles and makes gurgling sounds ■ sounds of one syllable evident, e.g. da da da ■ laughs and chuckles
6–12 months	■ sounds are directed to gain attention rather than crying ■ babbling now clearer and tuneful in some cases, e.g. more than one tone used to express needs ■ at 10 months understands about 17 words, e.g. hello, goodbye, mum, dad, drink ■ uses gestures to ask for things, e.g. pointing, waving
Linguistic stage	
12–18 months	■ first words spoken but may only be clear to main carer, e.g. 'gink' for drink ■ **holophrases** evident (i.e. one-word expressions which convey several meanings by changing sound and using gestures), e.g. 'up' to mean any of the following: 'up there', 'you get up', 'I get up' ■ at 15 months, a toddler may have a 10-word vocabulary
18–24 months	■ telegraphic speech appears (characterised by two-word phrases, e.g. 'drink now' ■ vocabulary increases with children learning approximately 10 to 30 words a month ■ some children have achieved 200 words by age two
2–3 years	■ new words are learnt more quickly ■ plural words are used with more accuracy, e.g. two cats ■ starts to ask questions, e.g. 'Who that?' ■ starts to use negatives, e.g. 'You no go out' ■ some grammatical errors evident in phrasing, e.g. 'Me go down here'
3–4 years	■ speech is understood by strangers ■ sentences contain four or more words and are grammatical, i.e. matching adult speech patterns for this age and stage ■ will make occasional grammatical mistake, e.g. 'You ated it' ■ vocabulary shows wider range with knowledge of names of things and objects more evident ■ understands and knows short stories and rhymes ■ more confident asking questions
4–7 years	■ vocabulary by five is approximately 5000 words ■ uses complex sentences ■ able to tell and understand stories, jokes, rhymes ■ uses language as social communication tool ■ stimulation of language development contingent on adult and learning environment, e.g. reading, conversations

A dialect is a regional variation of a language, with differences in vocabulary, grammar, and pronunciation. In Scotland, for example, the way English words are pronounced is different depending on the region a person comes from. Vocabulary and grammar also varies between the east and west coast, Edinburgh and Glasgow, between highlands and lowlands, between the islands and the mainland. Dialect is specific to each region and can even vary between towns relatively close to each other. For example, compare the cockney English spoken in central London with outer London or the shires. Dialects are also influenced by the prevailing or dominant culture in the country. Even pure dialects, such as rural Yorkshire or Dorset, have been influenced by cultural variations.

Slang is the term used for informal words and phrases that are more common in speech than in writing. Slang is most often used by a particular group, for example by people in a localised area or with a shared interest or background. Words may shortened or abbreviated from the usual common word or phrase, for example:

- hello: hiya, hi, hey, yo, what's up, peace, sup
- thank you: tanks, ta, cheers, 'ears mate, thanx, thankage

Find more slang on www.urbandictionary.com

---

case study 1.2

Language learning

Liz Horn is a nursery teacher at John Hayward School. She has a class of 25 five-year-old children and they are about to have story time. Story time is an excellent opportunity for the children to learn new words and to see how they would fit into conversation. Today's story is called *The Hungry Caterpillar*. It is about what the caterpillar likes to eat and also about growth and changing into a butterfly. Each day, the hungry caterpillar eats its way through various fruit and vegetables. Miss Horn asks the children to repeat after her the key phrases to that they can learn about different fruit and vegetables. They will also learn about the stages of a larvae and metamorphosis into a butterfly. A story sack containing several props is a good way of helping the children connect to the words. The sack contains a caterpillar, a butterfly and various plastic fruits and vegetables. Sometimes Miss Horn will bring in real fruit for the children to try. On another occasion, the children might go shopping to make a fruit salad. As she holds up the fruit or vegetable, Miss Horn asks the children to say the word, for example 'strawberry'. She pronounces the word slowly, almost spelling it out phonetically – 'str…aw…be..rry'. The children copy her and then speed up pronunciation. The word is repeated three or more times. After the story, Miss Horn reinforces the children's new learning of fruit and vegetables by playing a game called 'Sally went to market to buy…' (at this age the children should remember about five to ten items depending on complexity). During the day, a worksheet with some of the letters formed by dots will be used to practise writing and spelling skills.

Fig 1.10 Word association

Children can write the word by themselves and practice the correct up and down strokes by joining the dots or filling in the blanks.

Strawberry
St _ _ w _ err _

Flash cards are also another useful way to practice word association and spelling.

---

activity
INDIVIDUAL WORK

1 What might affect our ability to learn new words? Does age play a part in this?

2 Why is it that when we learn a new word we then hear it repeated more than before, for example hearing it on the news or hearing someone else use it? What new words have you learned recently?

Jargon is language used by a particular group, profession or culture, often in the form of an abbreviated short form for specific terms, phrases and words. Use of jargon can be inclusive when the vocabulary is common to a particular group, but it may alienate people who are unfamiliar with the vocabulary, if the jargon is not explained or it is assumed that everyone knows what is being said. For example the sentence: 'Mrs Farrell needs an MSU, WBCs, RBCs and to be NBM before EUA tomorrow' means 'Mrs Farrell needs the following investigations before Examination Under Anaesthetic in surgery tomorrow: a Mid-stream Sample of Urine; full White Blood Count; full Red Blood Count. She is also to be Nil By Mouth (i.e. have nothing to eat or drink). If you were the member of staff you would prefer the short version. If you were the client you would probably prefer the longer version.

It is important to avoid jargon in health and social care settings when talking to clients. Jargon can cause confusion and misunderstandings to occur and make people anxious.

Jargon can also be misinterpreted by professionals and new staff too so it is important that messages are clearly understood and repeated if necessary. On the other hand, jargon can be useful if you need investigations to be carried out promptly without further increasing anxiety for a client.

Non-verbal communication

Non-verbal communication consists of all the ways we pass on information that is not spoken, for example by:

■ use of body language

■ use of visual media

Body language falls into the category of para-language which describes all forms of human communication that is non-verbal language. Body language may be voluntary or involuntary. Voluntary body language occurs where we are consciously aware of our movements and use these in gestures and poses, for example, smiling, hand movements and imitation. Involuntary body language occurs when we are not aware of our own body movements, although someone observing our interactions might notice particular gestures or movements we use. Involuntary body language may be influenced by the person we are communicating with, when we mirror the other person's movements or are repelled by the other person's movements. For example, when we know someone really well, we might let them come within our own body space area and still feel comfortable, but if a stranger were to invade our personal space, we might move away because they are too near. Cultural differences may explain why we feel some people are invading our space when they might be feeling we are being distant and aloof.

Edward T. Hall (1963) a social anthropologist (someone who studies people and interactions between peoples) raises the question of personal body space, more commonly known as **proxemics** by describing unintentional social distance rules. He noted that people unintentionally position themselves as follows when communicating:

Fig 1.11 Distances and acceptable social spaces

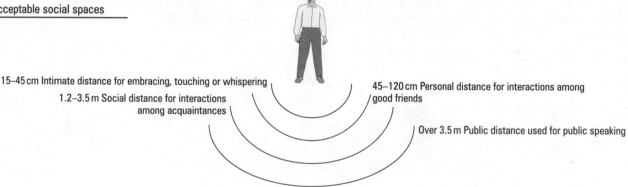

15–45 cm Intimate distance for embracing, touching or whispering

1.2–3.5 m Social distance for interactions among acquaintances

45–120 cm Personal distance for interactions among good friends

Over 3.5 m Public distance used for public speaking

Cultural differences also allow for variation to Hall's social distance findings. Proximity to another person may be affected by such cultural beliefs e.g. under Islamic law (Sharia), proximity known as *kalwat*, is forbidden between a man and a woman who are not married and who are not *mahram* (those people that would be forbidden by law to marry each other). If this law is being observed and is broken, punishment might take the form of being sentenced to receive whips or lashes. Of course, comfortable personal distances are also influenced by factors such as gender, social situations and individual preference.

Think about the distance at which you position yourself when you talk to:

■ your friends

■ your family

■ your tutor

■ your colleagues

■ clients or patients.

What factors are influencing interaction and proximity? What might you consider when talking to clients? Are you invading their space or are you being friendly?

We use body language to complement and reinforce the sharing and giving of information. It has been said that speech is only a small part of how we communicate to another and that body language gives us far more information than the spoken word.

Research shows that people pay far more attention to facial expressions and tone of voice than they do to spoken words. 93% of their attention is focused on non-verbal signals, of which 55% is through facial expression, posture, gesture and 38% through tone of voice.

Fig 1.12 Three elements of communication

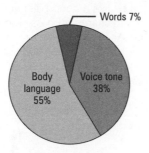

Words 7%

Body language 55%

Voice tone 38%

Uses of body language

Posture	how we sit, stand, position our shoulders, hands, head, feet
Facial expressions	using our eyes, mouths, eyebrows, cheeks, whole face
Touch	light, gentle, hard, aggressive use of hands, body, feet
Silence	head gestures, nodding, without sound
Proximity	using space, close or far, leaning in or away
Listening	tilting head to listen, acknowledging with prompting gestures, words

Other non-verbal ways of communicating with people occur through visual imagery, media and art, such as:

- posters
- photographs
- pictures
- books
- films

Visual media may be direct or indirect communication, because the message conveyed might be clear to one person but might mean nothing to another. Information conveyed in a variety of visual formats is useful especially where language might be a problem. For example, emergency or warning notices tend to use symbols and few words to convey meaning.

Fig 1.13 Emergency exit sign

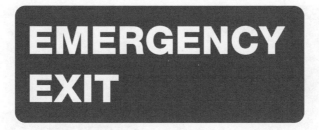

EMERGENCY EXIT

Listening and reflecting back

How often during a conversation with someone do you not really pay attention, only to get caught out because you have been asked a direct question and you answer it wrong because you weren't listening? Conversation can be like a good ball game, in which all players have contributed and successfully taken turns to share and pass. There is a rhythm of movement that flows from one person to the other. As in a good game, conversation is a process of sharing and being unselfish through not taking over. Do you notice that sometimes when you talk to people that they do all the talking and you do all the listening? Do you find yourself wishing you could get a word in edgeways?

Fig 1.14 Communication isn't happening when the person we are talking to isn't listening!

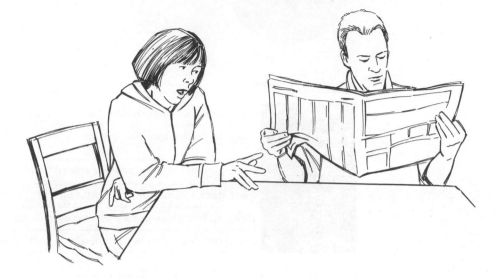

Effective listening means active participation in a conversation, only interrupting to acknowledge understanding and give appropriate feedback. **Active listening** incorporates several features of a conversation. It involves active verbal feedback including specific answers, prompts to conversation, such as 'Yes, I understand what you are saying', and short acknowledgements, such as 'uh huh' or 'carry on'. One visual clue to show that active listening is going on is 'mirroring', when one person in the conversation copies the body language behaviour of the other person. For example, if one person leans backwards the other person may lean forwards. Other body language clues to listening can be the use of eye contact; head nodding and verbal paraphrasing. These skills are used commonly in counselling situations.

Becoming an effective communicator can sometimes take time. These skills can be learnt and practised, for example, in role-playing scenarios. It's a good excuse to keep talking and of course to keep listening!

Fig 1.15 Effective listening

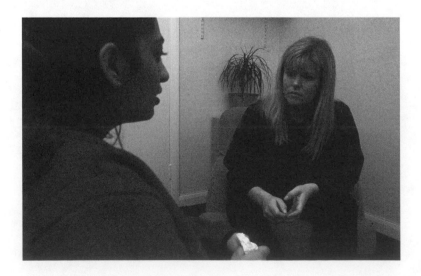

If the interaction and outcome is to be successful, the needs of the client should be met as appropriate and the staff should feel that these and the needs of other clients are met in a satisfactory way. In your role play and discussion, you might mention that the client may wish to discuss this matter in privacy; so that the client is given the opportunity to explain how he is feeling and why, for example, he threw his food on the floor. The staff member should sit facing the client at their level and should talk and listen in a calm manner. The staff member may discover the cause of the outburst and offer another way of dealing with the situation that does not result in food being thrown on the floor. Has the client had opportunities to discuss their unhappiness with anyone else? Has the client felt that they have been listened to? The conversation should close with some reflection and summary and of what might be done so that the situation does not occur again.

Effective listening skills

Paraphrasing	■ summarising what the person has been saying and repeating it to them ■ used to clarify understanding
Prompts	■ use of verbal and non verbal cues to encourage conversation, e.g. 'yes'; 'uh huh'; 'hmm... .'; 'carry on..'
Proximity	■ the distance from the person is important especially if the other person has hearing problems or is unable to see your face clearly ■ listening is difficult when someone is shouting or too loud ■ listening is difficult when the room you are in is noisy and the person is sitting too far away
Reflecting	■ feeding back what the client has been saying and asking them to look at things in a different way, from another viewpoint or, e.g. 'Have you considered looking at this another way?'
Silence	■ can help people to collect their thoughts, so that they do not feel rushed or hurried ■ used effectively, it can act to stimulate more conversation
Visual cues	■ encourage conversation by nodding head, tilting head to side, maintaining eye contact, smiling

The communication cycle

The pattern of interaction that occurs between one or more people is described as the communication cycle. Communication is initiated or started by a person known as 'the sender' which is received by another known as the 'receiver'. Between the sending and receiving of the message, the sender looks for visual clues to show that the receiver has understood and the receiver interprets the information that has been sent in order to give a suitable reply or response. This communication cycle goes backwards and forwards between the people communicating with each other. During a conversation, each person will be a sender and a receiver.

Fig 1.16 The communication cycle

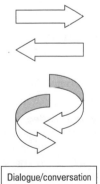

Sender

What do I want to say?

How am I going to say it?

Are they listening?

Do they understand?

Receiver

What are they trying to say to me?

Do I understand?

Am I ready to listen and respond?

Can they understand what I am saying?

Sender

Asks/gives information (encodes)

Ms. Ford what do you think you would like to eat today?

Receiver

Receives message; thinks about reply (decodes)

What did she ask me? What would I like to eat today?

Dialogue/conversation

Receiver:
Tell me what is on the menu?

Sender:
Vegetable Soup

Receiver:
I don't like soup.

Sender:
What would you like instead?

and so on …

case study 1.3 — Begum Sharmin

Nafeesa Sharmin is a 24-year-old Muslim woman who is a university graduate working in the City of London managing a small financial firm. She is an excellent communicator. Her mother Begum, aged 64, was admitted to a mixed medical ward having suffered from a perforated ulcer. Begum Sharmin can understand English but does not speak it very well. Her husband is out of the country. On visiting her mother, Nafeesa finds her in a distressed state and in obvious pain and discomfort. She appears to be the only female in the bay. When Nafeesa talks to the staff on the ward, she finds that her mother has refused to speak at all and that she insists that the curtains are permanently drawn around her bed. The staff including the consultant have found her quite difficult to manage. Nafeesa who is normally a calm and authoritative person gets very angry with the staff and tells them that they have treated her mother with a lack of respect. The staff say they did their best, but pressure on beds and short staff meant that they did what they could in the circumstances.

activity
GROUP WORK

How could this situation be handled so that the following client needs are met:

- communication needs
- cultural awareness
- personal safety and comfort
- staff training and development
- support for relatives.

You may need to consider:

- family pressures and responsibilities
- religious and cultural roles and practices
- mixed wards and female clients
- attitudes to pain and discomfort
- the role of advocates, translators.

The cycle of communication proceeds through a series of stages in which the interaction involves sending and receiving messages. Effective communication is a two-way process between sender and receiver.

Stage 1: Ideas occur

Ideas occur and a conscious decision is made to send a message. This could be verbal, typed or written. Sometimes unconscious actions occur where the message is conveyed without previous intent and is given away through body language, such as when a person unintentionally signals that they like or dislike you.

Stage 2: Message coded

The sender decides in what format to send the message so that the receiver can understand. Part of this process might involve moving nearer to the person or positioning the body so that the face, mouth and lips can be seen. The appropriate tone of voice, language and meaning is also considered. Most people do not consciously think about this as it occurs naturally, however, in new situations, you might find that you pay a good deal of attention to how and what you are communicating, such as when you are in an interview, giving information to someone in authority or speaking to a child.

Stage 3: Message sent

The information is given to the receiver.

Stage 4: Message received

The response will depend on a number of factors such as whether the receiver is in a position to hear or to listen or is able to interpret the information being sent.

Stage 5: Message decoded
The receiver processes the information.

Stage 6: Message understood
The receiver decides on a suitable response if appropriate.

Roles reverse and the receiver becomes the sender starting at stage 1 while the original sender becomes the receiver. A conversation occurs when sender and receiver understand and relay information and communicate from one to the other. The effectiveness and value of the conversation is dependent on the interaction between the two parties or group.

---

activity
INDIVIDUAL WORK
1.2

P2

M1

1 Describe the stages of the communication cycle using your own examples from work placement where you have experienced communication of information and checking for client/patient understanding.

2 Give examples of communication in health and social care settings where difficult, complex and sensitive information may need to be communicated. Explain how the communication cycle assists this communication process.

---

case study
1.4

Kevin Clark

Kevin Clark is an 82-year-old man who has severe hearing difficulties. He is a full-time resident in a retirement home situated in a rural setting. He shouts to be heard but is not really interested in the replies. Several clients have complained that he has his television turned up loudly at all hours of the day and night. When Mr Clark's relatives come to visit, it is disruptive for staff because they also shout. Mr Clark refuses to wear a hearing device. Staff have shared concerns that his privacy cannot be maintained because he repeats at the top of his voice every aspect of his care and his feelings about it. Otherwise he is quite content and prefers his own company. There have been suggestions that perhaps he should be moved to another home.

---

activity
INDIVIDUAL WORK

1 As manager for the care home, explain how the communication cycle may be used to communicate in helping to find solutions for the following problems:

■ maintaining Mr Clark's right to confidentiality

■ dealing with the complaints of the other residents

■ solving staff concerns regarding communication issues with Mr Clark and relatives

■ resisting pressure to move Mr Clark because he has specific individual needs that are challenging at times.

2 As the care home manager, explain how you would:

■ develop and review strategies for overcoming barriers to communication in the care setting

■ implement staff training and development, e.g. role-playing challenging situations

■ seek expert advice, e.g. audiology specialists.

Factors that influence communication and interpersonal interactions in health and social care settings

Link See page 54 in Unit 2 for more information about individual rights.

Communicating is a simple activity for some people. Yet for some it can be a strange or uncomfortable activity that can cause fear, frustration and embarrassment. Some people have trouble communicating on a daily basis. They may have a physical disability which affects communication. Others may be unable to communicate their thoughts and ideas because of mental health issues, illness or disease, or simply due to wear and tear on the organs of communication, such as the ears, eyes, mouth or teeth. The aim of this section is to help you examine the common factors that can affect communication with others.

Communication and language needs and preferences

Communication may be spoken, written, signed or carried out using a combination of methods. We communicate in the language that is most familiar to us depending on our physical and mental ability and capability.

An individual's preferred spoken language

Most people speak one language. Some people are able to speak several languages and are fluent communicators. The first language that a person speaks is usually the one in which their parents or main carers speak. If both parents speak the same language the child learns first to speak in what is known as the 'mother' tongue. This first language is then influenced by regional dialect, culture and outside influences. A child is capable of learning several languages but this ability decreases with age. An older person can learn another language but it takes time and perseverance. If the parents speak different languages, a child may learn to speak both languages, for example, a child with an English mother and a French father will become fluent in French and English with help and opportunities to practise.

Fig 1.17 Factors that influence communication and interpersonal interactions in health and social care settings

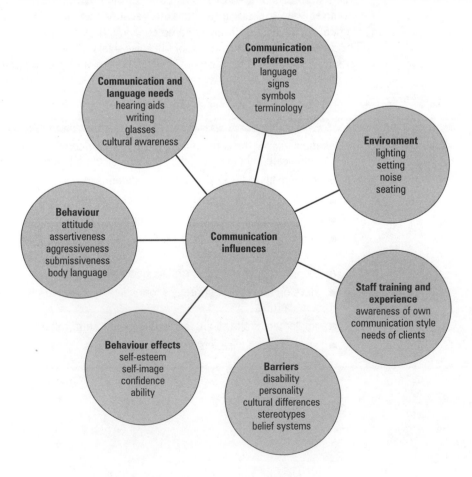

Regional dialects also influence the spoken word. Some words are specific to an area. People can make an educated guess about where you live by the accent you speak. Today, with people moving from one area to another, there is more opportunity to understand and learn new dialects and gain better understanding of communities. Presenters on television and radio with strong regional accents are often heard and understood. This was not always the case. In the past, television and radio presenters were only broadcast if they spoke what was known as 'the Queen's English', with no distinctive accent. In some parts of the country, English is not spoken and the regional dialect is actually the original language, such as Welsh and Gaelic.

In a care setting, it cannot be assumed that everyone speaks the same language. Culture and parental influences will determine the first language of choice.

According to the Central statistics census carried out in 2001, 95% of people in the United Kingdom speak English. Welsh is spoken by around 610,000 people (21% of the Welsh population). 60,000 people in Scotland speak Gaelic but the dominant language in Scotland is Scots which is spoken by 1.5 million people. In Northern Ireland, English is predominantly spoken with 30,000 people also speaking Gaelic.

First languages spoken in the UK

Languages	Number using this language as their first language
Angloromani	90,000
British Sign Language	40,000
Cornish	500
English	55,000,000
French	14,000
Gaelic, Irish	95,000
Gaelic, Scottish	58,650
Romani, Vlax	4,100
Welsh	508,098
Scots	100,000

The use of signs, symbols, pictures and writing

Spoken language is just one aspect of communication. Language and meaning can be conveyed in other formats, such as signs and symbols.

Everyone understands these five positive common hand signals:

- Hand wave – hello
- Beckoning hand wave – to summon someone
- Open palm – stop
- Circle with finger and thumb – meaning ok
- Thumbs up – meaning good

The universal use of signs, symbols and pictures can often promote effective communication and reduce barriers to interaction. Universal signs and signals are used to convey information to people who may have hearing problems, where the national language is not their first language; for people who have difficulty speaking. The most common formal communication methods using sign language in this country are:

- British Sign Language (BSL)
- Sign Supported English (SSE)
- Makaton
- Braille.

Symbols and signs are used specifically to help people who have hearing or speech difficulties. Sign language is a visual means of communicating using gestures, facial expression, and body language. Sign language is used mainly by deaf people and people with hearing difficulties.

Fig 1.18 Common road and safety signs

Signing

In Britain the most common form of sign language which is used by 50 to 70,000 people is known as British Sign Language (BSL). It is commonly thought that the same symbols and gestures are used throughout the country but each region as in language has its own 'dialects' and variations. Many countries have their own sign language system that is completely unrelated to BSL. BSL was recognised as an official minority language in Great Britain in 1993.

Fig 1.19 British Sign Language

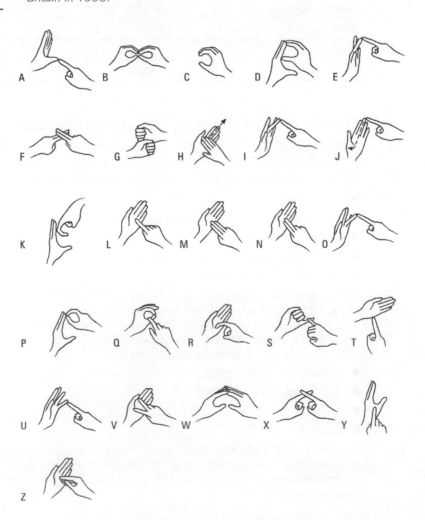

Signing uses two hands (in America it is possible to sign using one hand). The finger tips of the left hand (if you are right-handed) are used to denote the five vowels (A, E, I, O, U) and are pointed at by the right hand. Therefore the thumb equals A; the forefinger equals E, and so on. An easy way to remember the alphabet is to note that the finger shape mostly resembles the lettering. Notice C, D, J and L for example. Regular practice and learning to sign out names is a useful way of remembering the finger spelling alphabet. Words and gestures also have their place in sign language. Not all words are spelt out in full and the more common words have their own specific signs used with gestures and facial expressions.

Sign Supported English (SSE) is another variation of sign language used in this country. SSE mirrors the way English is spoken through symbols and is used where hearing people and non-hearing people work together, e.g. in fully integrated schools where children are learning grammar.

Makaton

Makaton is a combination of sign language, speech and gestures. It developed in this country from a research project which looked at the most common words used in the British language and developed as a set of symbols and gestures linked to speech. The Makaton Organisation says that Makaton is an internationally recognised communication programme, used in more than 40 countries worldwide. They also say that most Makaton users are children and adults who need it as their main means of communication. Everyone else who shares their lives will also use Makaton, including the families, carers, friends and professionals such as teachers, speech and language therapists, social workers, playgroup staff, college lecturers, instructors, nurses, and psychiatrists.

Fig 1.20 Example of Makaton using symbols and signs

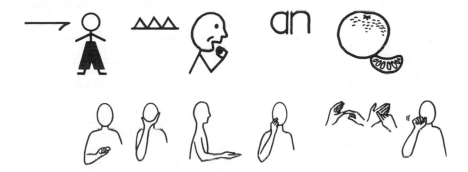

Braille

Louis Braille, a cobbler's son born near Paris in 1809, lost his sight in early childhood after an accident with one of his father's tools. He went to school in Paris where he learned to read embossed type and, remaining there as a teacher, perfected a system that could be both read and written by blind people. The Braille system he invented is based on six dots, like the design on a domino. It consists of 63 symbols made up of all the possible variations of these dots. Twenty-six of these represent the letters of the alphabet and ten punctuation marks. They can be used simply to produce a letter-by-letter copy of print. This is known as Grade 1 or uncontracted Braille. It is seldom used, as it takes up a lot of space and is comparatively slow to read.

Grade 2 Braille was developed to reduce the size of books and make reading quicker. Other symbols are used to represent common letter combinations, for example 'ow', and 'er', and words such as 'and' and 'for'. Combinations of two symbols are also used to represent some words, such as 'through'. Some characters may change their meaning, depending on how they are spaced.

Some people, particularly if they lost their sight later in life, find Braille too difficult to master. However, they may be able to read Moon, a system made up of lines and curves. Dr William Moon invented his system in 1845. He was partially sighted as a child and became blind when he was 21. He soon mastered all the systems of embossed writing available and found that none was really satisfactory. Moon uses some ordinary letters in simplified form, while others consist of straight and hooked lines, angles and half-circles. The alphabet consists of only nine characters, their meaning depending on which way they are used.

Objects of reference

Some people who are deaf-blind learn to use objects which symbolise a particular significant activity. A towel may indicate swimming, a fork may be used to show that it is lunchtime. This method allows people who are deaf-blind to choose activities, as well as other people to let them know what is planned.

Communication passports

A communication passport is a detailed document or booklet that uniquely states what the communication needs of an individual person are. They are written to support young people and adults to communicate and show how others might communicate more easily with them. The passport gives specific details of how the person prefers to communicate, especially where they have difficulty speaking for themselves. The communication passport is used to:

- describe the person's preferred method of communication

- present the person positively as an individual

- provide information from different sources to enable staff and others to understand the person and aid successful interaction

- give an outline view of the person's specific needs and personality and definitely not to be used as a set of problems or disabilities.

Human and technological aids to communication

Communication can be greatly enhanced by the use of technology but this is no substitute for what people can do themselves to help communication. Observing facial expressions, having visual cues, speaking and signing clearly all serve to help people 'talk' to each other. It is vital to make sure that a service user has all the assistance they need in order to communicate effectively.

See page 37 for more information about human aids to communication.

Technological aids are devices used to promote communication either by amplifying, interpreting, translating or transmitting information so that a person can carry on with normal activities of daily living as independently as possible.

The Royal National Institute of the Blind (RNIB) gives comprehensive advice and details about the wide range of equipment which can be used by blind and partially sighted people to help them access information, for example:

- glasses

- hand-held magnifiers

- closed circuit televisions (CCTVs) which magnify print up to 48 times the original size

- speech software which can read the computer screen to the user

- Braille translation software which can translate information on a computer screen into Braille that the user reads on a specially adapted keyboard

- screen enlargement software that enables the user to magnify the text on their screen to a suitable size.

Royal National Institute for the Blind   www.rnib.org.uk

There is a wide variety of equipment available for deaf and hard-of-hearing people. In the home there are alarm clocks, baby monitors, doorbells and smoke alarms that are specially designed for deaf and hard-of-hearing people. They use flashing lights or vibrating pagers or pads to get the person's attention. Equipment can be used separately or it can use a multi-alerting system that draws attention to a whole range of different sounds or events in the home. Telephones adapted for people who are hard-of-hearing, a text phone and even a mobile text phone will enable people with hearing difficulties to keep in touch with friends and relatives. There is also a range of equipment to help people hear conversations, for example, in the home, in a pub, in cafés or during meetings. These are called conversation aids. They work by helping to amplify spoken sound and reduce background effects.

Fig 1.21 Signs used to
show the availability of
communication technologies

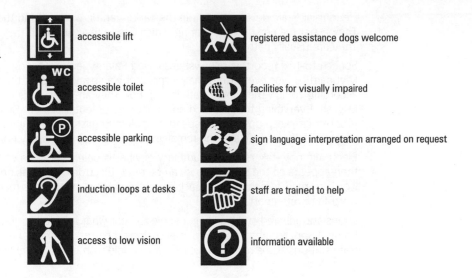

accessible lift

registered assistance dogs welcome

accessible toilet

facilities for visually impaired

accessible parking

sign language interpretation arranged on request

induction loops at desks

staff are trained to help

access to low vision

information available

The Royal National Institute for the Deaf (RNID) list these technology-based devices to assist communication for people with hearing:

- hearing aids
- speech to text reporters
- electronic note takers
- text phone
- mobile text phone
- conversation aids
- loop systems
- infrared hearing loops

Royal National Institute for the Deaf   www.rnid.org.uk

Fig 1.22 Text phone

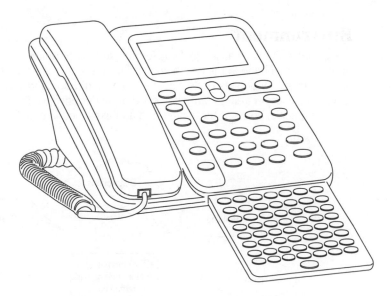

Hearing aids are devices that fit in the ear or can be work around the ear to amplify sounds. They assist the person with hearing difficulties to hear although they make all sounds louder. They are usually battery-operated.

Speech-to-text reporters use systems called Palantype® or Stenograph®. They use a special keyboard to type every word that is spoken by a speaker, typing the words phonetically, i.e. according to how they sound rather than how they are spelt. This is then converted back into English. Everything that is typed appears on a computer screen. By typing in this way, the reporter can keep up with the speed of spoken English. The resulting English is usually spelt at least 95% correctly and the remaining words are spelt roughly how they sound.

Electronic note-takers type a summary of what is being said on a computer. This information then appears on the screen, so it can be read. Electronic note-taking means there are fewer words to read compared to speech-to-text reporting, but it does mean you will not get a full word-for-word report.

Loops and infrared systems help people to hear what is on television, stereo or radio in the home. Loop systems in public places such as theatres, cinemas, banks, shopping centres and train stations also aid communication for people with hearing problems.

Fig 1.23 Loop and infrared system

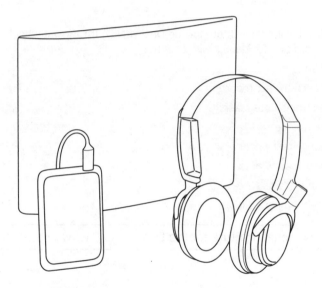

Environment

The environment can cause problems for people with communication difficulties. For professionals working in the health and social care sector, it is vital that they acknowledge how the everyday outside world can affect communication and interaction. Training today usually includes awareness of the factors that hinder effective interaction and communication between people. Some of these are listed and explained in detail below.

Fig 1.24 Environmental factors that hinder communication

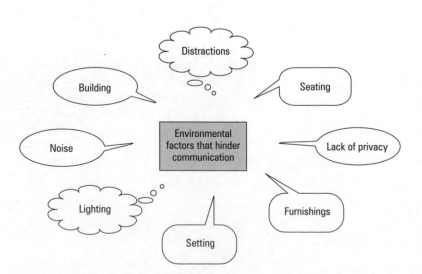

Setting

The care setting can greatly influence communication and interaction between carers and clients. Some settings can **inhibit** or prevent conversations due to their unfriendly and clinical appearance. Where there is a need for a clinical environment, staff may encourage and reassure clients through clear information-giving and reassurance to help reduce any anxiety that this type of environment can bring about. Clinical waiting areas usually have a liaison or link person who will assist people. Information is given regarding waiting times. Some clinical areas have calming background music, poetry, books, magazines and even a fish tank. These are excellent ways to distract people who may be feeling nervous. These measures aid communication in that they can help the person receiving care or investigations to relax.

Communication characteristics of types of care settings

Type of care setting	Communication characteristics	Example
Hospital	■ Formal	■ Explain hospital procedure, complete admission and consent form
Residential home	■ Formal	■ Medication routine
	■ Informal	■ Activities, games and conversations
Client's own home	■ Formal	■ Care planning
	■ Informal	■ Conversations
GP practice	■ Formal	■ Diagnosis and instructions for taking care of self
Social care office	■ Formal	■ Information sharing

Formal communication is usually to the point. Information sharing may be limited or prolonged but there is usually someone who controls the amount of time that is spent and in what way information is transmitted, for example, during a GP's interaction with a patient where there is a fixed appointment time. The patient will comment on what is wrong with them and the doctor will summarise treatment and or further investigation. The patient leaves. Medical notes are written, prescriptions are issued and a letter might be sent to relevant other health care professionals, such as consultants.

Informal communication occurs usually through mutual consent and agreement of both parties. A conversation may be on a variety of topics which could involve information sharing that does not have a specific agenda, for example, a carer talking to the client about the weather.

Large rooms are usually divided by chairs and tables arranged to make communication in a small group easier and less intimidating than in a large area. Rooms where there are rows and rows of chairs can restrict conversation. Who would feel comfortable chatting in a room where you might be facing thirty strangers?

The construction of the building can affect communication. A building made of bricks and steel is usually well insulated. However if there are high ceilings and glass windows and doors, the room can amplify sound making it louder and with echo. Wooden constructions can have the opposite effect of dampening or diminishing sound by making it appear muffled or dull. Buildings that are mainly of metal construction and that are not insulated, tend to reflect the environment outside, for example amplifying the sound of rain on a tin roof.

Soft furnishings for example curtains, carpets and furniture can affect the way sound is carried in a room. Soft furnishings absorb sound. They are useful not only in a decorative, privacy and comfort sense but also for reducing the sound effects of a noisy wooden floor, for example, or for reducing the echo effects in a large space. In a small room, they can create a more relaxed and cosy environment. All these can serve to promote communication.

Furnishings are used to great effect in places such as residential, nursing and respite homes. They help to promote a family atmosphere; a place where a person can feel relaxed and feel more able to talk and chat. Visitors feel reassured that they are leaving their friends and relatives in a setting that tries to promote communication. Hospitals where possible try to emulate this. Curtains around a bed promote a sense of privacy albeit a thin one. In reality, curtains unless cleaned regularly can be a source of infection, but they are kept because communication and maintaining dignity through privacy are considered equally important.

Where you hold a conversation greatly affects the quality of communication. Some people are less willing to share information if they feel their privacy is compromised or they are naturally quite shy. It is important that people are offered the opportunity to talk in a quiet and private environment if they wish to. People are less likely to talk to a person if they feel that their privacy and innermost thoughts and feelings are going to be broadcast too. It is important to reassure the person that information will be treated in a confidential manner if that is their wish.

Seating

Communication with another person is much easier when there are no physical barriers such as the way chairs are arranged or where there are tables in the way. Seating should be arranged so that there is an opportunity to face someone in order that they can see your face and body movements. The carer however, should not sit too close to the client as this can also prevent communication because they might feel crowded or claustrophobic.

Noise

Background noise such as people's voices, radios, televisions, and industrial noise such as drilling and building works greatly affect some people's ability to hear sounds and conversations. Background noise can inhibit communication because it can sometimes make it difficult to concentrate fully on what other people are saying. Think about the last time you tried to have a conversation at a party or club. Did you have to shout to be heard? For a person with hearing difficulties, even turning up a hearing aid may not make a difference when there is a lot of noise as the hearing aid amplifies all sounds.

Distractions

Noise can also be very distracting, as can people interrupting, a busy atmosphere or people talking very loudly. Such distractions can hinder communication because it makes it difficult to concentrate. Where there are constant interruptions especially to the person who is talking to you it is easy to feel less important. This can affect communication in that a dialogue or flow in conversation is hampered by other people interrupting. Sometimes it can cause a person not to want to speak at all.

Lighting

remember

For people who have cataracts, light is extremely important to enable them to read.

Lighting is necessary to aid communication. It is important especially for people who have sight and hearing problems. If you consider that the main form of communication may be through sign language and gestures then it is important that the other person can see facial expressions and hand signs. Lighting helps to facilitate this. Sometimes positioning a person with their back to the window can prevent them being able to read expressions because light is blocked.

Take a piece of paper and pierce a fine hole about the size of a pin through it. Try to read this text through the pinhole firstly facing the light and then away from the light. Imagine that this is what a person with cataracts experiences on a daily basis.

Behaviour

Behaviour is the result of the way in which a person responds to a certain set of conditions. In any interaction with another individual or group of people, we behave or react according to the attitudes, communication style, beliefs, ideas, self-image and identity, personality and feelings of ourselves and others. All these factors shape the communication and interaction we will have with another person. Interpreting these correctly is important to understanding how behaviour can influence communication both positively and negatively.

Understanding types of behaviour that affect communication and interaction will help clients express their needs much more effectively. A lack of understanding can severely restrict or undermine the rapport that is built up between care staff and clients. This will affect the care that a client receives and in some cases care that is offered and refused. Positive behaviour includes active awareness and working in a way which promotes the **care value base**.

Behaviour that fails to value people will hinder effective communication. Legislation that protects people such as equality, diversity and equal opportunities policies and procedures are used in health and social care to ensure that people are treated with dignity and respect.

Link   See page 69 in Unit 2 for more information about protective legislation.

Positive behaviour

Positive communication behaviours	Action	Example in care setting
Motivation	Using words and actions that stimulate and encourage	Communicating the benefits of a particular activity to the individual, e.g. 'This exercise will help you to walk unaided.'
Support	Encouraging through listening and being available	Listening to a client who is having a difficult time, encouraging them to share and solve problems together, e.g. when someone is grieving
Empowerment	Providing information that will enable client to become independent and make choices	Enabling a client to choose what they would like to do, e.g. choosing to learn a new skill
Promote self-esteem	Using language that promotes positive well-being	Ensuring that an individual receives positive feedback. Acknowledging a person's strengths, e.g. 'You are really good at helping people to understand this. Thank you.'
Make ideas become reality	Promoting communication of thoughts and wishes	Helping a client to overcome barriers such as low self esteem, e.g. 'You told me that you would like to be able to work again. Shall we work together to help you achieve this?'
Instil confidence in ability	Encouraging and support through successes and failures	Supporting client to keep trying even when it is difficult, e.g. learning to walk again
Promote feelings of self-worth	Encouraging individuals to express their feelings and be heard	Provide activities that give a person a chance to express themselves, e.g. through art or drama, group and one-to-one work
Make the impossible seem possible	Enabling clients and staff to remove barriers to personal goals and success	Support clients and staff to be innovative by thinking what can be done rather than what cannot be done, e.g. enabling someone who is paralysed to swim

Fig 1.25 Behaviour that influences communication positively

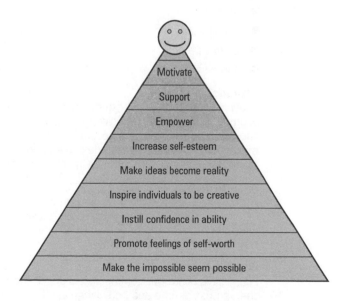

It is important when we communicate that we pay attention to the words we use. The question 'is the glass half-empty or half-full?' brings to mind that positive and negative influences are involved in the way we view or perceive things. The way we use language is an important part of this. Effective communication behaviour and the way we use our body language, surroundings, and so on, are also very important.

Negative behaviour

Negative communication behaviours	Action	Example in care setting
Lack of motivation	Using words and actions that discourage people from trying	Communicating the difficulties of a particular activity to the individual, e.g. 'This exercise will be hard to organise.'
Inadequate support	Being busy, not stopping long enough with individual to listen, not concentrating on what is being said because you are thinking ahead to next task	Not making time to sit with client and give them opportunity and space to talk to you
Lack of empowerment	Providing little or no information, carrying out task or activity so that choice is taken away from client which can lead to 'learned helplessness' and dependence on carer	Limiting or preventing a client's right to choose what they would like to do, e.g. choosing to learn a new skill
Diminishing self-esteem	Using language that is negative and critical, not using correct terms of address, e.g. Mrs O'Neil	'You are a lazy lump today.' 'You were rubbish at that, love.'
Overlooking the possibilities rather than helping to make ideas become reality	Concentrating on the negatives when people communicate thoughts and wishes	Providing excuses why something can't be done rather than reviewing how something can be done, e.g. 'You can't go there because your chair is too big.'
Conveying a lack of confidence in ability	Point out that person might not be able to do this before they have had a chance to try	e.g. 'You might go back to your old habits again if you do that.'
Not promoting feelings of self-worth	Making opportunities to express feelings and individuality limited or non-existent	Preventing individuals expressing their feelings and individuality by mocking or making fun of them
Making the possible seem impossible	Putting barriers in the way of individual's personal goals and success, not exploring the possibilities,	e.g. 'Alice can't go running because she is blind.'

We communicate behaviour through:

- attitude
- assertiveness
- aggressiveness
- submissiveness

Attitude
A person's attitude is the external demonstration of the way he or she is feeling, for example, through tone of voice, body language and language used. A positive attitude is shown through smiles, open posture and clear statements that show enthusiasm and are motivational. A negative attitude is the opposite, with forced expressions, closed posture (arms and legs crossed) and statements that might be sarcastic or surly.

Assertiveness
A person can express their opinions in an assertive way without being aggressive. For example, asking someone to carry out a task might be assertive, but telling them forcefully to carry out a task is more likely to be seen as aggressive. Assertive language spells out what is required but is not **patronising**.

Aggressiveness
Aggressive behaviour communicates anger and need for control. It may be threatening through use of tone and body language. For example, the tone of voice could be either raised or quiet but language used will be spoken through clenched teeth or shouted. Body language might include arm waving, close proximity to other person that invades personal space or short, clipped sentences.

Submissiveness

Submissive behaviour is where the person is overly eager to back down and not make a fuss. It is the opposite of assertiveness in that there is limited opportunity for the person being submissive to express their true feelings and opinions usually through fear of ridicule, shyness or being threatened.

Self-esteem and self-image of others

Responses to behaviour can make the difference between a person being able to express their feelings and how they are confidently, to not being able to be themselves or to fully experience what they are capable of. Behaviour can greatly affect people's perceptions of themselves and is particularly evident in communication that affects people's identity, self-esteem and self-worth.

A person's identity and self-image remains an important factor in maintaining self-esteem. For some people, other people's treatment of them, including respectful language, deference, listening to opinions and views is crucial to maintaining self-esteem. Such factors as age, injury, deformity, illness or loss can mean loss of identity, self-image and self esteem if the person has not developed their own internal sense of self-worth. The role of the health professional is to ensure that the client or service user is enabled to speak and to be heard. Opportunities to facilitate this should be available in a variety of formats from spoken conversations to written logs or comments. Sometimes people prefer to talk directly or indirectly through a third person, such as an advocate.

Martin Seligman (1965) in his research on animals identified the phenomena of 'learned helplessness'. He later found he could also attribute this behaviour to people. Learned helplessness occurs when a person in long-term care or with a chronic disability gives up or gives in because they have had negative responses or feel that recovery is hopeless. Seligman said that they learn to become helpless and therefore passive in their responses. This can happen quite quickly in care settings where everything is done for the client and responsibility is taken away. However little a person can do they still need to feel that they are in control of their situation to avoid learned helplessness.

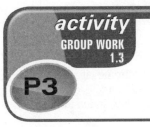

activity
GROUP WORK 1.3

P3

Describe the factors which may influence communication and interpersonal actions. Give examples from a variety of health and social care settings.

Barriers

Communication can be affected by many factors and the care worker needs to be aware of these so that misunderstandings are not made. Barriers can limit information being passed on or received and can cause people to become isolated if not correctly addressed. It should be remembered that the barriers that a client puts up may be a protective cloak and so communication needs to be sensitive and supportive.

Type of communication

Within health and social care settings, communication between health and social care professionals in interactions with **service users** tends to be verbal or using language that is appropriate, such as sign language.

Written information may also be given in the form of letters, leaflets or brochures that explain care routines and expectations. These can cause particular difficulties for some people. Barriers such as difficulty reading, writing or understanding specific terminology can hinder effective interactions. Latest studies report that one in five adults in this country have functional literacy problems. This means they have difficulties with day-to-day living such as filling in forms, understanding such things as bus timetables and understanding written language, e.g. prescription details. The implication of this in health care means some clients are only able to access information if it is spoken or signed to them.

Difficult, complex or sensitive information such as passing on news requires careful communication skills to ensure that the message is passed on and understood. It can be shocking to hear bad news and sometimes a person may react in such a way as to appear

Fig 1.26 Barriers to communication

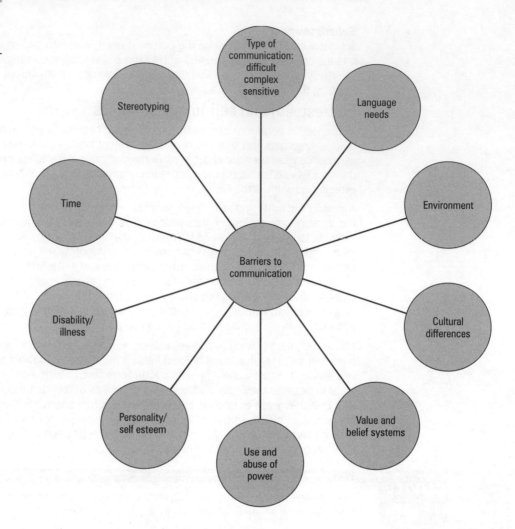

they have accepted and received the information, but find that a short time later they need confirmation or the message repeating. Consider how information that directly affects a person's health status, such as they need an urgent operation, may alter understanding.

Language needs and preferences

In a multi-cultural inclusive society it is good practice to provide equal opportunities and equality. This means that the person who speaks a different language or prefers to communicate in their own way should be respected. This can make the job of a care worker more challenging but it is one that can also be very rewarding. Barriers to effective communication can be created by making information inaccessible to different people, for example providing leaflets, posters and signs in one language only, lack of loop systems to assist with hearing difficulties, or lack of signage in Braille to assist people with sight difficulties. Awareness of potential difficulties can remove barriers linked to language needs and preferences.

Cultural differences

Cultural awareness and the needs of individuals due to personal beliefs may also cause potential barriers to communication. These can be overcome by asking an individual what they need and through education and information sharing. Knowledge of the potential client demographic will enable the care worker to **enhance** communication if they are aware of cultural and societal norms.

Disability

It is sometimes assumed that because a person has a disability they are ill and will have communication problems. Unless the person has specific problems with speech and hearing due to physical problems or intellectual problems, barriers to communication are usually a result of other people's perceptions and not the problem of the person with the disability. People who are assisted to use wheelchairs often talk of feeling invisible because people tend to speak to the person assisting them. It is worth noting that most people prefer to be spoken to as an individual in their own right which means talking to them first before making assumptions about ability.

Depression

Illness can lead to communication problems if the person is also affected by depression. This can lead to a person becoming withdrawn even after the illness has passed. Depression occurs when a person's expectations do not meet their needs and wants and they lose hope. It is more than feeling disappointed in themselves and situations; it is a feeling that can be overwhelming and all-consuming. In severe cases, a person finds it impossible to communicate anything. Depression can make people feel angry and defeated. Grief may be part of this process. The loss of something or someone or an inability to capture happiness will affect individuals in different ways.

Personality

What is it about personality that can attract or repel people? Some people are very easy to talk to and you might feel that you have known them a long time after even a few minutes. Some people you never find it easy to communicate with and conversations are hard work! In health and social care work, it is important that you consider what and how people are communicating. A person's personality can be a factor in this especially if they are quiet and introverted. It may be more difficult to obtain and receive information. Similarly a person with a very lively outgoing personality can hide behind a cheerful mask and obscure what they are really feeling.

Illness and disease can affect the way a person expresses themselves. For example, if a person is used to lots of social contact or prefers to keep their own company, a new situation can cause a reversal. A normally sociable person may feel that because they are ill they do not want to see anyone, or a person could feel overwhelmed by constant attention.

Value and belief systems

Value and belief systems help establish the rules and boundaries of communication and interaction between people. Shared values such as respect, dignity, equal opportunities, and so on, will help people communicate effectively because there is less chance for information to be misinterpreted or cause offence to the other person or group.

Belief systems can pose problems when communicating because not everyone can or does share the same belief system. However, in a professional environment, differences can be acknowledged and as long as both parties in the communication feel they can pass on information that is relevant and factual and people are able to express themselves without infringing another person's rights, then this should be positively encouraged. In a care setting, for example, a carer who is a Sikh might be looking after a client who is Christian. The carer has a professional duty to look after the client and not impose their own views or opinions unless asked to do so. The client has the right to refuse to be cared for, but respect should be shown to the carer and the client encouraged to receive care in the knowledge that the carer is a trained professional. The client and the carer have individual rights and neither should have the views of the other person's beliefs imposed on them.

Environment

Different types of environment will affect social interaction and communication. Formal situations may inhibit conversation, and it is the skill of the care worker that helps to put a person at ease and overcome this. When people are feeling comfortable and relaxed, they are more open to talking and interacting. In most health and social care settings, some formality is to be expected, but with detailed explanations and the provision of privacy where possible this should be reduced. Health and social care professionals are aware that when a person comes to see them or when they are visiting a person boundaries and rules should be observed to enable a person to understand and be understood.

Dr. Rob Hicks of BBC Health online says that around 80 per cent of the information your doctor needs to make a correct diagnosis comes from what you say. The remaining pieces of the puzzle are found when you are examined and from tests.

Time

Time influences communication. When a person feels that another person has time to talk they feel valued and appreciated. Within health and social care, this valuable tool can often be overlooked especially when there are pressures to meet targets and to see many people. However there is always scope for improving the quality of time spent with someone, even if this is reduced to a greeting and smile, until a mutually agreed time is more appropriate. Arranging longer appointment times will help, as will planning to spend more time with an individual or groups. It is important that a person does not feel rushed or hurried in conversation. Misunderstandings can occur and a person can be made to feel more anxious if they have not been able to say what they need to say.

Anxiety

Anxiety can cause communication difficulties, leaving people unable to speak through such factors as shyness, embarrassment, intimidation or fear. Physical signs can be experienced such as heart palpitations, racing pulse, dry mouth, perspiration and sweating. In extreme cases, people have been known to faint. Speech can become difficult or laboured and in some cases can cause stuttering and mispronunciation of words and sentences.

Abuse of power

Abuse of power occurs when there is an unequal relationship dynamic, i.e. one person unfairly exerts their will on another. In professional care settings, people should be protected by legislation and professional practice. Evidence shows that power is used to bully and harass people. It may happen to young and old alike. The common framework that facilitates abuse of power is an environment that looks the other way or has inadequate reporting facilities in place. In situations where people are vulnerable due to illness and disease, some people will take advantage. The only way that this can be prevented is to ensure that a person receiving care is given an opportunity to feedback their treatment and care to more than one person and on more than one occasion.

Assumptions and stereotypes

Consider the phrase 'we don't stereotype people here, we treat everyone the same'. What do you think might be wrong with this? If 'we treat everyone the same' it might mean that whoever the person is they will be treated the same as all the other people. What about individuality? We are not all the same so we should not all be treated in the same way. A person who finds it difficult to talk, for example, should be given individual treatment based on their needs rather than treatment based on assumptions. Stereotyping occurs where we attribute characteristics to people by making assumptions before finding out who they are individually. Taking a person's history to establish what kind of care is required, should rule out making assumptions about people.

Which of the following statements stereotype people?

- Old people enjoy playing activities, e.g. bingo.
- Young people enjoy music.
- Blind people can't see.
- Deaf people can't hear.
- Indian people eat curry.
- People with tattoos and piercings are extroverts.
- People who live on the streets are drug or alcohol addicts.

All of these statements stereotype people. Note that each phrase does not include any individual preferences. Some of the statements may be partially true but until absolutely certain you cannot assume that these statements would be all inclusive. Research and verification is one way of discovering the truth behind all encompassing statements.

In relation to the integrated workforce agenda

The NHS Plan (2002) for Modernisation of the National Health Service in the UK sets out how services will be integrated so that the needs of the national and local populace are met in terms of access to health and social care. The NHS Improvement Plan (2004) sets out how this will be achieved. For example, in the primary care sector the plan reads:

'The National Vision

The main vision for primary care services is to provide all patients with fast and convenient access to high quality care delivered by appropriate staff. This vision seeks to modernise the traditional role, whereby the GP has acted as a gatekeeper to secondary care, to make better use of the skills of other members of the primary health care team. It will exploit to the full the growing potential of information and communication technology. The vision will promote: self-help by patients and appropriate use of services; improved access to integrated, health and social care services; assured quality of care; manage demand for secondary care services through, for example, referral protocols, use of GPs with special interests and specialist nurses; and reduction in health inequalities in terms of service delivery and outcomes.'

Communication among health and social staff within settings and staff from other settings will be more integrated and connected as a result of this agenda for change.

Communication with professionals

Communication with professionals means the way in which information is passed on and shared between colleagues. This is usually formal and is based on information that concerns the client or patient. Within a care setting, this may occur through care planning and treatment carried out by various members of staff directly or indirectly. Records of care provided are written or typed. Access to this information and sharing information is protected by the Data Protection Act.

Multi-agency working

Some clients require help and care from several departments. For example, an elderly person admitted to hospital for an operation in addition to hospital services may require the help of the social services department, the occupational therapy department and the community care services department before being able to return home after treatment. The social services department may be responsible for helping with housing such as the need for a place in a social care setting as in warden-patrolled housing or a day care centre; the occupational therapy department may need to check the person's home to see if they need adaptations such as stair lifts or hand rails; the community care services may need to change dressings or bandages until full recovery is made. Co-operation between these services is important so that care is coordinated to aid the service user.

With the NHS Improvement Plan being implemented, closer liaison and interaction between departments and agencies should see less likelihood of people becoming 'lost' in the system. Agencies will communicate and share information to help track clients and patients.

Multi-professional working

In the Primary Care Workforce Planning Framework (2002) paper, David Amos, Director for Human Resources says that for many people their work or social patterns restrict access to traditional general practice. Primary care will be more flexible and responsive by, for example, providing accessible walk-in services to meet health needs that can be dealt with immediately. A range of clinical professions, usually GPs and nurses, but also others will provide hands-on care in all settings with appropriate skills (for example, counsellors, physiotherapists, mental health workers) in a convenient location. As primary care teams work together flexibly in new ways, they will be better able to provide responsive services. This will be supplemented by convenient access to medicines mainly through community pharmacies and increasingly through nurse prescribing. Tackling social exclusion will require the development of services aimed at those who are not registered with a GP and who do not use primary care services.

Primary Care Workforce Planning Framework (2002) www.dh.gov.uk
Search for *primary care workforce planning framework*

Knowing how patients and service users may be assisted by effective communication

Support services

People can be supported to communicate in health and social care settings through understanding of client's needs, appropriate training, use of communication aids and making good use of specialist advice and consultation. Effective communication can be taught and learnt. Understanding how this can help develop and encourage people is very rewarding as the results are a positive influence for all involved. It is one of the privileges of working in the health and social care profession to know that you have helped someone to tell you what they need and how you might help.

In order to assist communication, it is necessary to find out what the person needs. An assessment of individual communication needs is usually carried out at the beginning of any consultation. This assessment may be carried out in a formal way, characterised by some form of physical examination, completion of forms, referrals to specialist consultants, confirmed diagnosis and treatment. Alternatively, the assessment may be informal, through conversation where the client expresses a need or difficulty, such as not being able to hear people speaking on the telephone. When it is established what the communication need is a plan is formulated which will aid the person.

In health and social care settings, effective communication is supported by people who have had training in dealing with communication difficulties. These may be professionally trained specialists, people who have had some training in counselling techniques or people who are natural communicators and have useful experience which makes them useful as befrienders or advocates.

Advocates

Advocates are people who talk on behalf of or represent and support individuals who may find it difficult to communicate for themselves, for example, if the individual needs help completing a form because of reading or writing difficulties. An advocate helps the person to fill in the form but does not tell them what to say unless specifically asked for help.

Interpreters, translators and signers

Interpreters are people who translate or interpret the written or spoken word. Interpreters are used in situations where different languages are being spoken or different communication methods are being used, for example, where a client's first language is Greek but there are no staff who can speak Greek. An interpreter would be contacted to translate information on behalf of the client and the staff. Sometimes a client's own relative may carry out this service, or it could be someone who is a paid or an unpaid volunteer. Some large organisations have a list of interpreters who they can contact for this purpose.

Translators work in a similar way to interpreters but usually only speak or write what is being communicated word for word. They do not add their own thoughts or opinions to what is being said.

Signers are people who communicate using sign language, and may be brought in to assist communication with someone who can only speak using sign language.

Fig 1.27 Support services available in health and social care

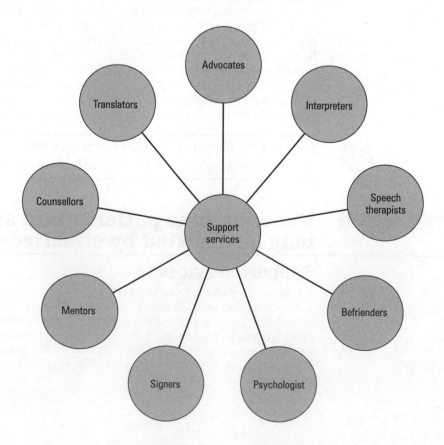

Speech therapists and other health professionals

When communication problems are a result of physical factors, such as wear and tear on organs, a person's GP may refer then to a speech therapist, or other health professionals such as audiologists (hearing specialists) and consultants who usually work in care settings such as clinics and hospitals. These professionals assess the client and recommend treatment which can vary from surgical procedures and fitting prosthetics (hearing devices) to therapy that involves learning how to speak, perhaps after an accident or due to a chronic condition, such as a stammer.

Counsellors and psychologists

Psychologists and counsellors work with people who have trouble communicating often due to psychological trauma, such as in cases of physical and mental abuse, or due to intellectual difficulties caused by memory loss as a result of illness or disease. Psychologists and counsellors work with the individual to unlock any barriers to communication where appropriate. In addition to talking and listening; they may recommend that the person try to communicate through creative therapies such as art, drama or music. Where traumatic events have occurred, this form of communication can help unlock hidden memories. The psychologist and counsellor will work together to put in place a programme of treatment to further support and assist the client to recovery.

Befrienders

If someone has no visitors or has no family or friends nearby, a befrienders will listen, chat, write letters and carry out small tasks for them. Befrienders offer the time that they can commit to and usually only work on a voluntary basis.

Mentors

Mentors are usually people who have experience of an illness or particular skills that they can pass on, such as someone who has learnt how to use Makaton. The client will be able to summon assistance from the mentor when needed. This might be frequent in the initial stages and then as time progresses and independence is gained less frequent.

Technology

Communication devices can support communication by enhancing sound, enlarging letters and helping people to process information using a variety of formats. The important point to remember in health and social care is that technology must be appropriate to the person's needs. They must be able to manage and understand how the device works, and know what to do if it breaks down and how to access other help when necessary. The client will be supported to learn how to use the device effectively through coaching and practice. Care workers also need to understand and keep up to date with new technology too.

Aids and adaptations

Many types of visual support aids are available, such as enhanced computer software to help with reading and writing, video magnifiers, talking books, voice translators, electronic note takers and telecommunications devices. For more information, contact your local GP surgery or look at the following websites:

Royal National Institute of the Blind	www.rnib.org.uk
Blind Business Association Charitable Trust	www.bbact.org.uk
British Computer Association of the Blind	www.bcab.org.uk

Examples of hearing support available are vibrating and flashing light watches, clocks and smoke detectors, mini-coms, loop systems, hearing aids, amplifiers and text telephones. The RAD (Royal Association for Deaf People) gives this advice to people who require a hearing aid: 'Talk to your doctor, family and friends and listen to their recommendations. Do not buy items described as "listening devices" or via mail-order. You may well end up spending a lot of money on something which proves completely useless and the HAC (Hearing Aid Council) will not be able to offer any help.'

Fig 1.28 Hearing aid

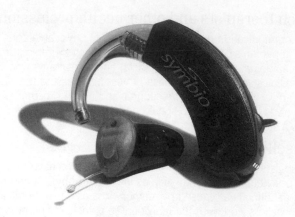

The hearing aid dispenser should carry out at least the following two hearing tests:

- an air conduction audiogram, where the client listens to a series of beeps through headphones and tells the dispenser which ones they can hear.
- a bone conduction audiogram, where the client wears a special headband which conducts sounds through the bones of their skull.

Royal National Institute for the Deaf	www.rnid.org.uk
Sign Community – British Deaf Association	www.bda.org.uk
The Royal Association for Deaf People	www.royaldeaf.org.uk
Hearing Aid Council	www.thehearingaidcouncil.org.uk
RAD Advice Service	www.radadvice.org.uk

A variety of speech support services are available, for example, feedback loops and electronic speech to text translators.

British Stammering Association	www.stammering.org
The Stroke Association	www.stroke.org.uk

Communication support available for mental health patients includes tapes, telephones and help-lines.

Mind (National Association for Mental Health)	www.mind.org.uk
BACP (British Association for Counselling and Psychotherapy)	www.bacp.co.uk

See page 24 for more information about technological aids to communication.

Preferred language

The caring role in supporting appropriate communication is first to establish what the communication needs of the client are. In a care setting where the client is newly admitted, they may arrive with a communication passport that gives details of the clients preferred communication method, for example, Makaton, signing, Braille or their first language. However this is not always the case so it is important to find out what the client's needs are and how these may be supported.

Refer back to page 21 for more information about formal sign language.

There is a difference between the client who has learned how to overcome communication differences and one for whom communication is a skill to be relearned. A person who has always been deaf will have developed communication skills over a number of years and will be an expert communicator. A newly diagnosed patient with sudden hearing loss or speech difficulties will experience other difficulties in addition to communication problems. There may be feelings of loss and grief to overcome. The person will have to overcome feeling helpless in order to communicate.

activity
INDIVIDUAL WORK

Imagine how you might feel if you were suddenly transported to a different country where nobody understood you. Then you also discover that you are unable to speak and that you will never regain the ability.

1   What do you think your first feelings might be?
2   How might you feel when you discover that you will never talk again?
3   What would you need to regain your communication skills?

You might now have a clearer idea of how a person might be feeling and the role of different types of support. Supporting the client to communicate again or to communicate effectively must take into account the feelings and needs of the client. The needs of the client may be physical, intellectual (linguistic and cognitive), social or a combination of all three.

Supporting

Clients in health and social care settings are supported through good working practice and training that ensures that clients are empowered and their needs are promoted through the care value base. The care value base will ensure that a client has the right:

■   to feel valued
■   to feel secure
■   to be heard
■   to be able to maintain dignity
■   to be able to be independent where possible.

In care settings this is achieved through:

■   training
■   qualifications
■   facilities and equipment appropriate for care
■   people who believe and want to make a difference to enhance other people's lives
■   a genuine ability to assist people to achieve their basic human needs.

Professional Practice

When supporting people with hearing difficulties:

■   ask the person what help they need, if any
■   ensure that the person can see full facial and hand movements
■   ensure adequate lighting is available
■   ensure background noise is kept to minimum as this can be distracting
■   talk clearly rather than loudly
■   ensure the person has access to aids to hearing
■   ask the person to switch on their hearing device if appropriate
■   ask the person if you are talking at right pitch, pace and with clarity
■   use the person's preferred method of communication, e.g. signing, cards, notes
■   seek training to learn how to communicate effectively
■   encourage regular check-ups to evaluate hearing.

When supporting people with visual difficulties:

- ask the person what help they need, if any
- ensure the person can hear your voice
- use touch to convey proximity and reassurance
- ensure adequate lighting is available
- describe the environment and people in detail
- be aware of safety and potential hazards to the person
- use the person's preferred method of communication, e.g. large text, Braille
- ensure the person has access to visual aids, e.g. glasses
- ensure regular check-ups to evaluate vision

Physical needs

Physical needs may be supported by ensuring the client has the appropriate aid to help them. This could involve helping the client to use these, for example, help with learning how to communicate using symbols, devices and aids effectively. In some cases, surgery may be appropriate , for example, cochlear implants to aid hearing or laser surgery to correct squints or remove cataracts to enable people to read.

Language needs

Communication can be supported through use of preferred language. It is usual to teach people the method that will give them the maximum communication choices. Age is a consideration in this and like all new languages, the methods used to teach will be a factor. For an elderly person who has had a stroke, it may be more effective to use existing symbols in the form of cards and signs rather than teach Makaton or sign language that might be too difficult a skill to learn. It is important that people are stretched so that they do not become dependent on carers but they should not be made to feel inadequate or incapable.

When supporting people with speech difficulties:

- ask the person what help they need, if any
- ensure the person can see your face and facial expressions
- ensure that you do not rush the person or appear impatient
- do not finish the other person's sentence for them unless they indicate that this is OK
- use the person's preferred method of communication
- enable the person to communicate in one-to-one and in group situations with support and confidence
- provide or seek training to enhance communication
- encourage the person to use speech aids as appropriate

Social needs

Social needs are met through having opportunities to communicate with people. In health and social care settings, it is necessary to organise activities that give people the chance to maintain and have contact with people. Care settings that acknowledge the importance of social activity to communication enable clients to see their family and friends, to make visits and to meet new people. A simple way of achieving this can be through seating arrangements that allow people to see and talk to each other, for example, at meal times in dining rooms, in lounge areas and in waiting areas. Activities that enable common interests, such as music, film, gardening, art, shopping and reading clubs, are also important. Carers can promote communication skills during day-to-day caring activities by having time to listen and taking a genuine interest in enabling the client to express themselves.

case study 1.5

Melcombe Day Hospital

Melcombe Day Hospital is a unit that provides therapeutic treatment for older people with various mental health conditions (specialising in dementia). The staff at Melcombe promote communication and interaction in an unusual yet innovative way through the use of role play. The underlying ethos is 'seeing the person behind the disease'. The staff have theme days where they dress up, cook meals that reflect the theme and displayed objects linked to the theme for clients to see and handle. The unit make good use of car boot sales to find inexpensive objects to use. During the day, clients are given the opportunity to explore and reminisce about their experiences or to gain new experiences. Staff promote and encourage involvement by assisting clients to handle an object from the past and by giving them the opportunity to talk about the past. Music from a particular era helps people to communicate where previously they might have remained locked inside their own particular worlds. Themes may be based on countries and food, local surroundings and jobs, or objects of special interest. For example, a doll's house could be used to talk about houses, how they are made, what goes in them, the houses that clients have lived in and the skills they have or have developed. Role play encourages communication by enabling staff and clients to have fun with a purpose.

For more information about this, contact lesley.benham@dorset-pct.nhs.uk Melcombe Day Hospital, Dorset NHS Trust, Weymouth, Dorset
http://www.northdorset.pct.nhs.uk

activity
INDIVIDUAL WORK

1　Why do you think people might be willing to talk about what they used to do?

2　How do you think using a prop such as a doll's house with a male patient might help him to talk about building or making things?

3　Role play, theme days and dressing up can have many positive benefits for people with mental health problems. Why do you think this is so?

Empowerment

Empowerment means enabling a person to be independent through choice, opportunity and understanding. Communication can empower people to express themselves positively. When people are unable to do this, they can feel helpless. Communication can be supported by providing choices, opportunities to practise communication in an encouraging and supportive environment, providing information and education appropriate to a person's individual needs.

Communication and empowerment

Empowerment actions	Example in health care	Example in social care
Choice	■ choosing what clothes to wear ■ choosing to make healthy choices ■ choosing type of care received	■ choosing help and how much ■ choosing action ■ choosing change
Opportunities	■ to learn or relearn ■ further training ■ adaptations to enable full participation in activities	■ advice and guidance ■ financial benefits ■ social benefits ■ training or education
Understanding	■ knowledge and information ■ application of skills ■ practising skills ■ acceptance and independence	■ how to access health and well-being ■ how to be independent

Promotion of rights

Communication can be made easier if the person feels that they can express their thoughts ideas and opinions without fear of ridicule or being made to feel insecure. In a caring community, staff will be able to help the client to express themselves. It is important that a person's right to be heard is valued. Agreeing rules and boundaries for communication will allow freedom of expression without offending others. Tolerance for others' views and opinions must be appropriate to the environment and all who will be using that environment. There are times when it is inappropriate to talk or discuss opinions especially if it is likely to cause offence to anther person. Where there are difficulties, clients should be able to discuss how they are feeling but will need to do so in private or agree to discuss strong feelings and opinions with the person concerned.

---

case study 1.6

Robert Brown

Robert Brown, aged 89, lives in Meadow Ridge Nursing Home and has been resident there for a number of years. He is quite deaf but can hear with a hearing aid when he remembers to switch it on. The resident in the room next to Mr Brown has complained about the loud noise of his television at night and has asked to be moved. There have, in fact, been several complaints about shouting and turning up the TV and radio in the lounge too.

activity
INDIVIDUAL WORK

1 How should Mr Brown be assisted to achieve his needs and rights?
2 How should the resident and other residents be assisted to achieve their needs and rights?

Maintaining confidentiality

Confidentiality means keeping something private or secret. In care settings, confidentiality about client's details may need to remain private in order to protect and enable the client to feel confident to communicate and trust the carers. Generally information is shared with the client's permission so that care staff can carry out appropriate and effective care. In health and social care environments, it is vital that the client feels that they can trust that the information they share with staff will be used to help them.

In extraordinary circumstances, information must be shared if the person or another person's life is at risk. If a client says they want to share information with you but they do not want you to tell anyone else, it is very important that you make it clear that you cannot do this. You may tell the client that you would need to discuss or ask them to discuss sensitive information with the appropriate professionals.

See page 78 in Unit 2 for more information about legislation and confidentiality.

---

activity
INDIVIDUAL WORK 1.4

P4

M2

1 Identify how the communication needs, including non-verbal communication, of service users may be assisted in three different health and social care settings, such as a hospital, day care centre, a client's own home, a hospice or respite care or a GP's surgery.
2 For each care setting, explain the specific communication needs of service users and the support they might require from staff to include the use of technological aids to communication, such as adapted telephones.

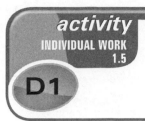

activity
INDIVIDUAL WORK
1.5

D1

1 Write a detailed analysis to include research on how people receive health information and the best way of sharing important information between health care professional and clients.

2 Describe in detail the benefits to the client of understanding the information that is given to them about their health by at least three health care professionals.

Demonstrating own communication skills in a caring role

Communication skills

In this unit, we have looked at communication difficulties and experiences of clients and how these are assessed. This section will be looking at your own communication skills and the communication skills of professional health and social care workers and other key people.

Verbal and non-verbal communication skills

Skill	Factors to consider	Hints and tips
Tone of voice	■ Do you talk loudly, softly, aggressively, passively? ■ Do you vary the pitch (high and low)?	■ Varying tone of voice helps communicate variety and interest. ■ It can be used to gain attention causing people to listen or switch off.
Eye contact	■ Do you look directly at someone while they are speaking? ■ Eye contact conveys interest in what someone is saying.	■ It is also used to assess understanding of communication. ■ Maintaining eye contact should be natural and not forced. If a person stares for too long it can feel intimidating. ■ Try to ensure that eye contact is at the same level e.g. sitting down next to client if in bed or chair
Prompting	■ Do you prompt further communication through the use of acknowledgement to demonstrate you have heard and are listening to the other person?	■ Encouraging sounds, such as 'yes' 'hmm' 'uhuh', and nodding are useful to help the communication 'flow' without interrupting what is being said. ■ They should not be used as an excuse for not listening!
Body proximity	■ Do you think about where you position yourself? ■ Position influences communication. You may wish to sit opposite, to the side, near the person, maintain a distance depending on type of communication.	■ Remove physical barriers to conversation where possible. ■ Do not stand over people when talking to them.
Reflecting	■ Do you reflect back what the person has said to ensure that you and they have understood the information that is being shared? ■ Reflecting is used to clarify communication and give people time to think about what is being said usually after long chunks of information sharing.	■ Allow enough time in a conversation for reflecting on what is being said. ■ Do not hurry the person or fill in gaps in conversation. ■ Silence is useful to help people reflect and give them time to think.
Paraphrasing	■ Do you give a summary of what is being said or communicated?	■ Try to ensure that you have summarised communication accurately. ■ Check understanding with the other person(s)
Body language	■ Do you think about how you are positioned in relation to the person you are communicating with? ■ Your body position, includes facial expressions, open and closed postures such as arms open or folded, legs crossed or uncrossed, turned towards or away from person, head up or looking down, avoiding eye contact, fidgeting and remaining still.	■ Consider whether your body language reflects what you are feeling or thinking? ■ Is this helpful or limiting the conversation with the other person?

The way to develop communication skills and awareness is to practise and train. Most professionals are offered training so that they can communicate effectively with clients and patients in health and social care settings. This may take the form of one-to-one or group sessions. Observations are made that can be taped, written or videoed.

Methods to help communication skills might involve some of the following:

Role plays

These involve acting out scenarios. Each person takes a part and is observed. Feedback is given through discussion or written notes.

Case studies

An individual or group is invited to discuss how information can be shared or situations handled using real-life case histories.

Counselling

This is used to help people reflect on their own personality and individual differences and behaviour. It is used in therapeutic training particularly for therapists in psychotherapy and psychiatric environments.

Self-reflection and analysis

Reflecting on one's own behaviour is quite difficult. It is useful to think about how you view your interactions with different types of people and how they are influenced. You might then consider how you would do things differently next time situations arise. Sometimes you can analyse your own communication styles by feedback from others. Some organisations carry out what is known as 360 degree profiles where the views of all the people surrounding (hence the term '360 degree') the individual are put together and analysis is made of strengths and weaknesses. Another method which you can carry out for yourself is a SWOT analysis (Strengths, Weaknesses, Obstacles and Threats). Under each heading you write down your analysis. When this is completed, the overview gives you an idea of your goal and what the obstacles are in the way of achieving this. It is usually used for defining problems, but could be used in assessing own communication skills. An action plan is then made to achieve the desired outcomes.

Fig 1.29 SWOT analysis to assess communication skills

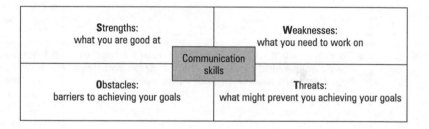

Strengths: what you are good at	**W**eaknesses: what you need to work on
Obstacles: barriers to achieving your goals	**T**hreats: what might prevent you achieving your goals

Communication skills

Interviews

In health and social care, interviews are used to gain information so that assessment of the client or service user's needs can be made. The use of questioning techniques to enable people to share information is a skill that requires practice. Appropriate use of open and closed questioning can elicit much information as can observation of client behaviour and body language.

Effectiveness

Assessing one's own communication skills requires feedback and evaluation. This may be written or oral. Communication is effective when information is shared, understood and feedback and responses are appropriate. In order to evaluate whether clients feel that they have had effective care and are able to communicate their needs, feedback and evaluation is given through a variety of methods such as questionnaires, surveys, opinion polls and interviews.

Key people

It is often the case that the client or person who requires help is unable to take all the information in one session. A key person, such as a relative, friend, or health or social care worker, should be included in the communication cycle. They can be made aware of what needs to be communicated and can support the client who requires assistance with communication. This key person can be a valuable source of help and comfort to the client and to the person sharing information. Sometimes the key person is able to explain things more easily than a stranger because communication requires a certain amount of trust and knowledge about the other person. For example, a daughter might attend a GP's surgery visit with her elderly father. The father might hear the first part of what the doctor is saying but miss other important part about medication and how to take it. The daughter can then explain the rest of the information to her father when he is ready to take it in.

activity

INDIVIDUAL WORK
1.6

P5

P6

M3

D2

1   Describe two examples from your work placement where you have used communications skills to assist clients or service users. Write a summary of the interaction, including examples where possible from your own work placement log or diary.

2   Review the effectiveness of your communication skills in these two examples using the communications skills checklist below to help you.

Communications skills checklist

Communication skill	Example used during activity or role play	Comment
Open questioning		
Closed questioning		
Pace		
Prompts		
Reflection		
Clarifying		
Summarising		
Tone		
Clarity		
Paraphrasing		
	Signature:	Date:

3   Review the communication checklist and explain how your communications skills could have been used to make the interactions more effective in these two examples.

4   It may be useful for you to be observed carrying out the interactions again. Make a comparison between your assessment and the observer's assessment of your communication skills. Analyse the factors that contributed to the interactions between yourself and the client.

Progress Check

1   List the different types of communication.

2   Describe what is meant by non-verbal communication.

3   Give an example of communication using visual technology.

4   What is a *phoneme*?

5   Describe the language development of a 3-month old child.

6   Describe the stages in the communication cycle.

7   What is a *communication passport* and how does it help the individual?

8   Name five environmental factors that can affect communication.

9   List barriers to effective communication.

10   Describe how these barriers can be overcome.

11   Discuss the advantages of formal communication methods.

12   What are the disadvantages of information communication.

13   Describe factors that will help effective communication.

14   How can anxiety affect a person's communication?

15   What is meant by cultural differences in communication?

16   What is the difference between a *translator* and an *interpreter*?

17   List aids that would help a person with hearing difficulties to communicate.

18   List aids that would help a person with visual difficulties to communicate.

19   How does the carer support the client to communicate using the care value base?

20   List the support agencies that help people communicate.

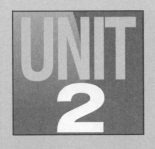

Equality, diversity and rights in health and social care

This unit covers:

- The concepts of equality, diversity and rights in relation to health and social care
- Discriminatory practice in health and social care
- How national initiatives promote anti-discriminatory practice in health and social care
- How anti-discriminatory practice is promoted in health and social care settings

Acknowledging and respecting diversity and the contribution this makes to British life is at the heart of health and social care practice. Health and social care workers need to have a good understanding of diversity and how they can promote equality and rights within their work to ensure that individuals are not disadvantaged and disenfranchised.

Health and social care workers also need to understand what constitutes discriminatory practice and the impact this can have on individuals, the quality of health and social care service provision and society as a whole. They also need to understand the legislation (laws) and guidance in place to support anti-discriminatory practice and how this underpins their work with others.

grading criteria	To achieve a **Pass** grade the evidence must show that the learner is able to:	To achieve a **Merit** grade the evidence must show that, in addition to the pass criteria, the learner is able to:	To achieve a **Distinction** grade the evidence must show that, in addition to the pass and merit criteria, the learner is able to:
	P1 explain the benefits of diversity to society Pg 50		
	P2 use recognised terminology to explain the importance of promoting equality, recognising diversity and respecting rights in health and social care settings Pg 57		

To achieve a **Pass** grade the evidence must show that the learner is able to:	To achieve a **Merit** grade the evidence must show that, in addition to the pass criteria, the learner is able to:	To achieve a **Distinction** grade the evidence must show that, in addition to the pass and merit criteria, the learner is able to:
P3 explain the potential effects of discriminatory practice on those who use health or social care services Pg 68		
P4 describe how legislation, codes of practice, rules of conduct, charters and organisational policies are used to promote anti-discriminatory practice Pg 78	**M1** explain the influences of a recent or emerging national policy development on organisational policy with regard to anti-discriminatory practice Pg 78	**D1** evaluate how a recent or emerging policy development influences organisational and personal practice in relation to anti-discriminatory practice Pg 78
P5 explain how those working in health and social care settings can actively promote anti-discriminatory practice Pg 81	**M2** explain difficulties that may be encountered when implementing anti-discriminatory practice Pg 81	
P6 describe ways of reflecting on and challenging discriminatory issues in health and social care Pg 81	**M3** analyse how personal beliefs and value systems may influence own anti-discriminatory practice Pg 84	**D2** evaluate practical strategies to reconcile own beliefs and values with anti-discriminatory practice in health and social care Pg 84

The concepts of equality, diversity and rights in relation to health and social care

The increasing visibility of racial and cultural diversity in Britain today can lead us to believe that multiculturalism is a relatively recent phenomenon. However, this is misleading. The United Kingdom (UK) has been a culturally diverse nation since the Roman invasions (55BC and AD41). Diversity increased with subsequent invasions by amongst others the Vikings and the Norman French. Throughout history, therefore, the UK has seen many people from many different lands come to its shores. Some have stayed and become part of our diverse heritage, so that many British people can trace their ancestors back to, for example, Europe, Scandinavia, the Indian subcontinent, Africa and the Caribbean. With history of an empire, colonialism and the British Commonwealth, it is not surprising that Britain is home to people from many countries and cultures. In fact, many people from Commonwealth countries always considered themselves British. The reasons why people come to Britain are as diverse as the people themselves. They have come for work, to escape persecution and for adventure, to name just a few. Each group has contributed something to the richness of British life and their influences are now a part of the fabric that is life in twenty-first century Britain.

Benefits of diversity

The social and cultural changes that have resulted from people from around the world settling or just passing through Britain has left a lasting legacy. Each group of migrants has left their mark and caused Britain to develop and progress as a society. Sometimes we have actively sought the help of people from other countries in order to fuel that progress economically. For example, in the 1950s when the demand for new housing was high and the numbers of available workers in short supply, Italians were encouraged to come to England to work in the brick-making industry and many stayed and settled in the Midlands. After the war as there was much to do and too few people to do it, so people came from all over the British Commonwealth to support Britain to rebuild the country, for example, those people who travelled from the Caribbean on the SS Windrush in 1948. In the 1960s, nurses were actively recruited from the Caribbean and more recently from the Philippines to fill vacancies within the NHS. Since the mid 1990s, people have come to work in the UK from European Union countries. They are working in areas as diverse as construction and dentistry, as Britain tries to meet the demands for new buildings, roads and housing, as well as skills gaps in health and other specialised areas.

We only have to visit our local supermarket or walk down the streets in our towns to see the influence of diversity on society. The variety of food available tells its own story as there are tastes and textures from around the world on our doorstep. We can eat food in our own homes that previously we would have had to travel far and wide to experience. Exotic fruits, vegetables and spices have been arriving in Britain for a long time but now more than ever before these are the basis of everyday food for many people rather than the privileged few. Much of the music we listen to has been greatly influenced by African music, mediated through black Americans whether it is rhythm and blues, jazz, hip-hop, soul or rock. Artists such as Picasso were, for example, influenced by African art while other creative arts including fashion and design demonstrate the diversity of ideas and influences that come from other cultures and experiences. Modern literature has become increasingly influenced by writers from diverse cultures, such as Alice Walker, Arundathi Roy, Zadie Smith, Ben Okri and Gabriel Garcia Marquez, all of whom contribute to increasing our understanding of life from different perspectives. The increasingly number of people from diverse backgrounds, cultures and races that are visible in public life, whether in the popular media of TV, music, entertainment and film, sport or in high profile jobs such as MPs, lawyers and academics have all contributed to second and third generation black British people finding an identity which confirms their position in society as one of equality. As part of the National Curriculum in schools, children and young people are taught to value diversity through exploring other cultures and world religions, as these are more representative of the population. As society changes, there is a need to develop a better understanding, one that engenders tolerance and acceptance of diversity.

A diverse society does, however, create its own tensions and conflict. Unrest and riots can result with cultural clashes being blamed for these. Often, closer examination will reveal that poverty and disadvantage are also significant factors, and these are not limited to any one social or cultural group. If Britain is to be a genuinely multicultural society, economic inequality that still exists must be addressed, otherwise the assumption that the white race and culture is and has the right to be dominant will remain and be reinforced and this will undermine integration and acceptance of diversity.

Fig 2.1 Diversity in British life

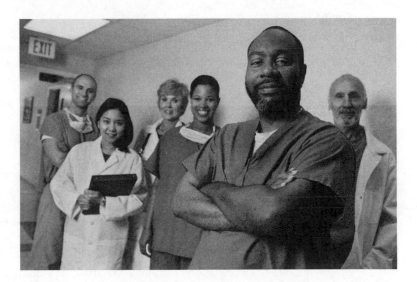

Fig 2.2 Influence of other cultures on British life

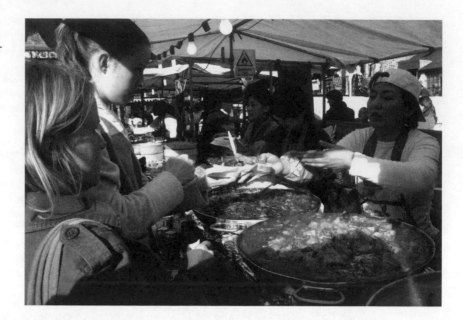

activity
GROUP WORK
2.1

P1

Explain, using examples, how the diversity of foods, cultural experiences, art, literature, and so on, are of benefit to you as an individual living in Britain today.

Terminology

To really understand what is meant by equality, diversity and discrimination it is important to firstly define these and related concepts.

Equality
Treating people with equality means treating them as equals, and providing them with the same opportunities and rights regardless of any differences they may have.

Equity
Treating people with equity means treating them with fairness and impartiality in a way that recognises and addresses the essential differences between individuals and groups to ensure their needs are met appropriately and they receive the same opportunities as others.

Diversity
Recognising people's diversity means recognising that people are different from one another and they have their own unique individuality, personality, identity and social and cultural background.

Rights
A person's rights are the things that they are entitled to by law.

Opportunity
An opportunity is a set of circumstances that enable an individual to do something that may prove to be useful or beneficial to them, such as being able to develop new skills, knowledge or qualifications.

Difference
Unique qualities or distinguishing features which make an individual unlike others around them, can be referred to as differences. This can relate to a diverse range of features, such as age, gender, race, culture, hair and eye colour, height, fitness level, educational background, job role.

Overt discrimination

Discrimination is the unfair treatment of people on grounds of differences, such as race, age or sex. Overt discrimination means it is open discrimination, for example, stating upper age limits in job adverts.

Covert discrimination

Covert discrimination is concealed or not clearly stated, for example, only promoting men to senior positions within an organisation.

Stereotyping

A stereotype is an oversimplified standardised picture or idea that is held by one person or group about another individual or group. Stereotyping, therefore, means considering people with similar characteristics to be exactly the same and not seeing them as unique, for example, the statement 'all older people are hard of hearing'. Stereotyping leads to making assumptions which then inform a person's decisions, attitudes and behaviour in the absence of knowledge or understanding about the uniqueness of the individual.

Labelling

We use labels as a way of naming, describing or categorising things. Labels applied to people usually relate to the person's appearance, behaviour or diagnosis, for example, 'Mr X is aggressive' ' Mrs Z is grumpy and uncooperative' 'the epileptic in bed 4'. If we use labels to describe individuals then we fail to see the uniqueness of the individual only the labels others have given them. Most labels have negative connotations which then lead others to make assumptions about the individual. This then may have a negative impact on their interactions with them.

Prejudice

Prejudice is an opinion that is formed without real or sufficient knowledge or understanding. It is based on irrational feelings, stereotypes, labels and assumptions which lose sight of the individual. Prejudice invariably leads to unfair and unjust treatment of the individual.

Disadvantage

To disadvantage an individual means to treat them less favourably than others and is often due to stereotypical images and ideas, labels, assumptions or prejudice. Disadvantage may take the form of blocking an individual's access or ability to access the same opportunities as others, such as access to good quality education, housing, employment or medical treatment. Equally, an individual may be disadvantaged if they are always immediately blamed for events without any consideration. For example, if they belong to a group stereotyped and labelled as criminals then they are likely to experience higher than average police arrests for questioning when crimes have been committed in their area.

Beliefs

A belief is a feeling that something is true or real, and is generally related to religious or spiritual doctrines (principles). Beliefs can also be considered in a wider context as a framework of ideas which underpin the way in which an individual chooses to live their life. This framework may well have been influenced by religion, but is not necessarily drawn totally from one religion. Instead, people's beliefs may be a mixture of ideas drawn from different sources, such as different religions as well as philosophy. Our beliefs are individual and underpin much of our attitudes and behaviour and moral sense of right and wrong.

Values

Values are the beliefs held by an individual that concern the difference between right and wrong. Like beliefs, values inform our intentions and motivations and underpin our actions. They are often closely aligned to our beliefs and as such are part of that framework by which we live our lives. Organisations and professions in health and social care work also set out and seek to adhere to a set of values. These are designed to describe to individuals accessing services what they can expect in terms of standards of behaviour and service.

Vulnerability

Vulnerability is the state of being exposed to emotional or physical danger or harm from others. Given the wrong circumstances, we can all be vulnerable, for example, standing alone late at night, in the dark on a deserted road in an unfamiliar area when our car has broken down. However, many of the individuals being supported by health and social services are particularly vulnerable due to the nature of their support needs. A **vulnerable adult** is an individual who is in need of the care services by reason of mental or other disability, age, or illness, and who is, or may be unable to take care of, or protect himself against significant harm or exploitation.

See page 362 in Unit 11 for more information on vulnerability.

Abuse

Abuse is physical, emotional or sexual harm caused to an individual, or the failure to protect an individual from harm.

See page 356 in Unit 11 for more information on abuse.

Empowerment

Empowerment is the action of making an individual or oneself stronger, more confident or more powerful by giving them more control over their life. It is achieved by becoming aware of and using personal and external resources to overcome obstacles in order to meet needs and aspirations. It also means having your voice heard in decision-making and being able to challenge inequality and oppression in your life.

Independence

We consider an individual to have independence when they are in control of themselves, their day-to-day life and decisions without being controlled by another person or organisation. Independence is connected to freedom in terms of choice and includes being able to make decisions without undue influence by others.

Interdependence

Interdependence is a situation where individuals are unable to survive or function in their daily living activities without mutual support, cooperation or interaction with others. To a great extent, we are all interdependent. This becomes evident when a group of workers, such as train drivers, go on strike. This causes disruption to services and many people are unable to go to work which may then impact on other areas of our lives. A society functions because we rely on one another to each play our part in making it work.

Racism

When the word 'race' was first used it referred to belonging to a family. It was then used to distinguish people of different nationalities and then by scientists to describe the physical differences between people from different parts of the world, for example, differences in skin colour, hair type and body shape. Racism is when individuals are treated unfairly and with hostility as a direct result of assumptions and prejudices related to these physical characteristics. Racism is often underpinned with ideas that one 'race' is superior to another in terms of abilities, rights and privileges. There is a tendency to think that only people who have different skin colours, for example white and black, can be racist. Recent history has shown this to be far from the truth with racism reaching an extreme through the ethnic cleansing in Kosovo, Rwanda, Iraq and the Sudanese territory of Darfur.

| Commission for Racial Equality | www.cre.gov.uk |
| Equal Opportunities Commission | www.eoc.org.uk |

Sexism

Discrimination against individuals due to their sex is called sexism. Both men and women can be subjected to sexism although there is evidence that this occurs more to women than to men.

Homophobia

Homophobia is an extreme and irrational aversion to homosexuality, homosexuals and lesbians. This includes everything associated with homosexuality, for example, gay culture.

Health and social care settings

As stated in the introduction, issues of equality, diversity and rights are at the heart of health and social care work and, as a result, all care settings will have policies and procedures in place to ensure that these are promoted and, if needed, poor care practice is challenged.

Residential care

There are a number of different types of residential care. Some individuals may be supported within a large residential care home with other people who have similar needs or of a similar age.

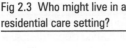

Fig 2.3 Who might live in a residential care setting?

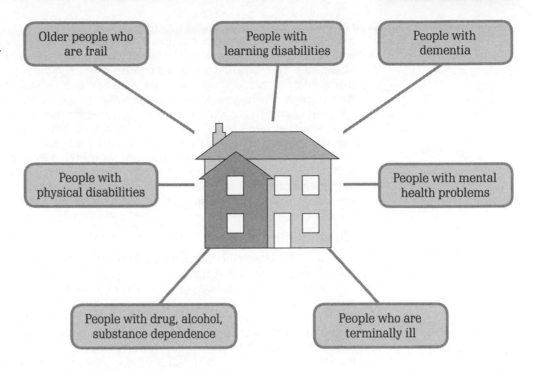

People who are identified as needing substantial support to manage their daily living activities often live in residential care homes as they are able to provide 24-hour, all-year care. Residential care may also be used for respite to give an individual's **carer** a break from caring.

There are three different types of residential care settings. These are residential care homes that provide support with social care needs, such as personal care and maintaining the individual's safety, nursing homes where the individual requires regular support from a qualified nurse or doctor, for example if they have long-term medical conditions that require regular monitoring and intervention, and duel residential and nursing homes which provide both types of care and support.

Children and young people may be supported within a residential care setting in circumstances where there has been family breakdown or the individual has specific needs such as physical or learning disabilities that require high levels of support 24 hours a day.

For individuals to live in residential care, their health and social care needs will need to be assessed. As a result of the requirements of the NHS & Community Care Act (1990), individuals have a right to a needs assessment. They can request this themselves or they can be referred for an assessment by someone else, such as a relative, their General Practitioner (GP) or community nurse. The assessment of needs could be undertaken by a social worker from the local authority social services department if the individual requires state funding for their care or by the registered manager of the residential or nursing care home if the individual is funding their own care. The purpose of the assessment is to establish the individual's needs and their wishes and preferences as to how these would be best met. It is essential that this is undertaken to ensure the individual goes to live somewhere that their needs can be best met and where they feel at home as far as possible. The individual's on-going care will be recorded in a care plan and this is used to meet their needs on a day-to-day basis providing the appropriate levels of support.

Day care

Day care can be provided in a number of different settings. It may be in a day centre, within the individual's home, a day hospital or a residential care home. Day centres can be found within the community. Some are purpose-built while others may be in converted houses. Some day centres are multi-purpose and have facilities that are designed to meet the needs of individuals with varying needs. Other day care provision is specifically designed to meet the needs of one group with similar needs, for example, people with dementia or adults with learning disabilities. Following an assessment of needs, it may be agreed by the individual, the social worker and others involved with supporting the individual, such as their carer, that some of the individual's needs (and the carers need for respite) could be met through attendance at a day centre.

remember

Respite care is a period of rest, or a break from caring for another person which enables the carer to recover from the physical and emotional demands of caring for someone who requires significant levels of support.

A carer is someone who looks after a relative or friend who needs support because of age, physical or learning disability or illness, including mental illness. They provide regular and substantial support for the individual.

For an adult with learning disability, attending a day centre provides an opportunity to develop new skills, develop or maintain independence as well as social interaction and leisure activities. For individuals with mental health issues, drug, alcohol or substance dependence, attending a day centre or day hospital provides them with the opportunity to participate in therapeutic activities, e.g. relaxation classes to help them manage their condition or change their patterns of behaviour. Many individuals who require health and social care support do not need or want to live within a residential care setting and wish to remain living in their own home. Day care supports and enables them to do this. Older people may receive day care within a local residential care home where they may also receive respite care. Some people may receive day care within their own home on a one-to-one basis with a support worker. Day care involves providing activities which will be stimulating for the individual while at the same time meeting their needs and suiting their interests and abilities, for example, gardening, playing games such as chess, quizzes, cooking, painting, craft activities, dancing, exercise or singing.

Nursing care

Nursing care is provided in either an acute hospital setting or within a nursing home. Nursing care involves not only providing support with personal care but also carrying out treatments and interventions as prescribed by medical staff or clinical nurse specialists. Individuals receiving nursing care are likely to have either acute or chronic (long term) conditions or illness, or to be recovering from accidents or operations. Nursing care is provided using the nursing process of assess, plan, implement and evaluate, along with a nursing model, such as Roper-Logan-Tierney (1983). Nursing care will also incorporate the Essence of Care framework which has been designed to improve the individual's experience and outcomes from health care support and interventions. Ten fundamental aspects of care have been identified as crucial to individuals receiving person-centred care.

NHS Modernisation Agency

www.cgsupport.nhs.uk

Essence of Care – Patient-focused benchmarks for clinical governance

Domiciliary care

This is where health or social care is provided within the individual's home. This usually involves support with personal care and the activities of daily living, such as washing, dressing, using the toilet, moving around and managing household tasks. Individuals may receive only personal care support or domestic support or both depending on their needs and the local provision of services. In some areas, individuals have to access and pay for domestic support themselves as only personal care support is funded by the local authority social services department. Individuals can access domiciliary care support independently or following a needs assessment. The purpose of domiciliary care is to support the individual to remain living in their own home and be independent for as long as possible while still having their needs met.

Active promotion of equality and individual rights in health and social care settings

Although people may be supported within a range of health and social care settings, it is important that a person is treated as an individual with a unique identity, needs, wishes and preferences and this individuality is acknowledged and structures are in place that enable a person to feel like an individual, an 'I' not just a 'we' of the group.

Principles of the care value base

These principles underpin how health and social care work is carried out. The care value base describes the attitudes and behaviours that constitute good care practice which values, respects, nurtures and positively supports individuals. These principles are often encapsulated within a health and social care worker's job description and the ethos or aims and objectives of their employing organisation. They are also within the codes of practice for health and social care workers.

General Social Care Council

www.gscc.org.uk

Codes of Practice

Care practice that is based on these values ensures that the individual is treated with respect, politeness and consideration for their diversity and individuality. This means considering language and tone of voice when addressing individuals as well as finding out the name they prefer others to use to address them. It also means providing care support which demonstrates the individual's choices have been considered and supported. Health and social care workers should support individuals in ways that promote their dignity, privacy and rights. For example, they knock before entering the individual's room; ensuring the individual's confidentiality is respected and maintained. If health and social care workers demonstrate these principles in their practice, they acknowledge the individual's right to a personal life and so individuals will learn to trust them. This trust underpins an effective working relationship.

Applying care values is also demonstrated through the worker supporting the individual in an enabling way which promotes and supports their independence and empowers them to manage their lives as far as they are able, for example encouraging them and valuing what they can do rather than focusing on what they are unable to do, taking time when supporting them and ensuring they are able to present their views and participate in decision-making.

Health and social care workers should work in a person-centred way as this shows individuals they value and respect their experience and knowledge as well as who they are as a person. This can be demonstrated by 'working with' them rather than 'doing things to' them and treating the individual as an equal partner in their care and listening to their views and opinions.

Health and social care workers also have a responsibility to ensure individuals are supported to realise, live up to or develop their potential. This may include supporting individuals to make their own decisions regarding risk by ensuring their decisions are informed ones, while at the same time ensuring they are also protected from abuse and harm. Making sure individuals are informed involves making them fully aware of the potential risks, the likelihood of these occurring, the potential outcomes; and the control measures to be put in place to reduce the risks as well as the potential benefits. At all times, the worker needs to demonstrate acceptance of the individual as a human being and a non-judgemental attitude, although the worker must avoid an acceptance or condoning of an individual's actions which may be hurtful or destructive.

Putting the patient or service user at the heart of service provision

Using a person-centred approach to supporting individuals means putting them at the centre of everything: assessments of needs, decision making, care planning, implementation, monitoring and review. To achieve this, workers need to spend time with the individual, and significant others if appropriate, to find out about them their biography (personal information and past history), their personality, interests, needs, choices, wishes and preferences so that these can be considered when providing support. Considering the individual as a whole person, what they want from their lives in the present as well as the future enables workers to encourage and maintain the individual's dignity, self-respect and positive self-esteem. Being person-centred also means working in partnership with those people whom are significant to the individual, such as partners, family, carers and other practitioners. Working in a person-centred way means focusing on the individual's strengths, needs and what is important to them and enabling them through active support to participate in a wider community life if that is their choice.

Person-centred approaches mean the health and social care worker promotes the individual's rights, choices and well-being. This may include ensuring the individual is able to participate fully in decision-making by supporting them to present their views effectively to others. For example, it might involve supporting the individual to make a video diary of their activities, views, wishes and expectations which can be shown to those who support them as well as in more formal settings such as a review meeting. **Advocacy** as well as augmentative communication strategies, such as pictorial exchange communication system (PECS) or BLISS symbols, should also be considered and accessed as appropriate. People with profound and multiple learning disabilities can use a multi-media profile (MMP) to help them communicate more independently with those who support them. A MMP is made up of video, photos, symbols and words and is accessed through using a computer. The individual is fully involved using their method of communication. This could be vocal sounds, gestures, facial expressions, body language, behaviour or any other form of communication. As this is captured on film, the individual can tell their story and show how they communicate. They can choose to share this with those who support them to enable them to have a better

remember

Active support means enabling individuals to participate in life activities to the best of their ability with or without support.

understanding of their needs and preferences and how they communicate these. Using any of these methods empowers the individual and enables them to be at the centre of the review, and supports their needs and right to have their say. This is particularly effective if the individual finds meetings with others difficult and overwhelming to the extent they feel unable to speak or really say what they want to say.

See page 3 in Unit 1 for more information on communication methods.

To put the service user at the centre of care activities, health and social care workers must also uphold the principles of anti-discriminatory practice in all they do, ensuring the individual is empowered to make their own decisions and choices. Empowerment means giving individuals meaningful choices and options that enable them to have more control over their lives and their circumstances. For some this can only become a reality when the impact of inequalities, oppression and discrimination are addressed. Empowerment takes time as often individuals can have a sense of impossibility, hopelessness and defeat about them as a result of internalising the discrimination or oppression they have experienced in their lives. This can, however, provide a way of helping individuals to understand and talk about how they have come to believe negative statements about themselves and consider them to be unchangeable parts of their personality. To support an individual to unravel the complexity of this damage and to move forward takes time and a trusting professional relationship.

Dealing with tensions and contradictions

Part of the health and social care worker's role and responsibility will be to manage the tensions that exist within the human relationships that make up this area of work. There are many situations where tensions and contradictions occur, for example:

- between identifying an individual's needs and working within resource constraints
- between promoting the individual's independence and protecting them from harm
- between empowering an individual to achieve their potential and managing risks
- between supporting the rights of the individual and the rights of the group
- between supporting an individual within their home and managing worker health and safety issues
- between the individual's perceptions of their needs and circumstances and those of their carer and the practitioner
- between the needs of the individual and those of their carer.

In order to actively promote equality and individual rights within these situations of tension or contradiction, it is important that the health and social care worker consults with and involves all those who are involved such as the individual, their carer, the worker's manager or supervisor and other practitioners. Unilateral (one-sided) decision making should be avoided, as often the views of others helps to create a realistic and balanced perspective and a shared decision is likely to have a better outcome for all involved because more people have a vested interest in a positive outcome. Unilateral decisions can also lead to an individual's rights being infringed, for example if the worker has a negative attitude towards risk taking and seeing their role as one of protector this will impact on their decision.

Professional Practice

Practice dilemmas, such as tensions and contradictions in supporting equality and rights, should be:

- discussed in supervision with manager or supervisor
- discussed with all involved
- fully documented at every stage of the decision-making process
- monitored and reviewed as decisions are put into practice.

Staff development and training

All health and social care workers are required to undertake induction training when they begin employment. Part of the induction training relates to issues of equality and diversity and the worker's role in the promotion of these as well as the individual's rights and choices. An increasing number of workers then progress to undertake a National Vocational Qualification (NVQ) in Health or Health and Social Care. This is where the worker demonstrates their knowledge, understanding and workplace competence in the practical application of the principles of care practice values, anti-discriminatory practice, a person-centred approach and service user empowerment in every aspect of their day-to-day work.

Specific courses and learning opportunities may be available to promote the worker's more detailed understanding, such as disability awareness training or person-centred planning. Another area where workers will receive specific training will be in record keeping and confidentiality.

Practical implications of confidentiality

The principles of confidentiality will have been clearly explained through the health and social care worker's job description and contract of employment, as well as the policies, procedures, aims and objectives of the organisation and the induction process. Understanding the implications of the practical application of confidentiality and the underlying principles is essential if the individual's rights to respect, privacy and dignity are to be promoted and maintained. When recording information, it is essential that this is factual, accurate, relevant, complete, legible, unambiguous, signed and dated. No records should contain value statements or judgements and, where possible and appropriate, workers should check what they have written is correct with the individual. The individual has a right to see their records and so it is important that written records reflect anti-discriminatory practice as much as direct work with the individual. When reporting information, it is essential this is carried out in a private area where those involved in giving and receiving the information will not be overheard. A verbal report should contain all the relevant information, be accurate, complete, factual, and unambiguous. In relation to information sharing, this can only take place with the individual's informed consent (i.e. it must be clearly explained to the individual what will be shared, with whom, when, where, how and for what purpose as well as the implications of not sharing information). Any limitations to information sharing the individual requires should be made known to all relevant staff in the care setting and these wishes adhered to.

When storing information, it is essential this is placed somewhere secure, such as a locked filing cabinet or drawer, or if information is stored electronically then this must be secure, for example, password-protected and regularly backed up. Only those who have a right to access confidential information should be able to access the computer-held records or keys to locked storage. When storing information, it is also essential that it is stored in such a way that it is easy to access and does not get mixed up with other information.

activity
INDIVIDUAL WORK 2.2

P2

Use examples from your own and work placement experience within health and social care services which you feel explain the importance of the following concepts when supporting individual with health or social care needs:

1 promoting equality
2 recognising diversity
3 respecting rights

Individual rights

Every individual has rights which protect them from harm and abuse by systems, organisations and other individuals. These rights enable individuals to achieve their potential and access the same opportunities as others. Individual rights are there to promote equality and value diversity. In the UK, each individual has the following rights:

Fig 2.4 Rights of individuals

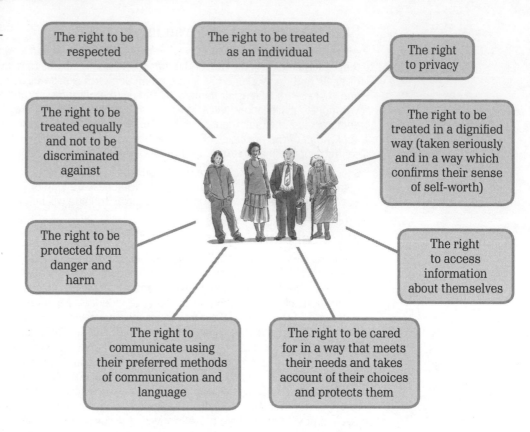

The right to be respected

The right to be treated as an individual

The right to privacy

The right to be treated equally and not to be discriminated against

The right to be treated in a dignified way (taken seriously and in a way which confirms their sense of self-worth)

The right to be protected from danger and harm

The right to access information about themselves

The right to communicate using their preferred methods of communication and language

The right to be cared for in a way that meets their needs and takes account of their choices and protects them

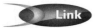

See page 355 in Unit 11 for more information on individual rights.

Discriminatory practice in health and social care

As described earlier, discrimination can occur against any individual or group who are different from the dominant and prevailing norm in that situation. With that in mind, it is useful to remember that, given the right circumstances, the potential for each of us to experience discrimination is there. However, there are a number of groups is society that are particularly vulnerable to discrimination.

Bases of discrimination

As individuals, our sense of identity forms in part due to our genetic inheritance, but perhaps more so from the influences around us that we use to construct and shape ourselves into the person we want to be. It is useful to remember that some people are not able to do this freely as their environment (external influences) is controlled by others for personal, cultural or religious reasons. Many would argue that few of us are totally free to construct our own identity, as we are subject to pressures from family, peers and society as a whole, so in a sense we too are socially constructed. The systems and structures within society, such as government, social status groupings, health and social care services, language, education (types, availability, eligibility criteria for access), socialisation (our relationships with others) and all forms of the media are all examples of factors that influence and reinforce the ideas we have about society, individuals within it, ourselves and our place within it.

Within any society, there are individuals and groups who are more powerful and influential than others, and as a consequence their needs and interests are viewed as more important than those of others with less power and influence. As a result of their power and influence, their view of society dominates and becomes the norm by which all others are measured and then integrated if found to be acceptable and advantageous or dismissed if unacceptable. All those individuals who hold the dominant views are then regarded as the norm and those who do not may be subjected to ridicule, unfair treatment and discrimination. The differences between individuals are constructed through the views of dominant groups being reinforced and presented powerfully and consistently as 'natural' and therefore constructing the norm.

Anything or anyone that is different is in comparison viewed as 'unnatural' and therefore abnormal, and so the social construction of difference is created. This process is sometimes referred to as 'othering', constructing a barrier between those who belong to the dominant norm group and those who are outside this group. Intertwined with this process are the processes of stereotyping, prejudice and the creation of ignorance and fear about anyone that is different in order to legitimise (to justify and make it appear reasonable and right) the attitudes and behaviour of members of the dominant group that are unjust, discriminatory and abusive towards individuals who are different in some way. Bound up with this is the idea that the dominant norm is superior and the only 'right way' to do something or behave. In the UK, the most powerful and influential group are white, middle class, employed, heterosexual, married, Anglican (Church of England) males. These people determine the dominant ideas of British society, and anyone who does not fit into any of those categories may be subject to discriminatory behaviour because they are considered different or inferior to this 'ideal'.

This process sometimes goes to extremes and the outside group are demonised so that the extreme discrimination, inhuman treatment or atrocities against them are viewed as justified. This is the case in any situation of genocide and ethnic cleansing, such as that carried out by Hitler against Jewish people during the 1940s, Cambodians under the Khmer Rouge in the 1970s, Bosnian Muslims in the former Yugoslavia in the late 20th century or the slaughter of the Tutsi minority by the Hutu majority in Rwanda in 1994. Less extreme but equally discriminatory was the idea of eugenics (selective reproduction to produce a race of people with desirable qualities and traits and no disabilities) and the 'othering' and segregation of individuals with physical or mental disabilities during the 20th century. Social construction is not static and changes over time and consequently between generations and social groupings.

Link   See page 242 in Unit 7 for more information on bases of discrimination.

Culture

Individuals from different cultures may experience discrimination due to the factors outlined earlier and as a result of people's lack of knowledge and understanding. Fear often lies at the root of discrimination as the idea of difference of any kind is viewed with suspicion and this makes people defensive. A lack of knowledge and understanding about cultural and religious customs, expectations and accepted behaviour can lead health and social care workers to discriminate against an individual unintentionally. Sometimes, however, individuals from a different culture are discriminated against because it is more work or costs more to provide appropriate support to meet their needs.

We need to consider culture in its widest sense too and not just align this with nationality or skin colour. There are considerable regional cultural differences across the UK in terms of how people relate to one another this is clearly demonstrated in the differences in how people greet and acknowledge others.

Many aspects of life are subject to unwritten rules. These norms are learned through socialisation processes as we grow up, such as what to wear in different social situations, how to greet someone you know or do not know, personal space, how to show respect for others. If we are unaware of these we can cause offence to others whose cultural norms are different from ours. Cultural norms could be viewed as 'the way we do things'.

Disability

The idea of disability is influenced by culture, religion and predominantly medical models which define and categorise disability in comparison to an idea of normality. All these factors have influenced society's responses to people with disabilities and how they should be considered and treated. As a result of social change, the way people with disabilities are viewed and supported in society has changed. During the 20th century, the majority of people with a disability were cared for either within the family or within large institutions often hidden away in the country. Parents were not encouraged to keep a child born with an obvious or visible disability. People who behaved in ways deemed be deviant by the dominant groups were often sent to a mental institution (a psychiatric hospital) even though they had no formal diagnosis of psychiatric illness. For example, unmarried women who had babies were frequently sent away and in some cases forgotten about (although interestingly men who had been party to the conception were not judged and segregated from society). When the long stay mental hospitals started to close in the 1980s, many of those who had been resident for decades were found to have had no physical or mental health problems at all.

However, the institutionalisation they had experienced made it impossible for many to regain their independence and they continue to be supported in various ways today. The processes of 'othering' that were discussed in the last section also apply as this group of individuals were seen as 'deviant' and less important that 'ordinary' people. An absence of people who were disabled in society reinforced the sense of difference and set them apart which made people fearful of what was unfamiliar and unknown.

With these historical and social attitudes as a backdrop, people with disabilities are viewed as different and consequently have experienced discrimination in all aspects of their lives and even, arguably, before they are born, such as in cases where genetic conditions are known and termination of pregnancy is strongly advocated by many as being the right thing to do. Access to equitable levels of health care, education, job opportunities and family life are all areas where people with disabilities may experience discrimination. Many people with disabilities have in the past reported inequitable access to health care especially if they have underlying medical problems which contribute to their disability. Poor or no access to education has meant that many people with disabilities have been unable to achieve their potential. Assumptions were made about their capacity to learn without real investigation or understanding on how to teach and assist them to learn. This has had the effect of reinforcing ideas that disability is total and a person is incapable of anything independently.

Changes to legislation have made it possible for many children to receive appropriate education opportunities and many are integrated into mainstream schools thus also breaking down the barriers that create the sense of difference. The Disability Discrimination Act (1995) (DDA) has also improved access to employment and areas of public life. The Disability Equality Duty (DED) which became law on 4th December 2006 applies to the public sector and takes this further with a code of practice and a duty to promote equality. The general duty requires public authorities to

- promote positive attitudes towards disabled people
- promote equality between disabled people and others
- eliminate discrimination that is unlawful under the DDA
- eliminate harassment of disabled people that is related to their disability
- encourage participation of disabled people in public life
- take action to meet the needs of disabled people even if this requires more favourable treatment.

Changes in social attitude and more recently the Human Rights Act (2000) has had an impact on the right to family life of people with disabilities, especially in terms of personal and sexual relationships and being a parent. For many years, it was customary that young women with learning disabilities were sterilised without their consent to avoid pregnancy as they were deemed vulnerable to sexual abuse and incapable of being a parent. Personal relationships of any kind between people with disabilities were discouraged and viewed by many as unnatural with parenting being out of the question because of issues of genetic inheritance. Attitudes have changed in many cases although not in all and resistance remains as individuals try and balance capacity and vulnerability with personal rights and choice.

remember

Institutionalisation or 'learned helplessness' occurs as a result of living in an environment with strict rules, routines and an inflexible approach imposed by those in charge. The individual loses independence of thinking and behaviour.

See page 72 for more information on legislation regarding disability. See page 255 in Unit 7 for more information on models of disability.

The Disability Equality Duty (DED)   www.dotheduty.org

Age

Both younger and older people can experience discrimination because of their age. What is appropriate for people of different ages to do is socially constructed and to some extent also subject to legislation. For example, in the UK there are legal ages when young people can do certain things such as age of consent and the legal age to vote. Until the advent of the Children's Act (1989), children were still regarded as 'belonging' to their parents. Decisions about children were made in what was considered to be the child's best interests with little or no involvement from the children themselves. In some cases this served not to protect but to increase the child's vulnerability to discrimination and abuse. Children and young people can still be discriminated against. In some circumstances they can be viewed as a homogenous group (all the same) and when this is underpinned with historical and social attitudes of vulnerability this can lead to stereotypical views which, as discussed before, can lead to discrimination. Negative images of young people are prominent today with young people being characterised as 'out of control', taking alcohol or illegal drugs, sexually promiscuous and involved in anti-social behaviour. To stereotype all young people in this way is as incorrect and misleading as it is to stereotype all older people as being grumpy, decrepit, demented, dependent and 'past it'.

There are many negative representations of older people within society and this has led to some of these stereotypical ideas. However, society is changing and the population is an aging one with life expectancy rising and more people over 80 currently living in the UK than ever before. Ideas of what is acceptable behaviour for older people are again constructed socially and historically, and some attitudes that predominate have led to prejudice and unfair treatment, such as the belief that older people are incapable of learning new things, or unable to travel alone. Many older people feel they are discriminated against in relation to access to health care because of their age, for example being told 'at your age what do you expect?' Older people are physically fitter than ever before and many do not want to retire at 60 or 65 years, but until the Age Discrimination Act (2006) many were forced into retirement regardless of their wishes or fitness to continue working.

Older age is not viewed the same by all cultures as in many older people are revered (treated with admiring respect) for their wisdom and their needs are supported well. Many people in the UK feel that this is not the case for older people, but that they are expected to be grateful for inadequate provision for their needs and interests. This is changing, however, as the post war 'baby boomers' now reaching their 60s and 70s are making their voice heard and are demanding better treatment in relation to working, pensions, concessions as well as health and social care support in recognition for their contribution to society. The recent Age Discrimination Act is testament to the strength of their voice and resultant activity. There are many more positive images of older people as a result of the 'baby boomers' getting older. There continue to be many examples of older people being discriminated against unfairly, however, often to the extent of abuse such as financial abuse resulting from financial decisions being made by family members without consultation with the person.

Social class

Social class is determined by the occupation of the main wage earner in a household. For many years this was always determined by the male or 'head' of the house, although this is no longer the case as the composition of families and households as well as traditional male/female roles have changed. Social class is closely linked to and largely determined by a person's family background, which in turn determines their education and achievements, where they live and the type of accommodation they live in.

National Statistics socio-economic classifications (NS-SEC)

1		Higher managerial and professional occupations
	1.1	Large employers and higher managerial occupations
	1.2	Higher professional occupations
2		Lower managerial and professional occupations
3		Intermediate occupations
4		Small employers and own account workers
5		Lower supervisory and technical occupations
6		Semi-routine occupations
7		Routine occupations
8		Never worked and long-term unemployed

Source: www.statistics.gov.uk

Individuals may find themselves discriminated against on the basis of their social class. For example, access to the more prestigious universities was traditionally through the fee-paying public schools where the majority of students were from the upper and upper middle classes. Now, however, universities are required to have wider access admissions policies and procedures to enable those students from the lower middle and working classes and state education to access places in an attempt to create a meritocracy, where social status is based on achievement and merit rather than inheritance or money and reduce inequality. Some occupations and organisations continue to be dominated by particular classes, for example the legal profession is dominated by the upper and upper middle classes.

Gender

As discussed previously, the dominant ideas within society have been controlled by men with women being seen and treated unequally as this was viewed as the 'natural order' described through the teachings of world religions. For centuries, women have come second in everything as their needs were considered less important than those of a man. Women have been excluded from many things we now take for granted, for example, girls were not educated, women had no right to the vote until the 1920s and women could not become medical doctors. The feminist movement in the 1960s challenged the dominance of male ideas. Coupled with the advent of the contraceptive pill, which enabled women to safely and effectively control their fertility, this movement changed women's perception and that of society about the role of women in society and their expectations for their life. Many women's lives are testament to the success of that challenge to patriarchal (male dominated) society as they participate in all spheres of life including government and industry. However, many women are still subject to social class, family and cultural pressure to conform to more traditional roles of wife and mother with little encouragement to actively participate and achieve in education or employment.

Strong ideas about what women and men should do also led to traditional work roles. Even today, many people find it hard to accept a male social care worker providing personal care as they view this as a female role. Stereotypical images of male and female roles are now unacceptable and this is one way of widening participation for both genders. Although the UK has had legislation in place for more than thirty years to address discrimination against women in the workplace, cases are still being brought under that legislation as women fight to be treated equally. Women still experience discrimination within more traditionally male areas of society. Research has shown that this is more to do with the ingrained male leadership styles and management models which are often in opposition to those that sit comfortably with women's values and beliefs. The world is changing however, and in areas of business it is the more feminine or androgynous (a mixture of masculine and feminine characteristics) leadership and management styles and models that suit those changes and bring success and its rewards.

Another factor that has affected the progression of women within the public sphere of work is the continuing gendered ideas regarding the natural care-giver role. Women are still considered to be natural care givers and with an ageing population women are predominantly trying to juggle work and caring responsibilities throughout their lives as they move on from caring for children to caring for older relatives.

See page 243 in Unit 7 for more information on gender.

Sexuality

The dominant ideas regarding sexuality are founded in religious belief and teaching of heterosexual partnership being 'natural' with other expressions of sexuality viewed as 'deviant'. Although there were periods in history when there appeared to be a level of acceptance of difference (such as the 'passionate friendships' of women in Victorian times) for the most part people whose sexuality differed from the heterosexual norm either denied this to themselves or hid this from public scrutiny, as to express this difference openly meant imprisonment, persecution or death. Sexuality is considered a private matter and so in most generations not a subject for open discussion and debate. However, attitudes towards this private aspect of an individual's life changed from the 1950s onwards with the emergence of the gay rights activists in the 1970s which created a positive identity for gay men and lesbians. Since that time there has been a growing acceptance of difference and this has been supported by legislation, such as the Human Rights Act. However, the act of openly expressing this difference in sexuality is still not accepted by all to the extent that individuals are treated with equity in all things. Gay people still experience discrimination because of their difference which some see as sinful, immoral, disgusting and shameful. Homosexuality is still denounced by many religious groups with some proclaiming they can 'cure' the individual. At times, this difference was constructed as presenting a danger to 'normal' people with homosexual men being constructed as predatory and likely to take advantage of and 'corrupt' young men. The social construction of homosexuality as deviant therefore, remains for many people an overriding one and one which has given rise to prejudice and fear.

This prejudiced view was reinforced and given further justification with the advent of HIV and AIDS in the 1980s which was first highlighted within the gay community as so many young men were dying of this previously undiagnosed disease. When it emerged that one of the ways HIV was transmitted was through unprotected sexual contact, the tide of condemnation against the gay community cited this devastating disease as judgement for their 'immoral, deviant, promiscuous sexual behaviour'. The reality of HIV infection and spread did not emerge and was not given the same prominence in the media until many people had already internalised these negative and discriminatory messages about gay men with the outcome that some people still hold these prejudiced views today.

Gay men, and to a lesser degree lesbians, continue to be victims of violent crime (physical assault, murder) with the perpetrator's only motivation for these attacks being the person's sexuality. Gay men and lesbians have however, fought through legal processes to achieve the same rights as heterosexuals especially in relation to rights that come with partnerships, such as pension rights, rights to register civil partnerships and equity with married couples.

Health status

As the demands for health care continued to rise throughout the 20th century, the need to ration or establish criteria for eligibility for services arose. In most cases, this rationing was covert or presented in a less contentious way to the general public, for example by viewing professional medical judgements as above question. Towards the end of the century, however, the debate about health and personal responsibility for health began to uncover these issues. Individuals who had disregarded medical advice relating to their health and well-being and continued what were considered to be unhealthy behaviours were experiencing restricted access to some areas of health care and treatment, for example smokers and people who were clinically obese experienced restricted access to surgical operations. The debate about lung cancer and the evidence from research of tobacco as a carcinogen led to debate and judgements about who was deserving or undeserving of treatment. The realisation that non-smokers could develop lung cancer due to 'passive smoking' (the effects of just breathing in tobacco smoke) further heightened this distinction.

Access to human organ transplants requires individuals to take responsibility for giving up their health-damaging behaviours in order to be considered a suitable recipient and placed on the waiting for organ donor list. A similar debate regarding access to expensive treatments arose in relation to HIV/AIDS with those viewed as deserving, i.e. heterosexual women, haemophiliacs and people who had received a contaminated blood or blood product transfusion, on one side as they had contracted the disease through no 'fault' of their own. The undeserving on the other side were homosexual men, prostitutes, and intravenous drug users, all of whom were considered by many as living on the margins of society and viewed as 'bringing it upon themselves' through their behaviour. Such was the ignorance and prejudice surrounding HIV status that until recently a declaration of HIV-positive status could potentially exclude individuals from getting a job in some areas, accessing a loan, life assurance or a mortgage. Equally individuals with mental health needs could often experience negative discrimination when seeking employment, housing or family life as a result of the social construction of mental health and the prejudice that created. People with mental health needs are often portrayed in the media as either 'mad' or 'bad' and a danger to themselves and others due their unpredictable behaviour.

Family status

As discussed earlier in relation to social class, the status of a person's family has a considerable bearing on how that individual is viewed within society and the opportunities available to them. The idea of family is driven by the norm of two adults of different sexes married to each other and living together, with one or more children who are the children of both parents. Any other type of family can be viewed negatively by some groups within society, and as a consequence may experience discrimination in terms of access to employment or housing. In addition, as the dominant group in UK society remains heterosexual, male, married and upper middle or middle class, it is the young, single unmarried mother who has in recent years been constructed as undisciplined, uneducated, a scrounger and irresponsible, particularly if the children have different fathers and the women has more children while receiving welfare benefits from the state. Some people would also consider an unmarried mother as immoral as well based on the dominant norm in society. For many years these judgments were directed at the woman and not at the absent father who had played a part in the child's conception. This came later when the government sought to force absent fathers to take financial responsibility for their children through the Child Support Agency. The social construction of young, single, unmarried mothers has led to stereotyping and prejudice and resulted in many experiencing discrimination in the form of abuse from other people and lack of access to opportunities, such as housing, education and training.

Cognitive ability

Individuals with impaired cognitive ability, for example, with learning disabilities or mental health problems, have been constructed in society in negative ways which has created a stereotypical view that they are unpredictable in their behaviour and unable to make reasoned choices. Both the stereotype and the vulnerability that results increase the likelihood they will experience discrimination. For adults with a learning disability, the situation of being talked over or ignored as a person addresses their carer and not them is one which probably all have experienced. Many adults with learning disabilities are now supported within their own home in the community with many employed and in relationships. Accessing a service such as a bank account has been an issue as staff often do not talk to the person and assume that because, for example, their speech or movements are different to those of others they also have a lack of cognitive ability to manage their own affairs. Older people with dementia often experience similar types of discrimination as their views are not sought regarding decisions that directly affect them and their well-being and their financial affairs being taken over against their will by, for example, a family member. The discrimination experienced is nearly always an abuse of power over the individual by another person. This person may feel their behaviour is justified due to the individual's lack of competence to make decisions, or that they will be able to get away with it because the individual's lack of capacity makes them unable to challenge decisions or that the individual's statements will be discounted as unreliable if they are able to tell someone.

See page 285 in Unit 8 for more information on cognitive ability

Discriminatory practice

From the discussion about what lies at the base of discrimination, it is clear that when a person discriminates against another they do so based on a judgement made in the absence of personal knowledge or understanding of the individual but more likely on a socially constructed, stereotypical view which has been influenced and reinforced by prejudice. If discriminatory views and attitudes are part of a health and social care worker's practice this denies the rights of those they seek to support and the worker becomes part of the problem and not part of the solution.

Infringement of rights

When an individual is discriminated against, their right to be treated with fairness and equity are infringed (disregarded). The examples given in the last section describe many of the different ways in which individuals have experienced this infringement of their rights, for example, with lack of access to those things in society considered by the majority as their right.

Covert or overt abuse of power.

Discrimination is also viewed as abusive as it is a misuse of power over another person. This can be either covert (hidden) or overt (open). Covert abuse of power is when, for example, the systems and structures (the way things work within society or an organisation) are set up to work to the advantage of the dominant group. For example, the dominance of male values in some business organisations (work first, family second) and the informal networks for decision making at senior levels (for example, on the golf course and in men's changing rooms after squash games) make it almost impossible for women with the skills and ability to break through an invisible 'glass ceiling' which excludes them from boardroom positions and authority. This lack of experience at senior boardroom level makes it difficult to compete on a level with men who have had no difficulty accessing this level of senior management. Therefore, when a company appoints yet another male to a senior boardroom position they justify this based on the differential in suitable experience, creating a situation which is difficult to challenge. Another example of covert abuse of power is bullying or sexual harassment which happens as a result of one person having power over another. This may be because the person is older, is in a senior position, is physically bigger or has information about the person they can use to intimidate them into doing what they want and not reporting the unfair treatment. This intimidation and abuse of power more often than not takes place in ways that are subtle and difficult to prove.

Overt abuse of power is more likely to be challenged and proven if challenged when the evidence to support it is unashamedly in the open for all to witness. Overt abuse of power means excluding groups or individuals from accessing facilities or services, such as members clubs and public places on the grounds of their gender (in the 1990s women were excluded from many golf clubs), disability (adults with learning disabilities being excluded from pubs or restaurant in case they frightened other customers away) or race (exclusion of Irish and black people from bed and breakfast accommodation in the 1960s).

The ability to challenge both covert and overt abuses of power depends on the power (in terms of strength and type), status and credibility of those opposing it.

Prejudice

As described previously, prejudice results from preconceived ideas about an individual, group or subject that are not based on knowledge or understanding. These ideas are often based on stereotypes and the assumptions that result from this. Prejudice leads people to disregard an individual, group or subject and treat them unfairly, for example excluding them for public facilities or activities, abusing them or blaming them for everything that goes wrong. This may be through direct discrimination or by indirect means, such as ignoring them.

Stereotyping

As stated earlier, stereotyping is holding an oversimplified idea of an individual or group and as a result making unfounded assumptions about everyone that appears to be part of that group. When an individual is stereotyped, this is likely to result in discriminatory and abusive actions which are damaging to the individual's well-being. Some examples of stereotyping can be seen on television, in books, advertising and other media, for example nurses are always women and doctors men, men are always engineers, and so on. This leads people to become fixed in their thinking that this is the norm, and discourages individuals who wish to be in such a role from trying to achieve it, as it appears out of their grasp and somehow an unnatural aspiration. Advertising campaigns for charitable organisations for people with disabilities are faced with a dilemma over stereotyping. In order to raise funds, the best images are those that may engender pity and guilt and so encourage people to contribute, but negative images reinforce a negative stereotype that disability equals dependency. This is a stereotypical assumption that people with disabilities and others are fighting hard to change as it is in opposition to current thinking and practice around valuing diversity and empowering disabled people to exercise their rights like any other citizen.

Stereotypical ideas are also shown to be part of the dehumanisation and demonising processes that accompany systematic oppression which if left unchecked can lead to genocide, for example the systematic blaming and negative stereotyping of all Jewish people in Nazi Germany.

Labelling

Applying a label focuses on one aspect of an individual and this label then acts like a filter through which we view that individual, seeing that aspect of them foremost rather than considering the individual. Using labels to guide our actions means we make assumptions and this will almost always be incorrect and misleading. When a label is applied to an individual, for example, 'Mrs S is ungrateful and demanding', this label gives us a preconceived idea about that individual based on our understanding of what those terms mean as well as our past experience. This preconception predetermines our response to the individual rather than allowing us to make up our own mind about them. Therefore, when we meet Mrs S, instead of trusting our own ability to respond and apply our own judgement with regards to Mrs S, we have already accepted someone else's judgement and so are led to respond in a way that lacks understanding of Mrs S as an individual, along with her needs and circumstances and which is likely to reinforce the label. For example, if we respond to Mrs S by ignoring her or not listening to her or dismissing her requests for help because we have already been told that she is 'demanding' which suggests that any request she makes is excessive, then it is not surprising that Mrs S responds by making repeated requests until someone listens and when they do finally respond she appears ungrateful. Applying labels is therefore, unhelpful, discriminating and potentially abusive, as it changes our response to a person and leads to treating them unfairly and in a judgemental manner as all we see is the label and not the individual.

Bullying

Bullying is a form of psychological abuse that involves intimidation and threatening behaviour. A bully will always choose a target who is vulnerable in some way and over whom they have power, such as being in a senior position or having greater physical strength. Their victim often either lacks credibility or is unlikely to speak out against the bully, for example due to limited cognitive ability or isolation from other people. Being subjected to bullying denies the individual's rights and means that they are being treated unfairly and not receiving equity of service provision.

Abuse

Abuse is a form of discriminatory practice which involves an individual being treated unjustly and denied their human rights. In addition to this, verbal abuse means using language which is insulting, offensive, derogatory and discriminating, such as name calling, using swear words, racist, sexist words, and so on.

See page 356 in Unit 11 for more information on bullying and abuse.

Effects of discrimination

Being judged not on your own merit but on ill-informed ideas attributed by others leaves a person with negative feelings about themselves and their worth as well as a loss of faith in justice and fairness. When an individual experiences discrimination, it is likely to reinforce negative feelings they already have about themselves if they identity themselves with a group in society which are socially constructed as different and as a result lack power in effecting change. This sets up a cycle of oppressive behaviour. The oppression the individual experiences reinforces the idea of the dominant norm, i.e. that their treatment by others is natural. This oppressive treatment therefore becomes accepted and legitimised and a stereotype develops based on the assumptions, labels and beliefs about the individual or group. This stereotyping becomes justification for further discrimination and unjust treatment.

Marginalisation

Marginalisation means being placed on the edge, outside or excluded from belonging or participating. If an individual is discriminated against due to assumptions, prejudice or stereotyping then this is likely to lead to their exclusion from activities that others are involved in. For example, if sexist attitudes prevail within an organisation it is likely that women's ideas are marginalised or they are excluded from opportunities to progress.

Disempowerment

Marginalised individuals feel isolated from others. They become disempowered as a result of this isolation and oppression and feel unable to challenge the discrimination they are experiencing as there is no one else able to support them and substantiate their claims.

Low self-esteem and self-identity

Marginalisation further decreases an individual's credibility, as their personal power is diminished as are their feelings of self-worth, self-identity and self-confidence. The power balance is such that marginalised individuals can begin to believe the assumptions and unfair judgements of others as the weight of evidence appears to be in favour of these judgements especially if the images, ideas and constructions surrounding the individual appear to justify

Fig 2.5 Effects of discrimination

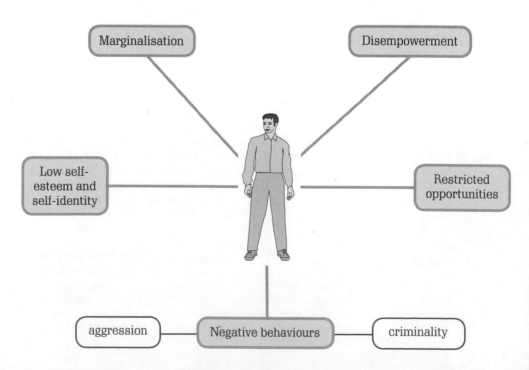

Fig 2.6 Gender
discrimination

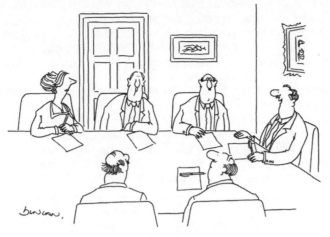

*"That's an excellent suggestion, Miss Triggs. Perhaps one of
the men here would like to make it."*

and legitimise the discriminatory treatment they are experiencing. This further compounds
the discrimination and isolation they feel and creates a downward spiral of low self-esteem
and loss of self-belief and self-worth. This further increases their vulnerability to attack and
ill treatment by others as well as disregard for their own well-being which may lead to risky
behaviours and unconsidered risk taking.

Restricted opportunities

The lack of self-confidence is likely to affect an individual's performance and achievement
as they will feel that no matter what they do they will never be treated fairly and have the
same opportunities as others. They may also experience direct discrimination in the form
of restricted opportunities, such as access to education, training, employment, housing
or leisure facilities. For example, a person with a physical disability might be denied the
opportunity to discuss their sexual needs if workers assume they are incapable of having a
sexual relationship because of their disability. As a result of this avoidance the individual may
believe their feelings and desires to be abnormal and this will impact on their sense of self,
their confidence and well-being.

Negative behaviours

For some, being subjected to unfair treatment on a day-to-day basis becomes intolerable and
leads them to have little regard for themselves or others. They may find their feelings become
impossible for them to manage and their anger, hurt and frustration may be expressed in
negative behaviour such as aggression, as this is one way they know people will take notice
of them. Behaviour is a form of communication and one that requires a considered response
rather than just an automatic reaction such as the use of power and control, as this may
escalate the aggression. If negative behaviours are expressed it is important to deconstruct
this to understand the underlying cause.

The sense of disempowerment, marginalisation and low self-esteem caused by discrimination
can create a situation where the individual loses not only a sense of self but also a moral
sense of right and wrong. Instead of their experience of society being one of fairness and
justice, they are surrounded by social constructions that reinforce the dominance of a group
from which they are excluded. The sense of injustice they feel as a consequence may be such
that it leads them into criminality as a way of trying to exert some power and lessen their
feelings of powerlessness and show disregard for a society that they consider has disregarded
them and in which they have no legitimate place.

Loss of rights

The impact of discrimination is most profound in terms of the loss of individual rights that
results. Discrimination and discriminatory practice is able to thrive when power is misused
and an individual's rights are overridden, for example, denying an individual access to an
appropriate assessment of their needs or making decisions which directly affect them without
including or consulting them. Legislation changes, such as the Mental Capacity Act (2006),
will change this and provide a measure of protection to avoid this occurring and to challenge
it legally if it does happen.

Incidents of institutional abuse have always included the inappropriate or excessive use of power and force over both staff and service users in order for it to continue. Behaviour management techniques have been criticised as having the potential to be abusive by overriding individual rights, especially if health and social care workers are not adequately trained in appropriate use and technique, are inadequately supervised or a culture of discrimination and control exists. Vulnerable children and adults can have their rights overridden on a daily basis if they are denied access to choice and their views are not sought, listened to and acted upon. The 1996 Beech House Inquiry was an internal inquiry set up by Camden and Islington Community Health Services NHS Trust to investigate the mistreatment by staff at Beech House, St Pancras Hospital, between March 1993 and April 1996 of the 12 mentally ill older people who had been transferred there from Friern Hospital (a long-stay psychiatric hospital). Recommendations from the inquiry helped to shape future adult protection policies and procedures.

Adults with mental health needs and children and young people who are subject to statutory powers, such as detention under the Mental Health Act or being made a Ward of Court, can have their rights restricted for a period of time in their best interests. However, regular reviews are required to ensure the individual's rights are not infringed. As a result of reviews, such as the Bournewood provisions, legislation is in place to ensure that vulnerable people with mental health problems are supported in the least restrictive way possible, while maintaining their safety and rights. The aim is to prevent arbitrary decisions being made about detaining an individual and to ensure they have a right of appeal against such decisions.

Department of Health

www.dh.gov.uk

Department of Health Briefing Paper explaining the Bournewood case and resulting rulings in the European Court of Human Rights (ECoHR).

case study 2.1 — Ronnie and Ben

Ronnie is a young man in his late 20s who has a learning disability. He lives in a supported tenancy with three other young men all of whom have learning disabilities. Ronnie has formed a close emotional and physical relationship with one of the other tenants, Ben, and they want to move in together. Jim their support worker feels that efforts should be made to stop this 'unhealthy' relationship and move one of them to a new tenancy. Jim is supported in his views by both Ronnie and Ben's families who do not agree with same-sex relationships. They have made their feelings and wishes known to the learning disability service provider.

activity — GROUP WORK

1   What reasons may the support worker have for not supporting Ronnie and Ben's choices regarding their relationship?

2   How is the opposition from others to Ronnie and Ben's relationship discriminatory?

activity — INDIVIDUAL WORK 2.3

Use examples to explain how discriminatory practice could adversely affect individuals who are supported by and use health or social care services.

P3

How national initiatives promote anti-discriminatory practice in health and social care

Conventions, legislation and regulations

There are numerous widely accepted conventions and legal requirements in place to promote, support and uphold the principles and practice of equality and diversity within not only health and social care but in society as a whole. The following table describes the main legislation relating to issues around equality and diversity.

Legislation relating to equality and diversity

Legislation	Outline and relevant section
European Convention on Human Rights and Fundamental Freedoms (1950)	This states fundamental civil and political rights and freedoms of individuals. (Human Rights section)
Sex Discrimination Act (1975)	The Act makes it unlawful to discriminate against a person on the ground of their sex or marital status. This legislation applies across all areas of life in education, as a consumer and particularly in relation to the recruitment, selection, promotion or training of personnel. In this context, there are two areas of exception: ■ Positive Action s48(1): Where work is carried out exclusively by men or women or where the numbers of one sex (minority sex) is small compared to the total, it is lawful for the employer to offer training for that work to the minority sex only to encourage members of the minority sex to take up opportunities for that work. ■ Genuine Occupational Qualifications (GOQ) s7 =(2)(e): Where the worker provides individuals with personal services promoting their welfare, education or similar personal services and those services can most effectively be provided by a woman (or a man), e.g. a male outreach worker for gay men who are HIV positive. Employers can introduce a 'supplementary' GOQ covering e.g. physical searches, work in private houses, live-in premises and provision of welfare services to vulnerable individuals. On 1st May 1999, an addition to the original Act included a section on gender reassignment which makes it unlawful to discriminate on the grounds of gender reassignment. On 6th April 2007, the Gender Equality Duty comes into force. This means that all public authorities must demonstrate that they are promoting equality for women and men and that they are eliminating sexual discrimination and harassment.
Mental Health Act (1993) & Codes of Practice	The provisions of this Act are designed to ensure an individual's rights are not infringed and they are treated in an equitable manner in terms of access to objective assessment and treatment. The Act outlines the arrangements for the compulsory detention of people with mental health needs for assessment or treatment and also include the guardianship of individuals with mental health needs in the interests of their welfare or for the protection of others (Section 7).
Mental Health Bill 2006	This provides more safeguards in relation to detention and more independent checks, rights to appeal and the appointment of a representative to look at an individual's rights (the Bournewood provisions)
Mental Health (Northern Ireland) Order (1986)	Part 11 of the Order sets out the circumstances in which, and procedures through which, a mentally disordered individual can be compulsorily admitted to and detained in hospital. It also outlines the principles of these processes. This includes respecting the individual's qualities and social, cultural and religious background.

Legislation	Outline and relevant section
The Convention on the Rights of the Child (1989)	This is the first piece of legislation to focus on children and is the most comprehensive and widely agreed internal human rights statement and guidance to date (only the USA and Somalia have not signed). It includes civil, political, economic, social and cultural rights and provides details of what every child (regardless of sex, religion or social status) needs in order to have a safe, happy and fulfilled childhood. It establishes a norm in terms of the expectations, rights and freedoms of children everywhere. It also takes into account the vulnerability of children and their need to have special assistance so this is not violated. Included in the convention are the following: ■ General human rights principles: including the right to life, survival and development, the right to non-discrimination, respect for the views of children and to give consideration to a child's best interests, and the requirement to give primary consideration to the child's best interests in all matters affecting them. This is particularly important in relation to assessment, care planning and decisions regarding their care and welfare. ■ Civil rights and freedoms: including the right to a name and nationality, freedom of expression, thought and association, access to information and the right not to be subjected to torture. ■ Family environment and alternative care: including the right to live with and have contact with both parents, to be reunited with parents if separated from them and to the provision of appropriate alternative care where necessary. ■ Basic heath and welfare: including the rights of disabled children, the right to health and health care, social security, child care services and an adequate standard of living. ■ Education, leisure and cultural activities: including the right to education and the rights to play, leisure and participation in cultural life and the arts. ■ Special protection measures: covering the rights of refugee children, those affected by armed conflicts, children in the juvenile justice system, children deprived of their liberty and children suffering economic, sexual or other forms of exploitation.
The Children Act (1989)	This is designed to help keep a child safe and well and, if necessary, help the child to live with their family by providing services appropriate to the child's needs. The Act imposes a general duty on local councils to provide a range of services to 'children in need' (e.g. a child who is disabled, is 'at risk' from harm or abuse, has experienced developmental delay or inequality of opportunity) in their area if those services will help keep a child safe and well. Local councils are responsible for identifying those children who may be in need and the extent of their need and decide how to support them. It also reforms the law relating to children and amends this in relation to children's homes, community homes, voluntary homes and voluntary organisations as well as making provision with respect to fostering, child-minding and day care for young children and adoption, and related purposes.
Race Relations (Amendment) Act (2000)	This strengthens the earlier legislation and extends to all public bodies who now have a duty to eliminate unlawful racial discrimination as well as enhancing the powers of the Commission for Racial Equality.
Disability Discrimination Act (1995)	The Act defines a person as having a disability where they have a physical or mental impairment which has a substantial and long-term adverse effect on their ability to carry out normal day-to-day activities. The Act establishes rights for people with disabilities to be treated fairly and without discrimination and to be afforded the same opportunities as others. This relates to all organisations and to all services provided, e.g. access to buildings, employment and leisure facilities. In addition, information regarding services must be available in a variety of languages and formats, e.g. in Braille.

Legislation	Outline and relevant section
Human Rights Act (1998)	The Act meant that the European Convention on Human Rights became incorporated into British law. The definitions under that law also widened to provide social and economic rights as well as the original concepts around basic human rights. There are eight main articles of particular significance to health and social care work: ■ Article 2 The right to life ■ Article 3 The right to freedom from torture and inhuman or degrading treatment or punishment ■ Article 5 The right to liberty and security of person ■ Article 6 The right to a fair trial ■ Article 8 The right to respect for private and family life, home and correspondence ■ Article 9 Freedom of thought, conscience and religion ■ Article 12 The right to marry ■ Article 14 The prohibition of discrimination in the enjoyment of the convention rights
Data Protection Act (1998)	The Act came into force on 1 March 2000. It gives effect in UK law to the 1995 EC Data Protection Directive. The Act strengthens and extends the data protection regime created by the Data Protection Act (1984), which it replaces. It also incorporates the Access to Health Records Act (1990) and the Access to Personal Files Act (1987). The 1998 Act applies to: ■ computerised personal data (like the 1984 Act) ■ personal data held in structured manual files (new) It applies to anything at all done to personal data ('processing'), including collection, use, disclosure, destruction and merely holding data and it is an enforceable good practice code. Organisations processing personal data ('controllers') must comply with the data protection principles. These require data to be: ■ fairly and lawfully processed ■ processed for limited purposes ■ adequate, relevant and not excessive ■ accurate ■ not kept longer than necessary ■ kept secure ■ not transferred to non-EEA countries without adequate protection. The 1998 Act creates some express new requirements. Controllers must: ■ meet one of six conditions in order to process personal data; ■ meet further conditions in order to process sensitive data (i.e. data about a person's ethnic origins, political opinions, religious beliefs, trade union membership, health, sexual life and criminal history) ■ inform individuals when their data are collected. The Act strengthens individuals' rights to: ■ gain access to their data ■ seek compensation. It creates new express rights for individuals to: ■ prevent their data being processed in certain circumstances ■ 'opt-out' of having their data used for direct marketing ■ 'opt-out' of fully automated decision-making about them.
Nursing & Residential Care Homes Regulations (1984)	This sets out the regulations covering the registration and inspection of nursing and residential care homes. Within the regulations, there are a range of specific standards, e.g. for staffing levels and record-keeping. These regulations were used to implement the registration and regular inspections of homes to check standards of care by the local authorities. The use of terms such as 'sufficient' and 'adequate' were open to interpretation and this was seen as a weakness in the powers of inspection and registration as there was considerable local interpretation and inconsistency. In April 2002 this Act was replaced by the Care Standards Act.

▶

Legislation	Outline and relevant section
Care Standards Act (2000)	This Act was broader in its remit than the Nursing & Residential Care Homes Regulations and covers all areas where health and social care support is provided, including previously unregulated provision such as domiciliary social care providers, independent fostering agencies, residential family centres and boarding schools. The CSA continues to register and inspect all those services as before, i.e. residential care homes for adults, nursing homes and children's homes. However the powers of registration and inspection were removed from local and health authorities and passed over to a new national public authority called the Commission for Social Care Inspection (CSCI). The CSA includes a set of National Minimum Standards with the aim of being less ambiguous and open to individual interpretation. The application of national rather than local standards is an attempt to standardize provision. For example, the national minimum standards for care homes for younger adults and adult placements cover all aspects of care support including: ■ the choice of home (standards 1–5) ■ individual needs and choices standards (standards 6–10) ■ lifestyle (standards 11–17) ■ personal and healthcare support (standards 18–21) ■ concerns, complaints and protection (standards 22 & 23) ■ environment (standards 24–30) ■ staffing (standards 31–36) ■ conduct and management of the home (standards 37–43) ■ the requirement for social workers to be registered with the Care Councils and undertake a mandatory 90 hours professional training each year.
The Children Act (2004)	The Act provides the legal framework for the wider strategy 'Every Child Matters: Change for Children', which sets out the requirements for improving children's lives. This includes the services that every child accesses, e.g. health clinics and education, as well as more targeted services for those with additional needs. The legislation is intended to be enabling as opposed to prescriptive with some scope for flexibility resting with the local authority. It therefore aims: ■ to encourage integrated working between agencies and disciplines (including the planning, commissioning and delivery of services) ■ to avoid duplication of activities ■ to increase levels of accountability ■ to improve the coordination of individual and joint inspections in local authorities. In addition to these changes, the Act places a new duty on local authorities to promote the educational achievement of looked after children.
The Disability Discrimination Act (2005)	This Act extends or amends the existing provisions in the DDA 1995 and the majority of these changes came into force in December 2006. In relation to health and social care this includes making it unlawful for operators of transport vehicles, private members' clubs (with more than 25 members) and landlords of rented property to discriminate against disabled people by denying them access to those services. It also extends protection to cover people who have HIV, cancer and multiple sclerosis from the moment they are diagnosed (from December 2005). The Act now covers all the activities of the public sector and requires public bodies to promote equality of opportunity for and positive attitudes to disabled people. They will be responsible for eliminating unlawful discrimination and disability-related harassment and encouraging disabled people to participate in public life. It also removes the requirement in the DDA that a mental illness must be 'clinically recognised' before it can count as an impairment for the purposes of the Act.

Legislation	Outline and relevant section
Mental Capacity Act (2005)	This provides a legal framework to empower and protect vulnerable people who are unable to make their own decisions. It sets out whom, how and when decisions can be made. The Act is underpinned by five key principles: 1 A presumption of capacity: every adult is considered capable unless it is proved otherwise. 2 The right for the individual to be supported to make their own decisions: ensuring that people are given appropriate help to do this. 3 Adults retain the right to make what may appear to others as unwise or eccentric decisions. 4 Best interests: everything done on behalf of someone who lacks capacity must be in their best interests. 5 Whatever is done must have the least restrictive impact on their basic rights and freedoms. The Act also replaces current legal schemes for enduring power of attorney and Court of Protection receivers with reformed and updated schemes. It also includes provisions for vulnerable adults such as being able to appoint an Independent Mental Capacity Advocate, making advanced decisions regarding the refusal of treatment and making it a criminal offence to ill-treat or neglect someone who lacks mental capacity.
Age Discrimination Act (2006)	This Act came into force on 1st October 2006 and for the first time gives legal rights to those, old or young, against an employer who discriminates against them in the workplace because of their age, e.g. not employing someone because of their age, mandatory retirement below 65 years or not offering training. The impact will be from recruitment through to all aspects of employment.

Disabilities Rights Commission	www.drc.org.uk
Commission for Equality and Human Rights	www.cehr.org.uk
Commission for Social Care Inspectorate	www.csci.org.uk

From October 2007, a new body, the Commission for Equality and Human Rights (CEHR), will come into being. The CEHR will incorporate the work of all the existing equality bodies for sex, race and disability as well as extending its work to new areas of discrimination law including sexual orientation, religion and belief, age and human rights. The remit of the CEHR will be to promote equality of opportunity and human rights; challenge discrimination; and promote citizenship and social cohesion. The CEHR will be responsible for the following:

- encouraging awareness and good practice on equality and diversity
- promoting awareness and understanding of human rights
- promoting equality of opportunity
- working towards eliminating unlawful discrimination and harassment
- promoting good relations between different communities
- keeping discrimination and human rights legislation under review
- being a source of expertise on equality and human rights.

Codes of practice and charters
Codes of conduct established by professional bodies

The professional bodies that represent those who work in health and social care have all produced guidance for employers and workers related to promoting equality and diversity in practice. For example, the Nursing and Midwifery Council (NMC) Code of Professional Conduct includes the following:

- Respect the patient or client as an individual.
- Obtain consent before you give any treatment or care.
- Protect confidential information.

All of these underpin the promotion of equality and diversity as a key aspect of the nurse or midwife role.

Codes of practice and rules of conduct for social care workers and employers

The General Social Care Council (GSCC), the Care Council for Wales (CCWales), the Northern Ireland Social Care Council (NISCC) and the Scottish Social Services Council (SSSC) have worked in partnership to agree the Code of Practice for both social care employers and social care workers with the purpose of raising standards. As the Code is within the public domain, it is also intended to inform service users and members of the public about the standards of professional practice that they should expect when dealing with social care services. The Councils will take action if registered social care workers fail to meet the expectations of and adhere to the Code. The Councils expect employers to take the Code into account when making decisions concerning staff conduct.

See page 381 in Unit 11 for more information on codes of practice.

Fig 2.7 Code of Practice

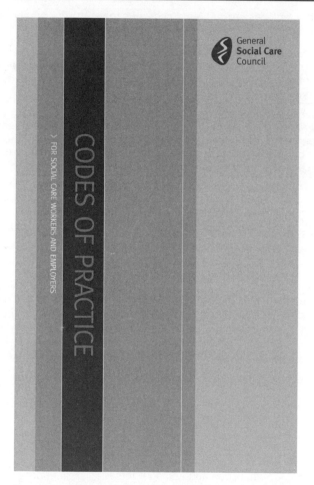

For employers, the Code of Practice sets out the responsibilities of employers in regulating social care workers and supporting workers to adhere to and meet the requirements of the Code and to take action should they fail to do this. The Code is intended to complement existing policies and procedures and enable employers to provide high quality social care services that promote public confidence and trust.

For social care workers, the Code describes the standards of professional conduct expected of them by their employer, colleagues, service users, carers and the general public within their day-to-day work activities. There are six standards which reflect current good practice and, although they all relate to promoting individual rights in some way, the first relates directly to a social care worker's responsibility to promote equality and diversity:

'As a social care worker, you must protect the rights and promote the interests of service users and carers. This includes:

1.1 treating each person as an individual

1.2 respecting and, where appropriate, promoting the individual views and wishes of both service users and carers

1.3 supporting service users' rights to control their lives and make informed choices about the services they receive

1.4 respecting and maintaining the dignity and privacy of service users

1.5 promoting equal opportunities for service users and carers

1.6 respecting diversity and different cultures and values.

See page 373 in Unit 11 for a complete list of standards.

General Social Care Council	www.gscc.org.uk
Scottish Social Services Council	www.sssc.uk.com
Care Council for Wales	www.ccwales.org.uk
Northern Ireland Social Care Council	www.niscc.info

Charters

The Patients Charter was replaced in 1998 by the NHS Charter which set out what patients should expect from the NHS as well as how to access the NHS and plans for the future.

All organisations within health and social care produce information for service users, carers and the general public about the services they offer, how to access these services in terms of physical access and eligibility criteria for services, for example receiving social care funding support from the local authority if appropriate. Leaflets, information on websites and local service centres are all ways in which individuals can access this information. Information is required to be in a variety of languages and formats to ensure it is accessible and in many places there may be additional support for workers to assist individuals with particular needs. All information will also include sections regarding how equality and diversity is actively promoted to provide an equitable service for individuals.

Fig 2.8 Information in different languages

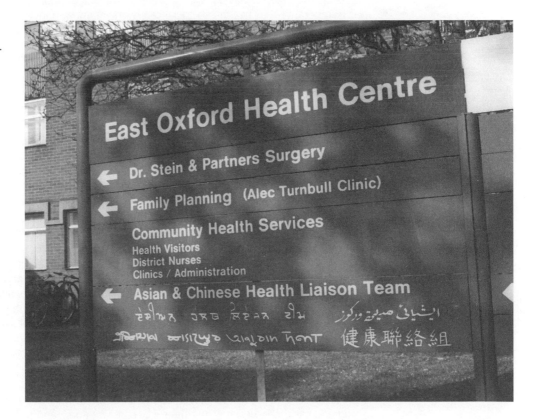

Organisational policies and procedures

Each organisation should have in place a number of policies and procedures related to the promotion of equality and diversity which are underpinned by the legal requirements, national and local guidance, professional codes and practice, outcomes of research and accepted good practice guidance.

Positive promotion of individual rights

Policies and procedures which promote individual rights and promote and maintain an individual's human rights should be part of the statement of purpose or aims and objectives of the organisation. This will describe the philosophy or ethos of the service as well as services and facilities provided. If an individual is living in a nursing or residential care home, they will also have a set of terms and conditions and a guide to the home which will include how their rights are promoted and upheld. The promotion of an individual's human rights will underpin all of the organisation's policies and procedures.

Advocacy

Within a service, there should also be information (i.e. contact details and what services are provided) as well as procedures which detail how an individual can access independent advocacy to ensure they can fully exercise their rights in any circumstance where decisions which directly affect them are being made. Some care service providers may ensure that all users have an advocate so that there is time to build up the relationship needed for this process to be effective in promoting individuals' rights and views.

Work practices

Organisational policies and procedures also ensure that workers carry out work activities in a consistent manner which is underpinned by evidence-based good practice and which uphold the principles of anti-discriminatory and anti-oppressive practice. Health and social care workers' work practice will be described with the organisations' general policies, such as health and safety, confidentiality, equal opportunities and anti-bullying, as well as the specific policies and procedures related to the needs of the specific service being provided, such as managing behaviour that challenges, running support groups, activities and outings. It is imperative that health and social care workers know, understand and work within the guidance these policies and procedures provide, as it is through adherence to these that the quality of services are maintained. The existence of policies and procedures that promote anti-discriminatory and anti-oppressive practice does not mean that this is the reality of an individual's experience. Every health and social care worker has a duty to implement these policies and procedures within their day-to-day work with individuals, others that are significant to them as well as with colleagues and other professionals.

Staff development and training

All organisations will have policies and procedures for recognising staff development and training needs and how these will be met. The policy should outline staff and employer responsibilities in relation to learning and development opportunities, for example, when a worker is entitled to access, commitment from both, and so on. The staff development and training procedures will describe the processes related to this area of employment. For example, it will include guidance on how workers access training, the application process and how they raise issues regarding their learning and development needs.

It is considered both good practice and in some areas a requirement (for example, within registered services) that all staff have regular supervision of practice as well as an individual development plan which contributes to the overall development and training plan of the organisation. Some staff development is mandatory in terms of health and safety training which is regularly updated, such as annual fire safety training. Other training relates to the achievement of qualifications and developing practice in terms of skills, knowledge, attitudes and behaviour. For example, developing person-centred approaches to working requires considerable attitude and behaviour change as many health and social care workers continue to work with a task-orientated model.

Staff development and training should also include issues related to equality and diversity. Skills for Care (SfC) is an employer-led organisation that aims to support employers to raise and address the issues affecting the social care workforce and in particular the development of skills and knowledge and the attainment of recognised qualifications.

> **remember**
> Advocacy is providing an individual with a means by which they an express and make known to others their wishes and decisions. It involves getting to know the individual well so that the advocate can understand the individual's values, beliefs, and so on, and so truly represent their views.

> **remember**
> A policy is a formal statement (structure or framework) of the guiding principles of a particular area of work. A procedure (or system) describes how those principles are put into action in practice.

Skills for Care   www.skillsforcare.org

In the wake of government enquires and reports, such as the McPherson Report into the murder of Stephen Lawrence on 22 April 1993 and the issues of institutional racism that arose, it is now considered best practice for equality and diversity training to be carried out by individuals with specialist knowledge. As a result of the benefits this has brought most disability awareness training is provided by an individual with disabilities.

McPherson report

www.archive.official-documents.co.uk

See page 220 in Unit 6 for more on staff development and training.

Quality issues and complaint procedures

Polices and procedures will also be in place which detail how the quality of the service provision will be monitored and maintained. This could be through regular feedback from those using the service, carers, staff, other professionals as well as regulatory processes, such as CSCI inspections. User and carer meetings as well as questionnaires may be used to achieve this. As part of that a complaints policy with accompanying procedures which details how to make a complaint should be available in appropriate formats. Having a complaints procedure which is accessible, understandable and usable by service users is essential if their rights are to be promoted.

Affirmative action and anti-harassment

Other examples of policies and procedures within the workplace may relate to taking affirmative action or positive discrimination. This could be one way of ensuring that individuals with diverse needs have their needs met in a way which does not discriminate. Examples of this may be policies regarding staffing rotas where there is a mixed service user group to ensure there is always a gender mix of staff available to support personal care activities especially if there are cultural or religious preferences. Anti-bullying and anti-harassment policies and procedures should also be in place to ensure that both service users and staff are not subjected to these forms of abuse. These polices should outline the organisation's definitions of these as well as their attitude and view of these situations. The procedures should describe what action is to be taken in the event of these occurring, reporting and recording processes and requirements, the support available to the individual being subjected to the harassment or bullying as well as the action that will be taken to investigate and, if the allegations are found to be true, the action that will be taken against those perpetrating the harassment or bullying.

Confidentiality and human rights

One of the cornerstones of good care practice is the promotion and maintenance of confidentiality. Organisations must have clear policies regarding confidentiality and procedures for maintaining confidentiality in the variety of circumstances that occur as part of health and social care work. Policies will include clear definitions, the roles and responsibilities of the organisation and those employed within it and the outcome if an individual is found to be in breach of the policy and procedures. All policies and procedures will be underpinned and comply with the legal requirements regarding personal data and other information, such as the Data Protection Act and the Human Rights Act. Procedures will include what actions are to be taken to promote and maintain confidentiality as well as what action is to be taken if there is a breach of confidentiality.

1 Using examples from your work within a health and social care service, describe how the following are used to promote anti-discriminatory practice within your day-to-day work with individuals:

■ legislation

■ codes of practice

■ rules of conduct

■ charters

■ organisational policies.

2 The Mental Health Capacity Act (2005) is a recent policy development in health and social care services. Explain how this will influence organisational policy relating to anti-discriminatory practice.

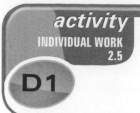

activity
INDIVIDUAL WORK
2.5

D1

Evaluate how the Mental Health Capacity Act (2005) will influence both personal and organisational practice in relation to anti-discriminatory practice.

How anti-discriminatory practice is promoted in health and social care settings

The very nature of health and social care work suggests that the individuals being supported are vulnerable. As we have seen through this unit, this vulnerability is often related to 'difference' in terms of capability or levels of independence. Vulnerability may be related to physical, emotional, financial or social well-being. Sometimes this vulnerability may include being vulnerable to discrimination, much of which is likely to be based on prejudice. Prejudice does not automatically lead to discrimination but views of this nature can lead to people being labelled, something which is particularly a problem within health and social care work. For example, staff can label clients as being 'difficult', or having 'challenging behaviour'. Even the label of a medical diagnosis, such as depression, dementia, autism, epilepsy or multiple sclerosis, can encourage assumptions to be made as opposed to finding out what that diagnosis means for that individual in terms of their behaviour, capability and attitude towards it.

Active promotion of anti-discriminatory practice

As discussed earlier, the effects of negative discrimination are likely to have an impact not only on the individual but also on the organisation and society as a whole. Promoting equality by treating everyone the same denies the reality that everyone is different and so we should be striving to promote equity where these essential differences are acknowledged and people are seen and treated as individuals but with an equal amount of care, respect and attention, i.e. the quality is the same but the responses are individual.

Ethical principles

Ethical principles are those which can be judged fair. Positive ethical approaches to health and social care practice are essential if individuals being supported are to be treated with equity.

Putting the patient or service user at the heart of service provision

Ensuring that every individual who comes into contact with any type of health or social care service is treated as a unique individual is essential if this is to be achieved. Health and social care workers need to take time to get to know and build relationships with individuals if they are to be effective in providing active support which is consistent with the individual's beliefs, culture and preferences. This will enable the worker to better understand the individual's past and thus their present situation, and will inform decisions regarding their future. This emphasis on the person being at the centre of health and social care processes, along with practice that is underpinned by the care value base creates real understanding of the individual's needs, interests, concerns and aspirations which enables workers to be more effective in supporting the individual in expressing their needs and preferences. As discussed previously, this may involve using an interpreter, advocate or a range of different communication methods.

 See page 3 in Unit 1 for more information on communication methods.

A positive working relationship which is mutually respectful with clear boundaries and understanding is one way in which a health and social care worker can empower the individual to make their own decisions and achieve their potential. Empowering individuals may include enabling them to access the information they need as well as supporting them to develop or use their skills in order to fully understand the information, the choices they have, the implications of those choices, such as the responsibilities that goes with the choice, and any dilemmas they represent. A major part of anti-discriminatory practice is the promotion of individual rights, choices and well-being. This can be achieved through understanding what rights individuals have and how they can access these. Not making assumptions about an individual's capacity to make choices is also important and this may challenge health and social care workers to find a range of ways in which to communicate with and understand the individuals they support, for example by using signs or pictures if they have limited verbal communication. To achieve this, workers may also need to support individuals to overcome emotional barriers such as anxiety, depression and low self-esteem so they can recognise their rights and feel confident enough to make their own choices.

Balancing individual rights with the rights of others

Having rights also means the individual has responsibilities and this includes not infringing the rights of others. Balancing individual rights with the rights of others can present health and social care workers with some difficult dilemmas, tensions and potential and actual conflicts. These can occur between service users, the service user and the organisation, and between the worker and the organisation. For example, if one service user has a hearing impairment and consequently when they listen to music it is louder than other service users would like it to be. The service user has a right to listen to their music but the others have a right to peace and quiet. This can lead to conflict. One way of easing this tension and avoiding conflict is to provide earphones for the service user.

Discriminatory behaviour, remarks, attitudes and actions are often not challenged as people have the view that 'everyone has a right to their own view'. However, to leave such behaviour unchallenged represents a failure in our duty to protect individuals and promote their rights. When dealing with conflicts where discrimination may or may not have been a feature, it is always important to spend time with all parties involved, and not fall into the trap of identifying one party as the victim and another as the perpetrator. Things are not always as clear as they may at first appear on the surface and to prevent similar occurrences in the future it is important to understand the triggers so that strategies can be put in place to minimise the potential in future.

Dealing with conflict

Conflict should be managed in as calm a manner as possible and, if possible, help from a colleague should be sought so that everyone involved can be adequately supported and listened to in order to avoid assumptions and judgements, which may be discriminatory, being made. An important part of anti-discriminatory practice is ensuring that health and social care workers have a shared understanding of what constitutes discrimination and how to identify and challenge discrimination.

Identifying and challenging discrimination

Challenging discrimination shows that in fact, you are not discriminating against those whose behaviour, views, attitudes and so on are discriminatory. If we fail to challenge such views or behaviours, it suggests that we have made a decision or assumption about that person's capacity to change, i.e. we assume their views are so entrenched that they are incapable of change, which in itself is discriminatory. The way we challenge is what is important. It is therefore essential to challenging the attitude, view or behaviour, and not the person as an individual.

Being respectful and assertive are key attitudes and values when challenging someone. The first step must be to try and understand the situation from their perspective and so we need to establish their interpretation of the situation, i.e. what is the intention behind their behaviour? This demonstrates a willingness to listen and not judge the person. Starting from a position of understanding rather than assumption is more likely to result in the change you are seeking to effect.

Getting the person to empathise (put themself in the other person's position) will also help to get them thinking about the other person as an individual and the impact of their behaviour on the other person. This will help to raise their awareness and is more likely to add impetus to any change. Showing respect by listening, being constructive and checking that the person understands are important when working to influence others. Once the person begins to understand the impact of their behaviour on others, it is important to offer them the opportunity to learn more including ways to change their practice, for example by explaining how to do things differently.

Challenging discrimination may not be just on an individual level but may be on an organisational or society level. Although individuals can feel powerless to change things outside their immediate sphere of influence, it is not impossible to challenge discrimination that is institutional or structural. This may involve canvassing support from others who have had similar experiences or share your concerns, as well as locating and involving others who hold positions of influence at these levels, such a managers, professional bodies, trade unions or MPs. Knowing an individual's rights and presenting real evidence and examples which demonstrate the impact of discrimination on individuals' lives are important when challenging the norm within an organisation or society. Discriminatory practice can become institutionalised and abusive to the extent that the organisational culture and behaviours have become overwhelmed. In this situation, such practice can be hard to challenge and often it is not until something significant, such as a suspicious death, occurs that concerns are raised, leading to an external investigation or a rigorous inspection by an external regulatory authority.

activity
INDIVIDUAL WORK
2.6

P5

P6

1   Explain what action you and other health and social care workers could take to promote anti-discriminatory practice actively within your care practice.

2   Use an example to describe how you would reflect on and challenge discriminatory practice within your workplace.

activity
INDIVIDUAL WORK
2.7

M2

With reference to the example you used in activity 2.6, explain what potential difficulties you may encounter when you try to implement change which reflects anti-discriminatory practice.

Personal beliefs and value systems

Our personal beliefs and values play a large role in our responses to difference. We are all unique individuals and our identity develops as we grow, learn and experience life and new things. Many different factors influence that process of growth and change. Some are positive while others are negative. The result of this is that we all have an individual view of the world which is unique and unless we share our view with other people it remains unknown to them.

Influences on personal beliefs and values

Socialisation is the process by which human behaviour is shaped through experience and being in different social situations. Through this process, individuals learn the values, beliefs, formal and informal rules or norms of the society in which they live and this in turn influences or reinforces their own values and beliefs. When we are young, it is our family or primary carers that are the greatest influence on the formation of our values, beliefs and views. It is here that we are influenced by our culture and traditions, such as our nationality and heritage that have been passed down through the generations. It is here too that the beginnings of our beliefs are sown. This could be through a shared family religion as well as through culture and family history. All of these things plus the experiences of our ancestors play an important part in developing our sense of belonging. For many people, their religion and culture are bound together and inseparable from who they are or how they live their life, and as a result this remains the dominant influence through their life. Past events may also play a part in shaping an individual's identity, personal beliefs and values. For example, a person who has been adopted can have a sense that something is missing as they have a different shared history from those who are blood relatives. For others, experiencing abuse, discrimination or oppression is likely to have a considerable impact on their values, beliefs and identity. They may be distrustful of everyone and have low self esteem which will impact on their choices and opportunities. For others, past events may bind them to other people with a sense of shared history, for example e.g. people who have lived through a war.

As we get older our horizons widen and we come into contact with a wider range of people with different backgrounds and experiences as well as having our own life experiences. Each of these will, to a greater or lesser extent, shape our unique view of life and may be the driving force in determining the choices we make about our life in terms of our relationships, job or aspirations. People around us, from our primary carers to teachers and colleagues, act as role models as do people we do not directly know, such as people in the public eye or from within our areas of interest, for example sports people, musicians, writers, actors or activists.

Other factors that influence our views and beliefs are, for example, friends at different times in life, school and other educational experiences, social groups, leisure interests, parenthood, work experiences and bereavement. There are considerable environmental influences including where we live, our education, television, music, films, newspapers and magazines which have all had an increasing influence on shaping peoples' views, values and beliefs. The internet is another more recent influence with the increased access to computers. It is through these means that role models are presented and the social constructions discussed earlier in this unit are created and reinforced. An individual's health and well-being will also influence their values and beliefs and sense of self.

Developing greater self-awareness and tolerance of differences

If individuals are given access to appropriate opportunities, such as learning about equality and diversity, personal experience of relationships with people from diverse backgrounds, beliefs and cultures, experiences that challenge them or constructive feedback from people they respect and trust, this can assist them to develop greater self-awareness and tolerance of difference. However, it is important to recognise that our views and beliefs can change as we travel through life and our experiences teach us new things about the world and about ourselves, so there is always the potential for change whatever someone's age.

Committing to the care value base

Deciding to become a health or social care worker will involve you considering your own beliefs and values and how these impact on your life, behaviour, decisions and relationships with others. Aligning your beliefs and values to those of the care value base is essential as this is the basis of effective care practice. It would be wrong to assume that this is an automatic process. We are often unaware of the prejudices and assumptions we hold as they are so ingrained in our thinking. We need to be open to challenging our thinking and to exploring these aspects of ourselves. If we are to be effective in developing supportive relationships with individuals then we must understand ourselves first, otherwise we are in danger of discriminatory action and becoming part of the problem and not part of the solution in that individual's life. To be an effective health or social care worker you need to internalise these values and demonstrate them in every aspect of your practice with service users, carers and other practitioners.

Careful use of language

When we write, we have time to consider our words and so often they are more measured and precise in their meaning. When we speak, we can often speak without thinking through the language we choose and this can create misunderstandings and possible offence. Language is powerful and the old adage that 'sticks and stones may break my bones but words will never hurt me' is not one that in my experience rings true. Words can be far more wounding than any physical blow, and the damage caused deeper and harder to heal. Harsh words and discriminatory language can cause damage to the individual's self-belief, self-image and self-esteem that no number of kind words can repair. For example, if another person tells us ten positive things about ourselves and one negative one, what most people remember is the negative comment. It is important to understand what is considered appropriate language in relation to difference such as racial differences as well as what is culturally acceptable. For example, many older people in their 80s and 90s may prefer to be addressed by their title (Mr or Mrs), as to them using first names is considered too familiar and there is a sense of identity and status loss. Addressing patients or service users using overly familiar terms such as 'dear' or 'love' is not appropriate as it is disrespectful and assumes a familiarity which is inappropriate. Often care workers defend this practice by saying the person does not mind. However, the service user may feel unable to speak out of fear of being labelled or marginalized, especially if they see this is the norm within the setting and appears to be accepted by everyone else. It is also important to use age-appropriate language. This means not using childish phrases and terms, such as 'there's a good girl' or 'who's being a silly billy?' with older people or adults with a learning disability as this is demeaning and disrespectful as well as increasing the power imbalance already in existence because of the individual's situation. Think carefully about the individual and if you are uncertain what is acceptable to them then find out by asking them or others that know them well or if this is not possible ask a manager for advice.

Working within legal, ethical and policy guidelines

Health and social care practice is underpinned by legislation, ethics and other guidance from research and government. All of these will be reflected within organisational policies. However, their mere existence does not guarantee automatic implementation and adherence. In reality, this can only be achieved through the day-to-day practice, attitudes and behaviours of all those who work within the care setting. Regular supervision of practice will support health and social care workers to ensure they work within legal, ethical and policy guidelines, while regular inspections and audits by regulatory authorities ensures adherence by organisations.

case study 2.2

Mindless discrimination

Sandra came to England from Ghana 30 years ago as a young woman and, between raising her children, took courses in chartered accountancy. At 51, she suddenly developed the features of a psychotic illness. She believed that cars would swerve to try to run her over. She was admitted to a psychiatric ward, where her behaviour was seen as loud, unpredictable and aggressive. So she was transferred to a psychiatric intensive care unit. Now she is almost fully recovered from her symptoms, but is adamant that this episode has irreversibly changed her life.

People treat her differently now, she says. 'My friends make me feel like a weakling.' She used to be a central figure in her community, and was heavily involved in her church. Although she tries hard to minimise the impact of her illness, she admits that it has damaged her. 'I used to be very influential in the local community, but I discovered that they do not involve me so much any more,' she says. 'I keep myself to myself more than before. I used to be someone who had leadership qualities. But I've lost confidence. I shy away from getting too involved. I used to socialise in my community, then they would be looking at me in a funny way, and for a couple of them, it's like you do not exist any more.'

But Sandra reserves her strongest feelings for the way she was treated by health staff. Although she says that the community psychiatric nurses who visited her at home were 'brilliant people', this was overshadowed by more negative experiences. When she was transferred to the locked, intensive care ward, she was forcibly injected with medication. This happened more than a year ago, but she is still very distressed when remembering the experience.

'I saw people surrounding me, holding me by the hand, by the legs,' she recalls. 'I do not think it was something they had to do. There was no talking. They would have helped better if they had more understanding, more talking – more respect. I felt really bad. While I was in hospital I tried to complain, but I do not know if anybody was listening. It was a nightmare.'

After leaving hospital, she felt physically unwell and consulted her family doctor. She says: 'I was feeling really tired and I thought I should see my local GP, and I said: 'Can you please do a physical examination?' He said: 'Have you had any mental problems before?' I was really angry with him. Was he trying to say that the reason I was coming to see him was because I had had a mental problem? I left the clinic that day feeling really bad.'

Sandra's mixed feelings about mental health care are common among people with mental illness, many of whom feel that they have been both helped and misunderstood by psychiatric services. It is a paradox that many mentally ill people do not speak highly of the mental health staff who are supposed to be there to help. Indeed, service users often rate mental health staff as one of the groups that most stigmatises people with mental illness.

The problem is not limited to mental healthcare. In recent years, it has become clear that people with mental illness also receive second-class physical healthcare. This process, sometimes called 'diagnostic overshadowing', means that a person with mental illness finds that doctors think that any physical symptoms are 'all in the mind', and so they decide not to investigate further.

by Graham Thornicroft, The Guardian, July 26th 2006

activity
GROUP WORK

Individually read through the above article and then in a group discuss the following questions:

1 What assumptions, stereotypes, prejudices and types of discrimination are being described in Sandra's account of her experience?

2 What impact did discrimination have on Sandra

3 What actions would you take as a health and social care worker to stop other mental health service users being treated in a discriminatory way?

activity
INDIVIDUAL WORK
2.8

M3

D2

1 Reflecting on your own experience, analyse how your personal beliefs and value systems may influence your own anti-discriminatory practice.

2 Evaluate the effectiveness of different practical strategies you could use to align your own beliefs and values with anti-discriminatory practice in health and social care.

Progress Check

1 Give four examples of the benefits of diversity to life in the UK.

2 Explain what is meant by *equity*.

3 Give four examples of how equality can be actively promoted in health and social care.

4 Name four individual rights.

5 Briefly explain the reasons why people may experience discrimination as a result of their age.

6 What additional protection does the Disability Discrimination Act (2005) provide for individuals?

7 What is the GSCC Code of Practice for social care workers?

8 Give two examples of organisational policies that promote individual rights.

9 Explain how you would support an individual in a person centred way.

10 Give four examples of influences on an individual's beliefs and values.

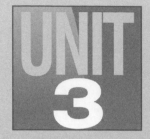

UNIT 3

Health, safety and security in health and social care

This unit covers:

- Potential hazards in health and social care
- How legislation, guidelines, policies and procedures promote health, safety and security
- The roles and responsibilities for health, safety and security in health and social care settings
- How to deal with hazards in a local environment

Places where people receive health and social care vary enormously and because of this patients, service users and staff can be in danger from many different hazards. Health and care workers have a responsibility to protect the people they look after from harm, for example from dangerous waste materials, chemicals, intruders and equipment hazards. Good carers anticipate hazards and make efforts to reduce the risks. Carers also need to be aware of the many legal requirements, regulations and guidelines that aim to promote safety in the workplace. They must be familiar with local polices and procedures and be confident in the knowledge of who has responsibility for safety issues in the care setting. Within this unit, learners will undertake a survey of a local environment used by patients or service users that will enable them to apply the theory of health and safety to practice.

grading criteria

To achieve a **Pass** grade the evidence must show that the learner is able to:	To achieve a **Merit** grade the evidence must show that, in addition to the pass criteria, the learner is able to:	To achieve a **Distinction** grade the evidence must show that, in addition to the pass and merit criteria, the learner is able to:
P1 use work placement experiences to explain a minimum of six potential hazards in a health or social care setting Pg 86		
P2 describe how key legislation in relation to health, safety and security influences health and social care delivery Pg 102		
P3 using examples from work experience describe how policies and procedures promote health, safety and security in the health and social care workplace Pg 102	**M1** explain how legislation, policies and procedures are used to promote the health, safety and security of individuals in the health and social care workplace Pg 104	**D1** using examples from work experience evaluate the effectiveness of policies and procedures for promoting health, safety and security Pg 104

To achieve a **Pass** grade the evidence must show that the learner is able to:	To achieve a **Merit** grade the evidence must show that, in addition to the pass criteria, the learner is able to:	To achieve a **Distinction** grade the evidence must show that, in addition to the pass and merit criteria, the learner is able to:
P4 examine the roles and responsibilities of key people in the promotion of health, safety and security in a health or social care setting Pg 106		
P5 carry out a health and safety survey of a local environment used by a specific patient/ service user group Pg 109	**M2** assess the risk associated with the use of the chosen local environment and make recommendations for change Pg 109	**D2** justify recommendations made for minimising the risks, as appropriate, for the setting and service user groups Pg 109
P6 demonstrate basic first aid skills Pg 114	**M3** demonstrate first aid skills on a critically injured individual Pg 114	

Potential hazards in health and social care

Hazards

A hazard is any object, substance, action or situation which is harmful or could become harmful.

In the working environment

It is easy to see that there are inherent hazards in some workplaces, such as factories and large warehouses where machinery and heavy loads are regularly moved around. However, it may not be so obvious that we are at risk from hazards in all environments, including care settings and in our own homes. In a setting where people are receiving care, there is by definition a group of vulnerable people. As carers, we have a duty to keep people safe whatever the type of building or type of client group we are working with.

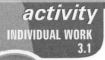

1   Make a list of at least six potential hazards present in your work placement.

2   Produce a poster illustrating a selection of these hazards.

3   Write captions on your poster to explain why these are potential hazards.

Poor working conditions

Poor working conditions for employees may lead to employees being unable to perform their jobs in a safe manner. Staff shortages may lead carers to cut corners in the care they deliver. For example, they may not follow **procedures** fully in order to save time. If staff do find themselves under pressure in this way, they must inform the manager so that more staff can be brought in to keep service users and employees safe. Staff also need reasonable breaks from duty during the day so that they are calm, refreshed and able to deal with all the challenges that a shift may bring. If a staff member is pregnant or ill, reasonable flexibility in duties should be afforded them. Access to first aid is essential and employers should make sure staff are trained in dealing with first aid emergencies. Working in clean, well lit, comfortable environments can greatly improve employee's working conditions.

Poor staff training

The health and safety of everyone in the workplace is paramount. Ignorance of a hazard, risk, proper action or procedure can lead to injury, disability and even death. It is important for staff to be trained in how to identify hazards, how to minimise **risks** and what to do if something goes wrong. If employees have confidence in their knowledge and abilities, they will work more efficiently and staff, service users and relatives will feel safer and more secure.

Poor working practices

Many people start out wanting to be good carers, but getting into bad habits is easily done. Familiarity with a procedure can lead individuals to rush and not carry out the procedure to the best of their ability. They may be tempted into doing just enough to get a task done rather than doing it well. New staff may learn these poor practices from experienced employees and pass them on as correct to others. Without vigilance and training, staff can become a danger to themselves and others.

Equipment

Many different types of safety equipment are available to carers today. Some are simple and cheap, such as a **slip sheet**, while other equipment is expensive and more complicated, such as a **hoist**. All types of equipment, whether simple or complex, require knowledge and practice before they can be used safely and with confidence. The correct application of safety equipment can reduce risks of injury to staff and service user alike. Staff should be able to ask their manager if they feel they need training.

Substances

Chemicals

In many care establishments, chemicals are used routinely. In large institutions, such as hospitals, pest control inspectors may use poison to keep rodent populations down and laboratory chemicals may be in regular use. In smaller care settings, cleaning chemicals, such as bleach, may pose a greater danger to staff and service users. However some substances can be harmful if they get into or onto the body. Some substances can cause problems years after exposure, while others can have an immediate effect. The Control of Substances Hazardous to Health Regulations 2002 (COSHH) state that employers must have carried out an assessment on the hazards of substances or, their ingredients in their workplace. Measures to keep all chemicals locked away and out of reach of vulnerable people, are imperative.

> **remember**
> Health and social care workers who are found to be not following policies, procedures or regulations can be disciplined, sacked or even be taken to court.

> **remember**
> The Management of Health and Safety at Work Regulations (1992) state that employers must train workers to use equipment correctly.

Fig 3.1 A hoist in use

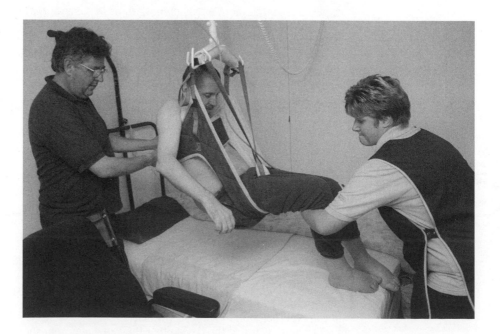

Potential effects of some chemicals:

- asthma
- lung damage
- liver or other organ damage
- skin problems: burns, **dermatitis**

Link

See page 109 for more information about first aid.

Pharmaceuticals

Any drug that is prescribed is potentially a danger to people. A nurse giving a drug to a patient has to make sure it is the right patient, the right medication and the right dose at the right time. A mistake in any one of the above requirements could have tragic results.

Some patients and service users may take medication improperly or take it when it is not meant for them. This might be because they are too young to know the dangers, have learning disabilities or are confused. The best way to avoid this happening is to assist the patient or service user to tale their medication if required and to keep all pharmaceuticals out of reach and under lock and key.

Fig 3.2 A drugs trolley

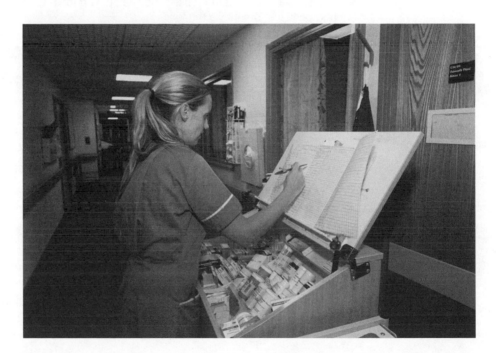

case study 3.1 Misadministration of pharmaceuticals

Eva lives in a residential home. The senior carer brought her tablets to her at 8 a.m. but Eva has to take them with food. She likes to have her shower before breakfast and so she left the tablets on her bedside table to take later. While she was out of her room, Pru, a confused resident, wandered in, took the tablets and swallowed them just as Eva walked back in. Eva was very upset and called for the carers who came rushing to see what the matter was.

activity
INDIVIDUAL WORK

1 What errors of procedure occurred that caused the wrong person to take the medication?

2 How could Eva's medication be delivered to her in a way which would suit her and still be safe?

Food

Food safety is important for all care workers who help prepare, serve or feed patients and service users. **Pathogens** such as bacteria can contaminate food that is handled, stored, prepared or cooked improperly. Other substances can contaminate food, such as viruses, moulds and natural poisons found in some foods, metals and chemicals that can also be absorbed into food. People of all ages can become unwell from eating infected food, but it is particularly dangerous for the very young, those already compromised by illness, pregnant women or elderly people.

Basic rules that all people should follow when handling food;

- Minimise food handling where ever possible. Reduce the risk of bacteria being passed on by using gloves or clean utensils.

- Keep cooked and raw foods apart. Raw foods are most likely to contaminate cooked food.

- Use separate equipment and utensils for raw and cooked foods. This cuts down on the chance of contamination.

- Clean all equipment and surfaces properly to remove pathogens.

- Keep food areas free from waste. Spoiled or rotten food is a haven for bacteria which could contaminate the fresh food.

- Prevent staff with health problems from preparing food. Germs can easily be passed from that person to others via the food.

---

case study 3.2 — Food hygiene investigation

In 1996, there was an outbreak of **E. coli** in Scotland. There were over 500 cases and 21 deaths. The outbreak was traced back to one butcher's shop. There cooked meats and cooked steak with gravy were identified as the culprits. A government investigation made the following recommendations to try and avoid this in the future:

- There should be better food hygiene controls in butcher's shops.

- Raw and cooked meats should be separated.

- All food handlers should be trained.

activity
INDIVIDUAL WORK

1 Find out who inspects butchers and other food retailers.

2 Research the training that a butcher or food handler needs for their job.

3 Produce a flyer advertising a job at a local butcher's or restaurant kitchen. Include training requirements in your advert.

See page 92 for more information about standard precautions for preventing and controlling the spread of infection.

The Food Standards agency   www.foodstandards.gov.uk

Incidents

Any incident that occurs must be reported in the correct way. For example, accidents must be recorded in the accident book with the time, date, name of the person involved and a description of the accident. If there was an injury it must be described and the treatment given must be documented. The disposal of the person must also be recorded (where they went for treatment after first aid, such as their GP or a hospital).

Working environment

The working environment is the place in which a worker carries out their job. In the case of health and social care workers, this may be within a health and social care setting, in the service user's own home or out in the community.

Within an organisation's premises

Safety within an organisation's premises must be a priority for everyone. Wet floors following cleaning or spillages, very hot water from the tap and dangerous broken furniture are just a few examples of hazards that can occur. The organisation has a legal responsibility for keeping everyone there safe.

In the premises of another organisation

If you have to visit another organisation, you can be assured that they are subject to the same legislation and regulations as your work setting. This ensures that health and safety measures are equally implemented and hazards are reduced in all workplaces.

In the service user's home

People in their own home are not required to meet legislation in the same way as workplaces, and it is worth remembering that 4000 people in the UK die every year from accidents in the home and another 2.7 million turn up at accident and emergency departments. If you see something that concerns you, alert the service user to the hazard and make a note of it in their care plan. If it is something that is very serious, inform your manager who may inform relatives or other agencies such as social services or even the police if appropriate.

Royal Society for the Prevention of Accidents　　www.rospa.com

Out in the community

Care workers increasingly visit people in the wider community. They have a responsibility to make their way to and from locations safely. They should always drive carefully, keep their car in good working order, wear a seatbelt and take out business insurance for their vehicle. A care worker should make it known where they are going and what time they expect to be back. Some employers supply two-way radios or mobile phones so care workers can contact their base easily. Some even give out personal alarms to their community-based workers in case they feel threatened.

Working practices

Working practices are the ways in which the tasks that make up part of a person's job are carried out.

Activities

Some activities used to stimulate or entertain those we care for can pose hazards. For example, craft and display work is common in nurseries and schools but nowadays the use of non-toxic paints and crayons is standard. Fun or educational trips for residents or pupils are very useful and enjoyable but can put them at risk of harm.

Procedures

There is usually a set of procedures for most tasks in a care settings. For example, there may be a written procedure for a school fire drill or for taking a blood specimen at a health centre. Procedures are necessary to give staff clear instructions and guidelines to follow to ensure consistency and safety in the job they do. If a procedure exists, it is the expected way of doing things. Any deviation from standard procedure can be measured and possibly lead to disciplinary action.

Storage and use of materials or equipment

Materials and equipment should always be stored according to manufacturers' instructions. If electrical goods, for example, get damp or are improperly put away they can malfunction or even cause a fire. It is important for staff to read instructions on how to use materials and equipment properly. They must also speak up if they feel unsure or worried about using something. If they lack the knowledge of how to use materials or have not been shown how equipment is used, there is a great risk of injury to service users or themselves.

Working techniques

Manual handling

All workers are at risk of injuries caused by moving heavy weights around, but in their daily work, health and social care workers often have to move people who are heavy and

case study 3.3   Always read instructions

Debbie is a new community nurse. One day Mrs Mackay, one of the patients she visited, required a shower and a dressing on her leg afterwards. Mrs Mackay asked her to apply a lotion to her scalp while in the shower. Debbie asked what it was for and she was told it was to stop dandruff. Debbie was pleased to help and she did as Mrs Mackay asked. Once Mrs Mackay had showered and her leg was dressed with new bandages Debbie left. Two days later, Debbie was called to see her manager who informed her that Mrs Mackay had put in a complaint that Debbie had burnt her head with the lotion. It transpired that it should have been washed off soon after it was applied. Debbie had to admit that she had not read the instructions on the lotion bottle before applying it to Mrs Mackay's scalp. Debbie had a written warning placed permanently on her file and Mrs Mackay received a few thousand pounds in compensation from the Primary Care Trust.

activity
GROUP WORK

Discuss the following:

1   Is Debbie at fault?
2   Discuss what steps Debbie could have taken to avoid this happening.

unpredictable. One out of ten serious work-related back injuries involves nursing personnel and about 12 percent of nurses leave the profession because of back injuries. Imagine hurting yourself so badly that you can no longer do your chosen job.

The majority of back injuries are preventable and care professionals can avoid them by following the correct procedures. Training in moving and handling people and objects safely should be available to all care staff on a regular basis.

The main rules when moving and handling a load are:

- Keep your back straight.
- Keep your head up.
- Use an appropriate grip.
- Keep close to the load (not at arms' length).
- Communicate with those around you (including the person you are moving).
- Keep your knees bent.
- Stand with your feet apart.

Food hygiene control
All workplaces where food is prepared and handled must ensure their staff are aware of the dangers of poor food hygiene. Training should be available so that workers are able to take the necessary precautions in order to keep the people who consume the food free from harm. A typical course that a worker might go on is a basic food handling course at the local college or the employer may have work-based trainers to assess them.

Risks

A risk is a situation which could be dangerous or have an undesirable outcome.

Possibility of injury and harm to people

Taking risks is part of everyday life. Just crossing the road each day, we are making a decision to take a risk. However in health and social care work as in other occupations, employees and employers have a responsibility not to put patients, service users and workers at any undue risk. Any possibility of an injury or harm to people is a risk. For example, if an unsteady patient may lose their balance and fall from a stool, then that is a risk.

Possibility of danger, damage or destruction to the environment and goods

The consideration of risk should not only include the possibility of danger to people, but to property or the environment. Possible causes of damage include fire, floods or explosions, for example from a gas leak. Most emergencies like this require care workers to raise the alarm and evacuate. In all cases, the safety of service users and staff is the first consideration.

Infection

Passing on contamination of germs is known as cross-infection and can occur through contact with people or objects. It is particularly important to avoid cross-infection when working with vulnerable people such as the elderly, the very young or people who are unwell. You can not know by looking at people what bacteria or viruses they carry, so it is always important to protect yourself and others by using barriers such as:

- disposable gloves
- disposable plastic aprons
- surgical masks
- protective clothing.

Care settings usually require staff to dispose of potentially infected protective gloves and aprons in designated plastic bags. These bags may be colour-coded, for example yellow for incineration.

Professional Practice

- Always throw disposable clothing away after each use.
- Avoid wearing uniforms or work clothes in public places, such as supermarkets.

A major way that care workers can prevent the spread of germs (pathogens), is by washing their hands thoroughly in between contact with each patient and after using the toilet themselves. Contact with your own or patients' and service users' bodily fluids can contaminate you and enable you to cross-infect another person.

Fig 3.3 Correct hand-washing technique

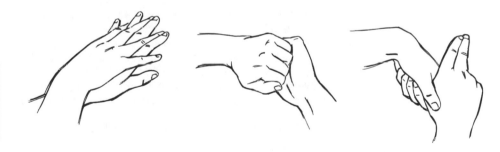

remember
People often wash their palms well but forget their thumbs, back of their hands and between the fingers.

Incidents

An incident is an event which is out of the ordinary, and usually undesirable, violent or dangerous. In health and social care settings, most incidents should be dealt with by following procedures and recorded using the appropriate channels, such as an incident or accident book.

Accidents

Accidents can happen to anyone anywhere but in health and social care the people who depend on care workers are often very vulnerable and at greater risk of having accidents if precautions are not taken.

Contamination risk

Once you have come in direct contact with a substance that is hazardous, such as a chemical or bacteria, you are contaminated. In health care, there is a great risk of passing contamination from one person to another because the job demands close proximity to other people and often requires staff to carry out intimate or invasive procedures when caring for patients or service users.

Chemical spillages

Most chemicals in care settings are in liquid form but there are substances, such as toilet cleaners, that can come in powder form. Chemical spillages can be dangerous in a number of ways:

- Liquid spilled on a floor can lead people to slip and injure themselves.
- Contact from a splash or fall onto a chemical can cause irritation to the skin or in some cases burns.
- If your skin is contaminated, you can pass the chemical on to others, for example when you touch someone.

Intruders

Intruders are people who enter places when they have no proper reason to be there. An intruder might walk into a private home, room, school or hospital ward, for example. In large institutions such as hospitals, surveillance cameras, identity badges and uniforms help to distinguish between people legitimately in the building and those who are not. In smaller care settings there might be fewer measures available to monitor people entering and leaving and so staff need to be vigilant.

If you see someone who you do not know, it is perfectly appropriate for you to ask politely who they are and what they have come to the care setting for. Most professional callers, such as GPs, health care workers and maintenance staff will carry identification tags showing who they are and who employs them, so you could ask to see identification if you were concerned. Unfortunately bogus callers may pretend to be a wide range of people in order to gain access. If you are unsure, check with a manager to see if the person is expected, or stay with them while they are on the premises.

Intruders might enter a service user's home to steal or hurt the person living there. Often people who are intent on committing a crime are very believable. They may wear work clothes to look like a genuine employee of a utility company, for example. Keep reminding service users to be alert to bogus callers. Advise them to check identity cards of any visitors before letting them into their homes and, if in doubt, ring the company to check. Genuine callers will be happy to show identification or wait until a call is made. Use of a door chain when answering the door is a good way to keep uninvited callers out. This gives the vulnerable person a physical barrier between them and the caller. It is also worth reminding service users to not buy things at the door, or let unsolicited salespeople in.

Aggressive and dangerous encounters

Aggression is violent or hostile behaviour or attitudes, and can be frightening and shocking to any witnesses. The most appropriate way to deal with aggression is to remain calm yourself and try to work out what has triggered this behaviour so you can diffuse it quickly, without further escalation. It is worth remembering that anyone may exhibit challenging behaviour of this kind. Patients, service users and relatives may verbally abuse staff, swearing and shouting at them. Some may even physically attack staff, spitting, biting and hitting them.

Where possible, anticipate challenging behaviour before it gets out of control. The body language of a person may give clues to the fact that they are tense, frightened or frustrated. They may have gritted teeth, avoid eye contact or their tone of voice might change. The care worker should check that their own behaviour is not making things worse, if so modify what they are doing, remain calm and try and diffuse the situation. If things do not improve and the care worker feels threatened, they should make co-workers aware that they need assistance and call security if available. In the community it might be necessary to call the police.

Fig 3.4 Opening the door to strangers

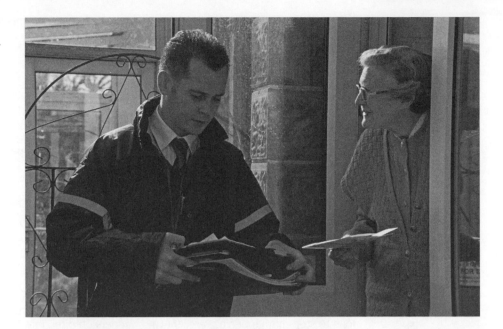

Fig 3.5 Why might people behave aggressively?

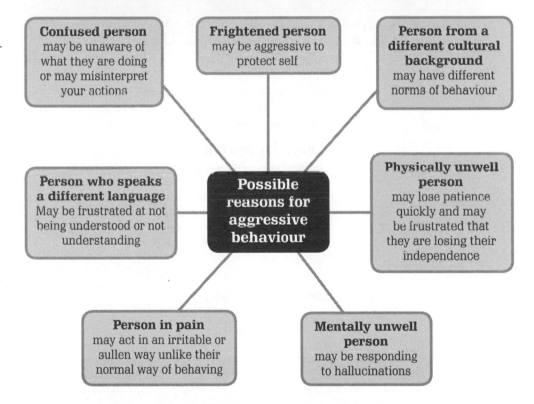

Lost keys, purses and other personal items

All workplaces have policies to follow in the case of lost or found property. If a worker, patient, service user or visitor loses something, they should report it in to the nominated person, for example, the receptionist or manager depending on the local policy, giving them a description of the item that is missing. Arrangements for contacting the person who lost the item should be made in case the property is handed in later.

Most workplaces advise people who find property to hand it in immediately. It is advisable not to look through a handbag, for example, for clues as to the owner's identity, on your own. Such an interest in the contents could be misunderstood and you could be accused of stealing.

Missing individuals

In large institutions, the chance of people going missing is high but this can happen in a small establishment or on an outing or trip as well. Care workers need to be aware, at all times, of exactly who should be in their care. Regular checks should be made to ascertain the whereabouts and welfare of patients and service users, as slipping out, getting lost, being forgotten or even left in the bath are all scenarios that could happen and all have potential health and safety implications. When someone goes missing:

- work out when and where the missing person was last seen
- ask others if they had heard the person discussing going somewhere
- search the area where the person should be, spreading out to the rest of the building and grounds
- check if the person has taken their belongings with them
- depending on the risk to the missing person, decide if you need to inform the next of kin and police.

Some clients often wander and you must complete a risk assessment to identify what can be done to stop this happening. A client who wanders off often may be confused or restless, unhappy or bored. You must never restrain a person by tying them to one place or putting chairs and tables in their way. There are much safer ways of dealing with this problem:

- Look at the immediate environment. Can a safe place to wander be designed?
- Distract the person with activities to keep them busy and engaged, such as helping staff complete tasks like washing up, or doing crafts, or stimulating activities such as quizzes.
- Do not be afraid (following risk assessment) to take the person outside to look at the garden or feed the birds or even go on accompanied short trips as this will keep them stimulated and busy.

Individuals locked out

Many care settings encourage service users to lead as normal lives as possible, to promote independence and integrate them into the community. This may lead them to be out of the premises at the time the building is secured for the night. A local policy for dealing with this situation should be in place in care settings where this is a possible occurrence. Preventing the situation is preferable. Staff could discuss with service users at what time they expect to return and be available to let them in straight away. Mobile telephones could be used to keep in touch and balance the need for the service users to exercise judgement and independence, with the care worker's responsibilities of care.

Fires within premises

All workplaces must have a fire assessment by law. This assesses the potential risk of a fire occurring in the premises by looking at a number of factors. These include:

- the building
- the materials kept there
- the equipment
- the type of person who is cared for there.

Care settings and other workplaces will have a procedure to follow in the event of a fire. Staff should have regular practice drills in order to make them familiar with what they have to do. Fire procedures will state what a person discovering a fire should do to raise the alarm, such as, operate the nearest fire alarm. It is important that all staff are familiar with procedures for their particular care setting. In some care settings, the fire service is automatically contacted when the alarm goes off. All staff must know whether they need to ring 999 in the event of a fire or not.

The procedure will also give instructions on what to do when people hear the alarm as well as the need for them to go to the designated assembly points. Some recently built care settings, especially those with frail or seriously ill patients or service users, do not evacuate clients outside, as safety zones have been constructed within the buildings. In such cases, residents and staff gather in a part of the building away from the source of the alarm.

Small outbreaks of fire can be tackled with fire extinguishers, hoses or fire blankets (depending on the type of fire). This should only be attempted by staff familiar with how to use the equipment and in situations where they are not putting themselves at risk of harm. Not all fire extinguishers are the same. Everyone should learn which extinguisher is for which type of fire, for example electrical fires should be fought with carbon dioxide or dry powder extinguishers.

Fig 3.6 Different types of extinguishers

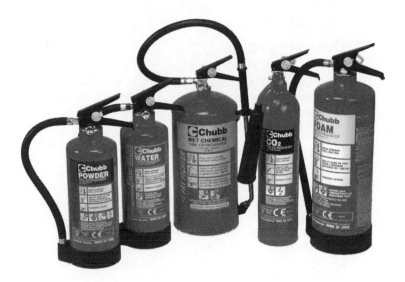

Bomb alerts

All bomb alerts should be taken seriously. If you are informed that there is a bomb at your care setting, you must follow the local procedure. Some workplaces have a different alarm sound for a bomb alert than for a fire alarm and staff should treat both alarms with the same degree of importance. Fire and police emergency services should be contacted. Often evacuation procedures are the same as for fire.

Accidents

An accident is a harmful event that occurs unexpectedly.

Due to falls

Falling from heights is a common cause of injury. Climbing up on equipment that was never meant to be used in that way can put you at risk. Standing on chairs, boxes and tables to reach up for something is extremely dangerous. Even the use of stepladders can be hazardous. They often are easily overturned, and the top step must never be used unless it has handles attached. The most common error people make is over-reaching instead of repositioning a stepladder. Other falls may be due to slipping on wet or uneven surfaces.

Due to hazards in the environment

The risk of accidents can be reduced if care workers are aware of potential hazards in the environment of their care setting and take steps to minimise the risk, such as locking away medicines and displaying warning signs when cleaning is in progress.

Due to poor manual handling

Moving any load can be dangerous. In health and social care, you may find that you are required to move heavy equipment or patients or service users with restricted mobility. All patients and service users should have details of their mobility problems in their care plan and the aids and equipment they require should be identified. It is important to monitor any changes in the person's ability and to update their care plan with any changes immediately, to reduce risks to staff and the person being helped.

See page 99 for more information about the Manual Handling Operations Regulations (1992).

Due to illness

When people feel unwell, they sometimes have symptoms that lead them to have accidents. A faint, a fall, dizziness or **lethargy** can all result in injury.

Due to weakness

Underestimating the weight or size of an object can mean that people try to move things beyond their capabilities. It is important that care workers know their limitations and take the time to assess their capacity to carry out a strenuous task before undertaking it. Both workers and service users who are ill can find that they are unable to carry out tasks as well as they could when they were fit.

Due to disability

People with disabilities often like to be as independent as possible and some take risks in order to complete tasks without help from others. Disabled people in your care should be encouraged to try new things, live as independently as possible and not rely on staff all the time. However, in a care setting risk assessments should be undertaken and measures put in place to enable the disabled person to live as independently as they can with minimum risk to themselves.

Due to frailty

Many older people are well and independent to the end of their lives, but some people become frailer as they get older. It can become harder for them to judge the hazards around them and they may take unreasonable risks. Frail older people may injure themselves more easily, for example, breaking a hip as the result of a minor fall.

Due to sensory impairment

Our senses help us judge where we are in space and let us know of impending dangers. People with sensory impairment, due to disability, illness or taking of prescription or non-prescription drugs, may be unable to judge the hazards around them.

Due to cognitive impairment

A person with a **cognitive** impairment may not have the optimum ability to think through an activity, assess the risk and plan to reduce the risk before carrying out the activity. A cognitive impairment could be due to a learning disability, an organic disease such as dementia or brain injury, for example following a car crash. People with these problems might act impulsively, unaware of the dangers around them and it is important that their carers anticipate hazards and risks around the person before they get hurt. Getting to know the individual, their patterns of behaviour and what they may do is vital to keep cognitively impaired people safe from harm. Sometimes, with support and practice, an individual with cognitive impairment may learn to avoid certain dangers but this would depend on the level and type of cognitive impairment.

How legislation, guidelines, policies and procedures promote health safety and security

Legislation and guidelines

Legislation means the laws agreed by the government which set out the way things should be done and which are enforceable by law. Guidelines are policies and procedures produced by an organisation which suggest the optimum way of operating in any given situation.

Health and Safety at Work Act (1974) (HSWA)

Every workplace is covered by this law, including health and social care settings. Until the mid-1970s, factories and shops had different laws relevant to their areas. This Act pulled all the laws together so that all places where people work were covered by the same legislation. The Act places obligations on everyone at work whether they are managers, suppliers, employers or employees. It was designed to reduce accidents at work. For example section 2 of the Act protects workers undertaking any manual handling task.

Health and Safety Executive	www.hse.gov.uk

Food Safety Act (1990)

The Food Safety Act was passed in 1990 in response to public concern over the safety of food. The Act aims to control safety at all stages of food production. The act also sets out powers of enforcement and penalties for those who do not follow it.

The Act defines what food is in order to prevent any misinterpretation of the law. The definition of food under the Act includes any drinks, articles and substances used for human consumption, or used as ingredients in the preparation of food, as well as chewing gum and similar products, and fish that are eaten live, such as oysters.

There are four main offences under the Act:

■ Making food injurious to health either deliberately or accidentally.

Sometimes people maliciously add things to food. This can be done for many reasons by people who want to get publicity or hurt people for their own pleasure. Accidental contamination is also an offence.

■ Selling food that does not comply with food safety requirements being unfit for human consumption or contaminated.

People may pass poor quality food off as good food to make money.

■ Selling food which is not of the nature or substance or quality required by the consumer.

Nowadays packaged food is clearly labelled to show the ingredients and 'display by' and 'use by' dates.

■ Falsely describing, advertising or labelling food and food products.

In order to make a profit, people might try to pass off food as something that it is not, for example, claiming a fruit juice drink contains 80% real fruit when it does not.

Local environmental health officers enforce the Act. They are given the power to enter food premises and take samples of food for analysis. Managers and employees have to co-operate with the officers. They can give warnings or close premises without notice.

Food Safety (General Food Hygiene) Regulations (1995)

These are the main regulations made under the Food Safety Act (1990). They incorporate rules set out in the European Food Hygiene Directive (93/43/EEC) which applies to all European Union countries. The regulations apply to anyone who handles food or works with articles that come in contact with food. This could be people who repair refrigerators or cleaners, not just people that prepare or serve food. Owners of businesses must ensure that everyone who handles food is trained and every step of food preparation, distribution and sale is carried out hygienically.

The main provisions are:

■ Premises, vehicles and equipment should be suitable, clean, well lit and properly ventilated.

■ Facilities for waste should be adequate. Waste should be removed from food-handling areas quickly and should be stored in closed containers.

■ Vehicles for transporting food should be specifically designed for the purpose and kept clean. If appropriate they should be refrigerated.

■ Washing and sanitary facilities should be adequate for staff. Suitable hand-washing and hand-drying facilities must be provided.

■ Food handlers should wear protective clothing and maintain high standards of personal hygiene. They should not be allowed to handle food when ill and should be trained and supervised.

Fig 3.7 Environmental health officers

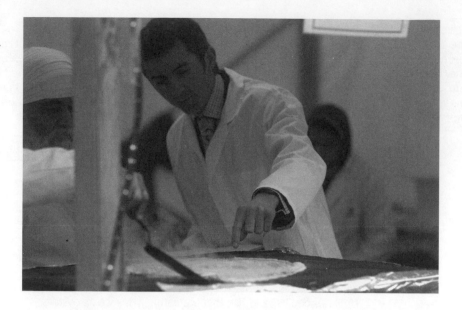

Manual Handling Operations Regulations (1992)

These were introduced to enforce safer moving and handling at work. They enhance the HSWA. The main provision is that staff should be trained in safe techniques of moving and handling loads.

Health and social care workers may need to move patients or service users in order to keep them independent, maintain their self-esteem and prevent injury by build up of pressure on the skin. Sitting or lying for long periods in the same position squashes the blood vessels and could impede the circulation of blood to the tissues. Frequent moving helps to prevent this happening. Well individuals change their position without thinking about it. If the blood does not circulate, a clot might form causing serious, even life threatening conditions. For example, a clot may travel and stick in the vessels of the lung (a pulmonary embolism), which can be fatal. People with conditions such as chest infections are usually more comfortable if they are sitting up rather than lying down.

Before you move anything it is important to prepare yourself mentally and physically.

- Check the area or route for hazards.
- Consider the weight. Do you need assistance?
- Use mechanical aids if possible.
- Wear appropriate clothing.
- Gain the consent of the person to be moved.
- Explain your actions.

Equipment to help with lifting comes in a variety of forms, from mechanical and electric hoists to trolleys to move heavy objects.

Fig 3.8 Aids for moving patients

Aid	Advantage	Possible health and safety consideration
Monkey pole	■ Independence	■ Must have strong arms and be able to bend knees
Transfer board	■ Independence	■ Must have strong arms
Moving belts 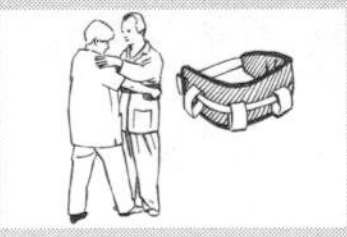	■ Service user can be assisted to stand without lifting and they can help with the procedure	■ Needs one or two staff
Glide sheet 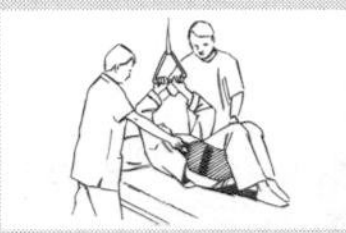	■ Enables service user to be moved and turned without lifting ■ Causes no body friction and is comfortable	■ Time consuming to put into place and position client
Turntable	■ Independence when turning	■ Can be unstable
Hoists or slings 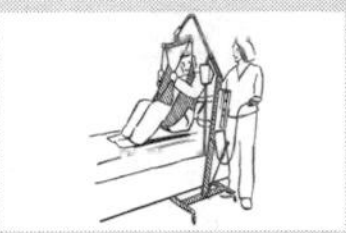	■ Ideal to transfer person from one surface to another	■ Service user can be frightened ■ These items are bulky to store ■ Different sizes of sling needed for different individuals
Tracking hoists 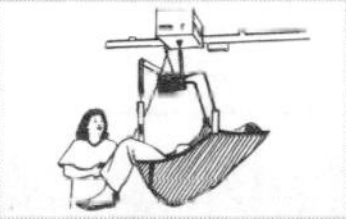	■ Ideal to transfer person from one surface to another	■ Service user can be frightened ■ These items are bulky to store ■ Different sizes of sling needed for different individuals
Wheelchairs	■ Independence	■ Can be difficult to drive, steer or push ■ May need strong arms
Walking sticks	■ Supportive ■ Can give reassurance and confidence	■ Can be used incorrectly
Walking frames	■ Independence, support and security	■ Can be used incorrectly and become unsafe
Grab rails	■ Independence	■ Sometimes bulky ■ Individuals can get knocked
Stair lifts	■ Independence ■ Easy to use	■ Expensive
Self-raise armchair	■ Independence ■ Easy to use	■ Expensive ■ Can be large and cause an obstruction

Reporting of Injuries, Diseases and Dangerous Occurrences Regulations 1995 (RIDDOR)

RIDDOR regulations require employers to report any major accidents or incidents occurring at a workplace, as well as serious diseases contracted in or likely to infect the workplace. If in doubt, the Health and Safety Executive (HSE) can advise. This information is used by local authorities and the HSE to identify where and how serious risks occur. These risks can then be monitored and managed appropriately.

Fig 3.9 Health and safety contacts

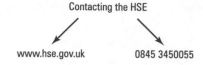

Contacting the HSE

www.hse.gov.uk   0845 3450055

Direct number for reporting incidents under RIDDOR

0845 3009923

Accidents need be reported only when they happen because of the work the people were doing. To be serious enough to report under RIDDOR, an accident would result in an employee:

■ dying

■ being absent from work or unable to do their normal duties for more than three days, for example due to an act of physical violence or because of back injury due to lifting heavy equipment

■ suffering a major injury, such as a fracture (except to the fingers, thumbs or toes), amputation, dislocation of the shoulder, hip, knee or spine, loss of sight, or loss of consciousness following an electric shock.

Which accidents should be reported?

Reportable accident	Non-reportable accident
A nurse opens a window on the upper floor of the hospital. The window frame gives way and he falls to the ground suffering serious injuries.	A social worker wears sandals to work and trips up on the corridor hurting her knee badly, where there were no obstructions or defects with the floor surface.

There are a number of diseases that people may contract as a direct result of their work, such as occupational asthma, occupational cancer and infections reliably attributed to work with body fluids or other biological agents.

Fig 3.10 Magnified tuberculosis bacteria

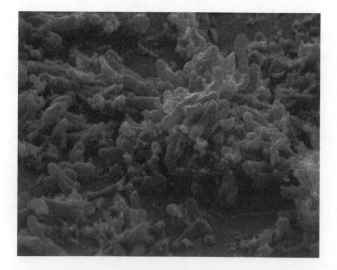

Which diseases should be reported?

Reportable accident	Non-reportable accident
A laboratory technician working with specimens containing Tuberculosis contracts the disease.	A day nursery worker contracts chicken pox as well as some of the children at the nursery and her own child at home.

Dangerous occurrences are not just those that lead to injury but those that potentially could have done. Examples are the collapse of lifting equipment such as a patient hoist or an accidental release of any substance that could damage health.

Which dangerous occurrences should be reported?

Reportable dangerous occurrence	Non-reportable dangerous occurrence
An electrical fault causes a fire at a residential home and it has to be closed for over 24 hours.	A bedpan containing urine and faeces is dropped and the contents spill onto the ward floor.

Employers should keep RIDDOR records carefully and securely, as with any other accident paperwork. Health and safety inspectors may visit the workplace at any time and request to see the forms. If any personal health information is contained in the paperwork, the employer is allowed to withhold this.

activity
INDIVIDUAL WORK 3.2

P2

P3

1   Divide into three groups. Each group should make a poster outlining the key legislation relating to:
   - Group 1: major workplace accidents
   - Group 2: major workplace incidents
   - Group 3: notifiable disease in the workplace
2   Each group should then discuss how the legislation they have listed influences health and social care delivery.
3   Add examples from your work experiences to the posters, to show how these policies and procedures promote health, safety or security.

Data Protection Act (1998)

The Data Protection Act was introduced to protect the peoples' rights concerning personal data stored in relation to themselves. The Act seeks to ensure that such data are stored in a secure and confidential manner, and outlines what may be done with these data, as well as allowing individuals the right to view data about themselves stored by organisations.

Link   See page 71 in Unit 2 for more information about the Data Protection Act.

i   Information about data protection   www.ico.gov.uk

Management of Health and Safety at Work Regulations 1999

These regulations require the employers to assess risks in the workplace. Employers have to keep records of these risk assessments, monitor any changes and re-assess as necessary. Risk assessments may be done, for example, concerning a part of a building, such as steep stairs, or potential risks on an outing or the needs of service users. Risks to individual service users are usually included in their care plan.

case study 3.4 — A question of mobility

Hugh is a service user of respite care at a care home. He usually stays for one week every three months. This helps his family have a break from caring full time for him and gives him a chance to socialise more.

Hugh has Parkinson's Disease which affects his mobility. He walks with a shuffling gait and uses a walking stick to support himself. His care plan states that his mobility is good and that he 'uses a stick for confidence only'. On Hugh's most recent visit, however, staff felt his mobility had deteriorated as he had stumbled and had nearly fallen a couple of times.

The care manager spoke with Hugh and said he had noticed a change in Hugh's mobility. Hugh agreed he did not feel safe using the stick anymore and wanted to try a different aid. The care manager wrote his observations in Hugh's care plan and spoke to the other staff to alert them to Hugh's mobility problems. The next day, the care manager contacted the community nurses at Hugh's health centre and they arranged for a physiotherapist to come out and assess Hugh for a new walking frame.

activity
GROUP WORK

1 How did the staff monitor Hugh's mobility?
2 Why is it important to tell the other staff of Hugh's deterioration?
3 In what form did the risk assessment take?

Control of Substances Hazardous to Health Regulations (COSHH) 2002

The use and storages of chemicals are regulated under COSHH. Any workplace could have a variety of substances that can poison or harm people, but in the care setting these are most likely to be cleaning products, for example bleach. An assessment of the potential risks of harmful substances at the workplace should be undertaken and a file of these should be on the premises. This should give information on the chemicals, what the dangers are and what to look out for if someone is harmed, as well as the required treatment if contaminated.

Policies and procedures

No two workplaces are identical and so organisations may have a set of instructions on what to do if there is a health and safety issue on their premises. Your placement care setting should have policies and procedures available to you and all staff. Familiarise yourself with these policies as you will have to follow your employers rules or guidelines if something goes wrong, for example an accident. Your employer will have written the policies in order to satisfy the requirements of the health and safety legislation and these are usually presented in a clear way so that all staff will act responsibly and legally.

Health and social care service delivery

All health and social care services have to ensure that their working practices are safe and will not harm the service user or care professional. They have a duty of care which means that they should not only care well for patients and service users but that they have legal obligations to predict and minimise risk at their care settings. Employers have to ensure risk assessments are undertaken whenever there is a potential risk identified and monitor this risk in case of changes occurring.

Link

See page 104 for more information about the roles and responsibilities of employers and employees in risk assessment.

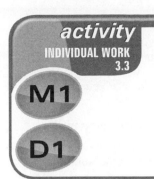

1   Make a list of all the health, safety and security legislation, policies and procedures in your work placement in a health and social care setting.

2   Explain how these promote the health, safety and security of individuals in that workplace, using examples.

3   Produce a presentation to explain your findings.

4   Using examples from your work experience, evaluate the effectiveness of these policies and procedures in promoting health, safety and security.

The roles and responsibilities for health, safety and security in health and social care settings

Link

See page 225 in Unit 6 for more information about service provision in the health or social care sectors. See page 98 for information about understanding methods of promoting and protecting public and environmental health.

Roles of employers and employees

The role of employers with regard to health, safety and security, is to ensure that their premises, equipment and working methods are safe for everyone and that they meet the requirements of the law. Employers should also make training available to their staff with regard to health, safety and security.

Employees must be vigilant and aware of risks, and make others aware of them. They should ask their managers for training if they feel they need it.

Responsibilities

All health and social care workers must follow legal and organisational requirements relating to their workplace, and should know how to deal with hazards when they occur.

Following organisation's safety and security procedures

In any workplace, things can go wrong and an organisation needs to be ready to deal with unforeseen events. A lot of time and effort will have been spent preparing for possible emergencies in order to meet legal obligations. The safety and security procedures that an organisation has written should be followed exactly by employees. An employee's actions at the time of an emergency may be judged later, comparing their behaviour and actions to the written policies and procedures.

Risk assessment

A risk assessment is a formal examination of things in work that could cause harm and the precautions needed to keep people safe. Employers have a legal obligation to identify potential hazards and undertake risk assessments.

There are five stages of risk assessment:

1   Identify the hazard.

2   Decide who might be harmed and how.

3   If there is a risk are existing precautionary measures adequate? If not, put new precautionary measures in place.

4   Record your findings.

5   Review the assessment and change it as necessary.

Checking rights of entry and take appropriate actions

You should stop visitors to the premises on their arrival. Check who they are and if they are expected. Alert the manager if you are unsure about letting someone in or not. A genuine visitor should not mind and may even be impressed that you are so vigilant. You must follow the care setting's procedure, be polite but firm and you should know what your employer expects you to do if the person is not allowed in.

Identifying and minimising health and safety and security risks

Always be on the look out for potential hazards and, as soon as you find one, let your manager know. Employers rely on their staff to be their eyes and ears in the workplace. Keep safety uppermost in your mind and your colleagues will be doing the same to keep you safe. It is not acceptable for you to think it is someone else's responsibility, even if you are there on a temporary basis, such as a placement.

Monitoring work practices

Working every day in a familiar work environment can make staff feel over-secure, resulting in them not following procedures properly. Supervisors and managers must monitor staff's practices to ensure that they are conforming to the organisation's set procedures.

Procedures must be reviewed regularly. Just because things have been done a certain way for some time does not mean that good, new, work practices should be ignored. An employer must monitor work practices and keep the procedures up-to-date as new ideas and legislation are introduced.

Respecting the needs, wishes, preferences and choices of individuals

Gone are the days when patients and service users had no say in their care. People were dressed in the same hospital pyjamas and nightdresses when they arrived in a hospital and the set meals were all that there was to eat. Today, health and social care workers take note of a person's individual needs and gives them choice in everything they do and the care they receive. A patient or service user may wish to wear certain clothes, have their hair done in their own style or have a choice at meal times. They will expect their preferences to be taken into account, from what activities they want to join in with, to accepting or refusing whatever treatment a doctor suggests they have.

Respect for an individual's choices must be balanced out by considerations about their health and safety. The carer may offer guidance and make the individual aware of potential risks, but individuals should be encouraged to make their own decisions.

Taking appropriate action to ensure that equipment and materials are used and stored correctly and safely

Health and social care workers have a responsibility to be aware of how to store and use equipment correctly and safely. You should be confident enough to speak up and tell your supervisor if you are unsure about how to use something. They should advise you or train you as necessary. The potential for major health and safety incidents will be vastly reduced if you know how to use equipment properly.

Dealing with spillages of hazardous and non-hazardous materials safely

Every health and social care setting will have procedures outlining the correct way to dispose of any materials that have been spilled. Some materials have specific cleaning needs due to their hazardous nature. Some materials may be harmless but if left could be a slip hazard. Be familiar with each material and the recommended way to clean up spillages.

Disposing of waste immediately and safely

Different care settings may have slightly different procedures to deal with body waste or clinical waste. However, they all will have strict rules in place for disposal of such hazards. Make sure you know which bag waste to be incinerated goes into, as opposed to general rubbish bags which often go into landfill sites with the rest of the area's household rubbish.

Fig 3.11 Sharps container

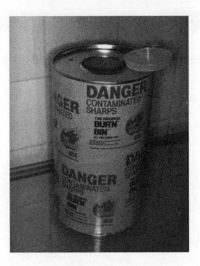

Following correct safety procedures

It is the responsibility of everyone working in a health and social care setting to follow safety procedures to the letter. Safety procedures exist to help protect everyone in the setting, and should not be ignored. Where necessary, you should support others in understanding and following correct safety procedures.

Following correct manual handling procedures and techniques

Every year, carers take risks and lift heavy loads in an unsafe way. Many of them receive back injuries that lead to them having to stop their chosen career as they become chronically disabled by their injury. Manual handling training should be offered to all employees and as new techniques emerge staff should be updated.

Reporting health and safety issues to the appropriate people

Usually procedures outline who to inform in your place of work when you need to raise a health and safety concern. The activity below will help you explore the people that may need to be informed.

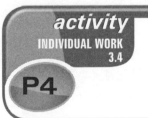

activity

INDIVIDUAL WORK 3.4

P4

1 Draw a flow chart diagram outlining the type of employees and managers at your placement or a local care setting.

2 Plot on the diagram who are the key people responsible for the promotion of health, safety and security and write what their responsibilities are.

Completing health, safety and security records

Records are vital to outline the sequence of events when an incident occurs. Clear records will help a carer explain what happened. It is always preferable to write things down as soon as you can, so facts are still fresh in your mind. Years later, your written records could be used in a court so it is important that you are objective, clear and neat when writing accident reports or in care plans. Never use liquid paper on mistakes and always cross out a mistake with a single line. If words are obliterated, it could lead to suspicion that records have been doctored for some reason.

Operating within limits of own role and responsibilities

In any workplace, there are clear boundaries between the ordinary worker, the supervisor and manager. It is important that you know the limits of your knowledge, expertise and authority. You should understand the right time to inform your line manager or when it is appropriate to go to a higher manager. Procedures can help you with this, but as a student on placement you may not have the experience to know when to speak to managers about your concerns. If you are unsure and it is not an emergency situation, you could discuss the issue with your teacher or lecturer and ask them for advice.

How to deal with hazards in a local environment

Environments

Health and safety must be considered even if you take service users out of the work setting, for example on a trip to a local park, tourist attraction, shopping mall or children's play area. The managers and employees at those places will have their own policies, procedures and responsibilities to keep visitors safe.

---

case study 3.5

St George's Primary School

The class of 28 year 5 students from St George's Primary School are on a trip to a local mere. It was not very well planned, since it was arranged on the last minute. They have been pond dipping with little nets and found some newts and frog spawn. The three members of staff with them are busy seeing to Rory who has waded into the pond and got his trousers wet. One of the pupils, Charlotte, then got separated from the group as she wandered away to look for a toilet. Mr Murray did not realise Charlotte was gone until he was informed by the Ranger that a little girl had slipped and hurt herself on the café steps.

activity
INDIVIDUAL WORK

1   What could Mr Murray have done in order to have avoided this?
2   Charlotte is injured. What paperwork is required?
3   Who should fill it in?
4   Is it necessary to inform Charlotte's parents?

Patient and service user groups

No matter what client group you care for the health and safety legislation applies. You should be aware of the type of risks any vulnerable people you work with may be at risk from.

Fig 3.12 Risks for vulnerable people

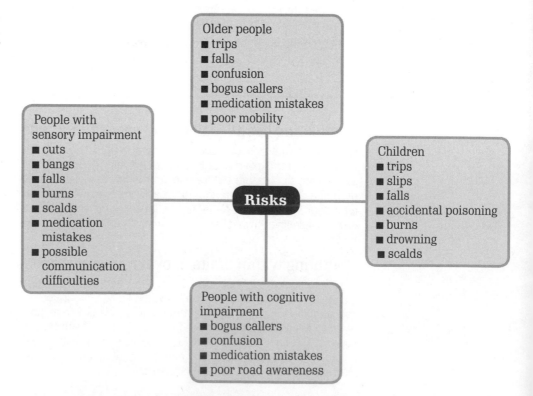

Older people
- trips
- falls
- confusion
- bogus callers
- medication mistakes
- poor mobility

People with sensory impairment
- cuts
- bangs
- falls
- burns
- scalds
- medication mistakes
- possible communication difficulties

Risks

Children
- trips
- slips
- falls
- accidental poisoning
- burns
- drowning
- scalds

People with cognitive impairment
- bogus callers
- confusion
- medication mistakes
- poor road awareness

Survey

Employers may have overall responsibility for risk assessments but good employee/employer communication will ensure the service meets the legal requirements. Workers often identify dangers that a manager may not be fully aware of, and may realise the limits of their client group to a greater extent and have a wider knowledge of the environment.

In activity 3.5, you will be required to undertake a health, safety and security survey of a local environment used by a specific patient or service user group, for example, older people, people with sensory or cognitive impairment or children.

To begin your survey, you need to be fully aware of the health, safety and security issues and demonstrate that you have identified the hazards and risks yourself.

- Inspect the area you have chosen.
- Look at the work or activities undertaken there.
- Obtain feedback from people who work in or use the area.
- Depending on which environment you choose, you might be able to ask if you can see evidence of past accidents.
- Examine instructions on any aids or equipment to understand any safety issues affecting that product.
- Examine directions for use on any substances.

Next, you need to decide who could be harmed and how. For example; colleagues, visitors, service users and students on placement.

Now evaluate the risks. To do this you need to consider:

- how likely is it that a potential hazard could cause harm
- are existing measures adequate
- what control measures could be put in place?

Evaluating a risk can be difficult, but if you work out the extent of the hazard, the amount of people exposed to it, how long they are exposed to it, the probability of it causing harm and the severity of possible injury, you can work out if a hazard is acceptable or requires action to stop it causing injury. In the care setting, dangers such as infection, injury from equipment or injury due to accidents are very high risks because of the vulnerable people you are caring for.

Fig 3.13 Carrying out a risk assessment

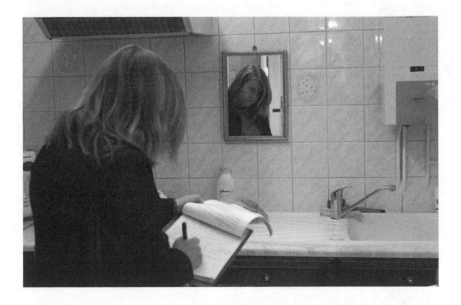

The following table outlines a typical risk assessment carried out in a residential home. Note that the hazards and people at risk are identified.

Risk assessment

Identified possible hazard or risk	Hazard? Yes/No	Who could be harmed?	Comment
Kitchen ■ Heat ■ Scalds ■ Cuts ■ Food hygiene	Yes	■ Chef ■ Staff serving	Not all food cooked on premises; some brought in and gets reheated
Lounge/Day room. ■ Cluttered furniture ■ Poor access (falls, trips)	Yes	■ All staff ■ All residents	Too many chairs and coffee tables
Stairs ■ Threadbare carpet (trip hazard)	Yes	■ All staff ■ All residents	–
Dining room ■ Residents eat together	No	–	–
Resident Jack ■ Allergic to tomatoes (rash, breathing difficulties)	Yes	■ Jack	Could have a serious allergic reaction
Fire safety ■ Fire door is propped open ■ Poor fire barrier	Yes	■ All staff ■ All residents	Manager going to explain why should not do this in next staff meeting

activity
INDIVIDUAL WORK 3.5

P5

1 Choose an environment that is used by a specific patient/service user group and carry out a health and safety survey of this environment.

2 Assess any risks in this chosen environment.

activity
INDIVIDUAL WORK 3.6

M2

D2

1 Make a list of your recommendations for change in light of this risk assessment.

2 Justify your recommendations for minimising the risks, as appropriate for the setting and service user groups.

First aid procedures

First aid is the first help given to a person who has sustained on injury or who has become ill. Knowledge of first aid is not only useful for helping in an emergency, but may even enable you to prevent the death of someone with a life-threatening condition. First aid procedures change from time to time as more up-to-date treatments are recommended, so it is important that you refer to recent first aid books and manuals when learning what to do. A practical first aid course is the best way to learn how to give safe, effective first aid.

St John's Ambulance   www.sja.org.uk

Action in an emergency

■ If you think there is a real emergency situation, you should dial 999 for an ambulance, or tell someone else to do it. If you ask someone else to ring 999, also instruct them to come back and tell you that the ambulance has been called, as sometimes people in a stressful situation may not follow instructions and the emergency services would be unaware that help is needed.

Fig 3.14 Making an
emergency call

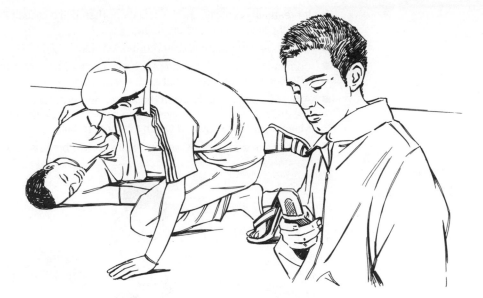

- You must give clear information to the emergency services, outlining the type of help required, such as an ambulance, a description of the accident, injury or serious illness, a description of the condition of the casualty and the location of the casualty.

- Try to be calm and speak clearly. If there are people around who can assist you, get them to go to where the ambulance will arrive in order that the paramedics are not delayed.

- If the situation is not an emergency, alert the person in charge of the area you are working in and inform the workplace's first aider.

- While waiting for help, it is essential that you do not panic. You may be worried or nervous if an emergency occurs, but if the casualty sees your anxiety it can make them upset and could make their condition worse. Reassure the casualty that you are with them and that help is on the way. It will help to keep them calm if you talk to them.

- Look for danger before you approach a casualty. The thing that caused them injury may still be there and you might be injured too if you rush in.

- Assess the nature of the injury or illness and ascertain whether the casualty is conscious (awake and aware) or unconscious (unresponsive).

- Never give a casualty any food or drink, even if they ask for it! It may make their condition worse or delay required surgery. Food and drink before an anaesthetic can put people at great risk and medical staff may prefer to wait for digestion of the food before embarking on surgery.

- You should be familiar with the location of the accident book and how to fill it in correctly.

Emergency first aid

If you come across a casualty you will need to assess what has happened and decide if emergency first aid is required. By finding out what has happened you can decide how severe the injuries may be. Ask the casualty or any other people present what decide.

Never underestimate the value of giving first aid in an emergency. If you are assisting a first aider, always follow their instructions exactly.

Life-saving procedures

- Keep safe. Check for danger before approaching.
- Check casualty's response 'Hello can you hear me?' Tap on their shoulders.
- If no response shout for help.
- Turn the casualty on their back.

The first checks to make on a casualty relate to their airway, breathing and circulation. Remember: A (airway) B (breathing) C (circulation).

- Make sure the person's airway is open by tilting their head and lifting their chin.
- Check for normal breathing for no more than 10 seconds

- If breathing normally, check circulation, then place casualty in recovery position, get help and check for continued breathing.
- If not breathing normally, send or go for help.
- Commence 30 chest compressions on centre of the chest to a 4-5cm depth at a rate of 100 compressions per minute.
- After 30 compressions, open the airway and give two rescue breaths (take a normal breath, hold their nostrils closed and blow into their mouth for about one second). Maintain open airway and watch for chest to fall.
- Continue at a ratio of 30 compressions to two breaths until help arrives.

Fig 3.15 Life-saving procedures

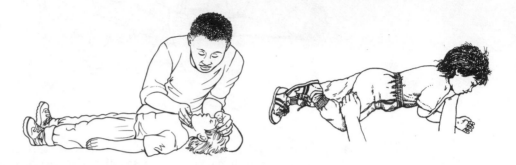

 Resuscitation Council   www.resus.org.uk

Dealing with injuries:

Fractures

Fractures are broken bones. They can be caused by direct force, such as a fall, or by being struck with an object in an assault. Fractures may be caused by indirect force and this type occurs away from the point of impact, for example people who fall with outstretched arms sometimes break their collar bone due to shock waves travelling up their arm. Closed fractures occur when the bone has broken inside the surrounding muscle and skin. Fractures that break through the skin are known as open because they are open to the world and infection.

The following signs may be evidence of a fracture:

- pain
- swelling
- inability to move the injury or lack of power or sensation
- abnormal appearance compared with the un-injured side
- symptoms of shock due to loss of circulation
- crepitation (the sound of the ends of the broken bones grating together).

The main aim when treating a fracture is establishing the priority it takes in relation to any other injuries. This means that if the casualty is not breathing and has a fracture, treat the breathing problem first. Treatment of breathing difficulties, bleeding and burns take priority over fractures.

1 Steady and support the fracture in the most comfortable position you can.
2 Immobilise the limb affected, for example by padding around it with a coat or blanket.
3 Raise the injury if you can do so without moving the fracture, for example lift the arm without moving the broken fingers.
4 Reassure the casualty.
5 Keep checking ABC.
6 Arrange transport to hospital.

Sprains

A sprain is an injury to a ligament or surrounding tissues. It is often caused by twisting a joint, such as an ankle.

The following signs may be evidence of a sprain:

- pain
- swelling
- discolouration.

The treatment of a sprain can be remembered by RICE:

Rest   Rest the injury in the most comfortable position.

Ice   Apply a cold compress, for example a bag of ice or frozen peas wrapped up in a tea towel, to the injury for about 5 to 10 minutes.

Compress   Compress (bandage) the injured part well above and below the injury to reduce swelling but take care not to restrict circulation.

Elevate   Elevate the injured part

Arrange for the casualty to be seen by medical staff as soon as possible as quick intervention can reduce healing time. Remember to keep reassuring the casualty.

Bleeding

There are different types of bleeding. Bleeding from an artery spurts out in time to the pumping of the heart. Bleeding from a capillary oozes out from the skin. Bleeding from a vein gushes out and can appear dark red because it has given up its oxygen and is returning to the heart.

To treat severe bleeding:

1 Apply direct pressure to the area of skin where the bleeding is happening. Wear disposable gloves if possible and apply a finger or the palm of your hand to the area affected.

2 To reduce the flow of blood to that area, elevate the injury.

3 Lie the casualty down in case they feel faint or go into shock.

4 Apply a dressing to the wound once the bleeding has come under control.

5 If the bleeding comes through the bandage, simply apply a new bandage over it without removing the first one.

If bleeding is severe, direct pressure alone may not stem the bleeding. In this case:

1 Apply indirect pressure to where the artery passes over a bone in a place away from the wound. This could be high in the groin for a leg and foot, or on the inside upper arm for the arm or hand.

2 Hold for no longer than ten minutes at a time, release the indirect pressure at ten minute intervals to allow blood to reach the limb.

3 Continue to apply pressure for the next ten minutes and so on.

4 Keep checking ABC.

5 Reassure the casualty

Burns

Quick action can prevent long-term pain and discomfort and scarring of a burns victim.

There are different types of burn:

Types of burns

Type	Causes
Dry burn	Flame, contact with hot object, friction
Scald	Steam, hot fat
Electric burn	Household electrical equipment, railway line
Cold injury	Frostbite, liquid gasses
Chemical burn	Bleach, industrial chemicals
Radiation burn	Sunburn, sun beds, radioactive sources

To treat severe burns:

1   Douse the burn with plenty of cold water. This will help the pain and stop continued burning.

2   Lay the casualty down.

3   Keep cooling the burnt area.

4   Monitor the casualty for deterioration in breathing.

5   Remove jewellery or anything that could restrict the skin if it swells.

6   Only remove burnt clothing if it has not stuck to the skin as you can do more damage.

7   Cover the burn with a sterile dressing, plastic kitchen film or a fresh clean pillowcase. You should avoid using anything with a 'fluffy' finish.

8   Keep checking ABC.

9   Reassure the casualty.

Asthma attacks

If a person is having an asthma attack they may feel anxious and have difficulty breathing.

To treat an asthma attack:

1   Reassure the person and keep calm yourself.

2   Sit the person down and ask them to lean forward a little. Do not lie them down.

3   Assist the person with taking their own medication. A mild attack should ease after about three minutes.

4   If symptoms go, then the person will probably know how to manage themselves following an attack.

5   If the attack is severe and normal medication does not work within five minutes, dial 999 for an ambulance.

6   Keep checking ABC

Epilepsy

There are two categories of epilepsy.

Minor epilepsy is known as petit mal. The signs of a petit mal are the person 'switching off' mid-sentence or going into a dreamlike state. Sometimes lip-smacking or fiddling can be observed.

Major epilepsy is known as grand mal. Sometimes a person feels they know a grand mal seizure is about to happen from a certain feeling or taste in their mouth. They may lose consciousness and fall to the floor and begin to convulse. This can last for three to four minutes.

To treat a person suffering an epileptic seizure:

1   Keep the person safe during convulsions, removing furniture from around them if possible. If you can, place something under their head, to stop them banging it on the floor.

2   Stay with the person until the seizure passes. Check ABC.

3   It is not always necessary for a person who has had a seizure to go to hospital. However if it is the first one they have ever had or it has gone on for a longer than five minutes, you must call 999.

4   Keep checking ABC.

> **remember**
> Do not put anything into the casualty's mouth. You might get bitten accidently!

Diabetes

A person who has diabetes is likely to wear a medical identification bracelet or carry a warning card. There are two possible conditions which may affect a person who has diabetes:

Hypoglycaemia is low blood sugar. You should look for the following signs:

- evidence that the casualty has not eaten after injecting their insulin
- pale, cold, clammy skin with profuse sweating
- deteriorating level of response
- occasional aggressiveness and confusion
- weakness and a fast heartbeat.

To treat hypoglycaemia:

1   Assist the casualty to a comfortable position.

2   Give a sugary drink, sugar lumps. The drink should not be hot and it must be sugary drink and not just sweet.

3   Usually the condition improves immediately. Continue to give sugary food, such as a biscuit.

4   Reassure the casualty. Advise them to eat a meal and see their doctor if necessary.

Hyperglycaemia is high blood sugar. This condition can develop over a number of days and there is too much sugar in the blood. It can lead to unconsciousness. You should look for the following signs:

■ flushed dry, skin

■ sometimes a smell of acetone (like nail varnish remover smell) on their breath.

There is no first aid treatment for hyperglycaemia save making the casualty comfortable reassure them and sending for an ambulance immediately. Check ABC until help arrives.

Bites
Treat as wounds in bleeding section.

Stings
Stings from bees, wasps or plants such as nettles can affect individuals in different ways. Some people will get a small localised rash, others can have a severe reaction called anaphylactic shock. This can lead to breathing difficulties and red blotchy skin and swelling of the air passage.

To treat stings:

1 Remove the sting if it is still there.

2 Apply a cold compress and reassure.

3 If the reaction is more severe, keep checking ABC and call 999.

Allergies
If people are allergic to something, their bodies react in a way that other people would not do. Different allergies have different symptoms or signs, such as rashes, severe itchiness, sneezing or, in severe reactions, breathing difficulties and anaphylactic shock. To treat allergies, reassure, monitor condition and keep checking ABC.

remember
Be prepared to put into recovery position if unconscious

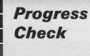

activity
GROUP WORK 3.7

P6

M3

1 In a group, demonstrate basic first aid skills on each other.

2 Take it in turns to pretend that you are a critically injured person. Now demonstrate your first aid skills (ideally by completing a first aid course or assessment).

Progress Check

1 List five potential hazards in a care setting.

2 Which type of extinguisher should be used to fight electrical fires?

3 Name three types of protective clothing used in care settings.

4 In which year did the current Health and Safety Law come into effect?

5 Describe three food handling risks

6 What does RIDDOR stand for?

7 What do the COSHH regulations cover?

8 Why is it necessary to complete risk assessments?

9 Why should you never give a casualty food and drink?

10 What does ABC stand for in first aid?

11 List four signs and symptoms of a fracture.

12 What is the treatment for a sprain?

13 Describe the two types of pressure you can use to treat bleeding.

14 Name two types of burn.

15 What is the treatment for hypoglycaemia?

16 Name one thing that can cause people to have anaphylactic shock.

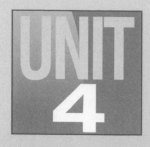

Development through the life stages

This unit covers:

- Human growth and development through the life stages
- How life factors and events may influence the development of the individual
- Physical changes and psychological perspectives in relation to ageing

Health and social care workers need to have a knowledge and understanding of human growth and development through the life stages in order to meet the needs of the individuals they support. They also need to understand the effect of expected and unexpected life factors and events on those they support and their families. This unit gives you an opportunity to gain an understanding of the different life stages and how people grow and develop, to reflect on the influence of a variety of factors and major life events on the development of individuals, and to understand the nature-nurture debate. It also allows you to gain an insight into the ageing process and to become familiar with both positive and negative perspectives of ageing.

grading criteria	To achieve a **Pass** grade the evidence must show that the learner is able to:	To achieve a **Merit** grade the evidence must show that, in addition to the pass criteria, the learner is able to:	To achieve a **Distinction** grade the evidence must show that, in addition to the pass and merit criteria, the learner is able to:
	P1 describe physical, intellectual, emotional and social development through the life stages Pg 130		
	P2 describe the potential influences of five life factors on the development of individuals Pg 135	**M1** discuss the nature–nurture debate in relation to individual development Pg 135	**D1** evaluate the nature–nurture debate in relation to development of the individual Pg 135
	P3 describe the influences of two predictable and two unpredictable major life events on the development of the individual Pg 137	**M2** explain how major life events can influence the development of the individual Pg 137	

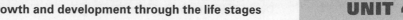

To achieve a **Pass** grade the evidence must show that the learner is able to:	To achieve a **Merit** grade the evidence must show that, in addition to the pass criteria, the learner is able to:	To achieve a **Distinction** grade the evidence must show that, in addition to the pass and merit criteria, the learner is able to:
P4 describe two theories of ageing Pg 139	**M3** use examples to compare two major theories of ageing Pg 139	**D2** evaluate the influence of two major theories of ageing on health and social care service provision Pg 139
P5 describe physical and psychological changes due to the ageing process Pg 147		

Human growth and development through the life stages

Life stages

The stages that an individual passes through during the course of their life are commonly described as conception, pregnancy, birth and infancy, childhood, adolescence, adulthood, older adulthood and the final stages of life.

Fig 4.1 Life stages

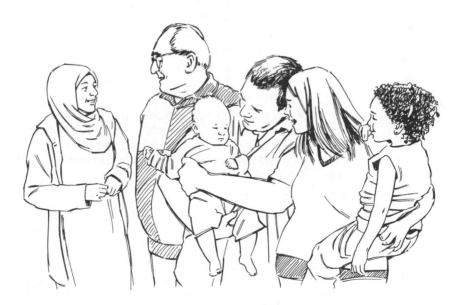

Conception

Conception or fertilisation is the term used to describe the penetration of an egg cell by a sperm cell and the fusion of their nuclei to form the first cell of a new living organism. Conception normally occurs in the fallopian tubes as a result of sexual intercourse. However, alternative means of conception are available in the event of infertility, which is when the ovaries do not produce eggs, the fallopian tubes are blocked, abnormal mucus in the cervix prevents sperm entering the uterus, too few sperm are produced, or sperm are not sufficiently active.

Alternative means of conception include:

■ fertility drugs, which contain hormones that promote the release of egg cells from the woman's ovaries. Use of hormones may cause the release of several egg cells, leading to multiple births.

- in vitro fertilisation, in which the woman's eggs are fertilised outside her body in laboratory conditions and then implanted into her uterus. Babies conceived this way are often known as 'test tube' babies.

- egg transfer, in which a fertilised egg from a female donor is inserted into the woman's uterus

- artificial insemination, in which sperm from a fertile donor is inserted into the woman's uterus at the time of ovulation

- surrogacy, in which a woman becomes pregnant through artificial insemination with sperm from the would-be father and gives the baby to the father and his partner for adoption when it is born.

Impotence occurs when a man has difficulty either getting or keeping an erection because of insufficient blood getting into or staying in the penis. Impotence can be treated with, for example, drugs such as sildenafil (Viagra), devices that trap blood in the penis, or surgery to correct blood supply to the penis.

See page 162 in Unit 5 for more information about the reproductive system.

Pregnancy

A fertilised egg is called a zygote. It divides rapidly to become a hollow ball of unspecialised **stem cells** called an embryo. In order to continue growing and begin the process of **differentiation**, the embryo needs to access a life-support system. Pregnancy begins when the embryo implants or embeds itself into the lining of the uterus wall and develops:

- an amniotic sac filled with amniotic fluid that surrounds the embryo and acts as a shock absorber

> **remember**
>
> The first few weeks of pregnancy are critical for the embryo and its development can be seriously affected by its mother's health and behaviour

- a placenta filled with the mother's blood, which attaches the embryo to the uterus and through which the embryo obtains nutrients and oxygen and eliminates waste

- the umbilical cord, which contains the blood vessels that transport nutrients, oxygen and waste products between the embryo and the placenta.

The mother's blood in the placenta does not mix with the embryo's blood but they are sufficiently close for dissolved nutrients and waste products to be exchanged, as well as some medications, alcohol, chemicals such as those in tobacco smoke, and infectious agents such as the virus that causes rubella (German measles).

The embryo continues to grow and develop rapidly, and as a result, is extremely sensitive to anything in its environment. For example, exposure to the rubella virus while the eyes and ears are forming can lead to severe defects, whereas the same exposure when they are fully developed would have no effect. The embryonic stage is therefore described as a critical period of development.

Birth and infancy

Between about eight weeks and birth (38 to 40 weeks after conception) the embryo is known as a foetus. Birth marks the end of the foetal stage and the beginning of infancy. Labour, or the process of giving birth, is divided into three stages:

1 Dilation: Strong uterine contractions cause the cervix to dilate until it is wide enough for the baby's head to pass through. This stage can take from two to 24 hours. The pain of uterine contractions can be managed using relaxation and breathing exercises, using a mixture of oxygen and gas such as nitrous oxide, using pethidine, a powerful pain reliever, or using an epidural anaesthetic, which blocks the nerves that transmit information about pain in the lower abdomen.

2 Delivery of the baby: The baby is expelled through the birth canal (uterus, cervix and vagina) to the outside world, usually with the help of the mother pushing down. The bluish colour of the baby quickly turns pink as he starts to breathe. Once breathing has commenced, the umbilical cord can be cut, separating baby from mother. This stage can last about two hours.

3 Delivery of the placenta (afterbirth): The placenta becomes detached from the uterus wall and is pushed out through the vagina. This stage usually occurs within 20 minutes of delivery.

Fig 4.2 Birth

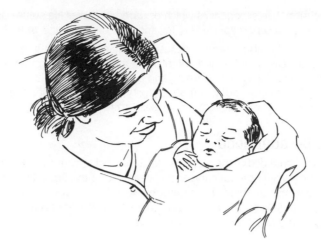

Birth complications include:

■ an overdue baby or when the health of mother or baby is at risk. In such instances, labour is started by artificial means, for example, through the use of a hormone drip or by cutting the amniotic sac to release the fluid (breaking the waters). This is known as induction.

■ breech birth, when the baby appears in the vagina buttocks first. The baby's spinal cord is put at risk if the vagina is not sufficiently wide.

■ weak contractions that fail to push the baby out, or a mother too anaesthetised to help the delivery by pushing. In such instances, forceps or vacuum extraction that eases the baby gently through the birth canal can be used.

■ a tight birth canal or danger to the mother or baby necessitating immediate delivery. Caesarian section is a surgical incision made through the mother's abdomen wall and uterus, enabling the baby to be removed.

■ anoxia (lack of oxygen), because the baby has difficulty breathing, for example, due to inhalation of **meconium**

■ low birth weight, either because the baby is premature, i.e. born before the 38 to 40 weeks of a normal pregnancy, or because there has been a slow-down of growth while in the uterus.

Infancy is the term used to describe the developmental stage between birth and three years, and like the embryonic stage is a period of rapid growth and development. Neonate is the term used to describe an infant during its first four weeks of life.

Childhood

Childhood is the term used to describe the stage between ages three or four and nine. Early childhood, from about three to five years, is the exploratory stage of life, when, through curiosity and because of countless new experiences, children develop a vast range of physical, intellectual, emotional, social and language skills. Later childhood marks the beginning of formal education, when children have an opportunity to develop and refine their skills in an organised setting. They also begin to be exposed to and influenced by different values, views and beliefs, which broaden their view of themselves and the world and enable them to begin to develop the skills necessary to cope with challenges in the future.

Adolescence

Adolescence describes the stage between about age 10 and 18. It is the period in an individual's life when physical growth is rapid and sexual maturity is triggered, and is a time for exploring sexual feelings, developing a sexual orientation, having a heightened self-awareness and developing relationships. It also marks the development of independence and an ability to think in more abstract terms, for example, to explore ideas, challenge authority, solve problems and develop personal values, views, beliefs and morals.

Adulthood

Adulthood is said to occur between the ages of 19 and 65. It is the stage of life during which individuals are able to assert their personality, autonomy and independence and make important choices, for example, in relation to occupation, family and friends, and lifestyle.

The formative experiences which occurred in earlier life stages are important in preparing adults to accept responsibility for and the consequences of their decisions.

Adulthood is also a time of exposure to many challenging major life events, both predicted, such as leaving home and parenthood, and unpredicted, such as divorce, redundancy and serious injury. The learning and understanding gained from life events and personal experiences gives adults an opportunity to further develop their personalities and their intellectual, social and emotional skills, to re-assess the choices they have made and to adjust the way they live their life.

Older adulthood

Older adulthood is the stage of life commencing with the 65th birthday. It is characterised by a decline in the function and appearance of the body, known as ageing, that can affect the way people think about themselves and their lives. But alongside this physical decline is a growth in wisdom and an opportunity to review life events and achievements with a view to enjoying a positive and productive old age.

Fig 4.3 Ageing

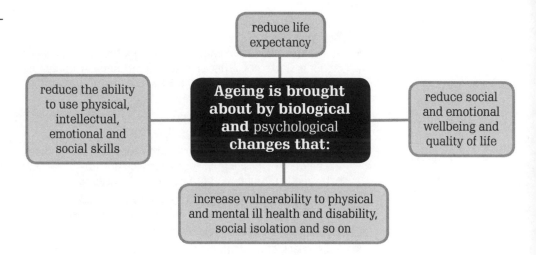

The final stages of life

Death or the final stages of life can occur at any age, for example, as a result of ill health or a serious injury, but it is most commonly linked with old age. Most people are aware of their impending death, unless they die suddenly as a result of, for example, an accident or heart attack. They may liken it to a long, peaceful journey, the beginning of a new life, or face it with fear, depending on their cultural and religious background.

Kubler-Ross (1969) proposed a five-stage process of dying:

1   Denial: where people react to the news that they are dying by denying the diagnosis: 'It can't be true.'

2   Anger: where people are outraged by the diagnosis: 'Why me?'

3   Bargaining: where people attempt to bargain, for example, with God or their doctor, in order that they may be spared death.

4   Depression: where people no longer deny their situation and their anger is replaced by a great sense of sorrow.

5   Acceptance: where people give up their struggle and, in some cases, welcome the peace that they expect death to bring.

Definitions

Growth and development

Each life stage has characteristic growth and development. Growth is to do with changes in body size, weight and shape, whereas development is to do with changes in complexity of the individual. Given appropriate conditions, human beings have the capacity for growth, to develop language skills and to develop physically, socially, emotionally and intellectually.

Developmental norms

The benchmarks against which an individual's growth and development can be assessed are called developmental norms. They are based on a range of measurements of a large number of healthy people. While everyone grows and develops at a different rate, developmental norms are useful gauges from which significant deviations generally indicate that growth and development are not proceeding normally.

Growth and development is assessed for comparison with developmental norms using a variety of procedures. For example, amniocentesis and chorionic villus sampling (CVS) are diagnostic tests that check the foetus for the presence of chromosomal abnormalities such as Down's syndrome and neural tube abnormalities such as spina bifida.

Urine tests are used to identify the amount of glucose in a pregnant woman's urine. An abnormally high level of sugar can be a sign of gestational diabetes, which can cause the foetus to grow too large. Very large babies are more likely to need delivering by Caesarean section; and Caesarean section babies are at greater risk of developing abnormalities such as jaundice and breathing problems.

Testing a pregnant woman's blood identifies her level of immunity to rubella. Should she be infected while pregnant, development of the foetus' heart, sight and hearing could be seriously affected. It also identifies the presence of:

- the hepatitis B virus, which if passed on to a foetus could seriously damage his liver
- syphilis, which if not treated could cause foetal abnormalities
- toxoplasmosis, an infection spread through cat faeces, undercooked meat and soil, which can stunt foetal growth and cause miscarriage and premature labour
- chemicals that indicate that the foetus has Down's syndrome
- hormones that indicate whether the placenta is functioning normally and keeping the foetus supplied with nutrients and oxygen
- HIV (human immunodeficiency virus), which causes AIDS (acquired immune deficiency syndrome). All pregnant women should be offered an HIV test as part of their routine antenatal care.

Ultrasound scanning can also detect Down's syndrome, as well as the age of the foetus and whether it is growing normally for its age and is in a normal position for birth. The foetus' heartbeat is measured using a stethoscope on the mother's abdomen to find out if it is beating between the normal values of 120 and 160 beats per minute.

The neonate's weight at birth is an important screening tool for detecting developmental defects. Like premature babies, babies whose birth weight is below normal (low birth weight babies) have a higher risk of poor health, delayed development and of dying within the first few weeks of their lives.

The well-being of the newly-born neonate is assessed using the Apgar score, at one minute and again at five minutes after birth. Its heart and respiratory rate, muscle tone, **reflex responses** (see Figs 4.4 and 4.5) and skin colour are assessed and each factor is given a

Fig 4.4 Reflex responses in the neonate

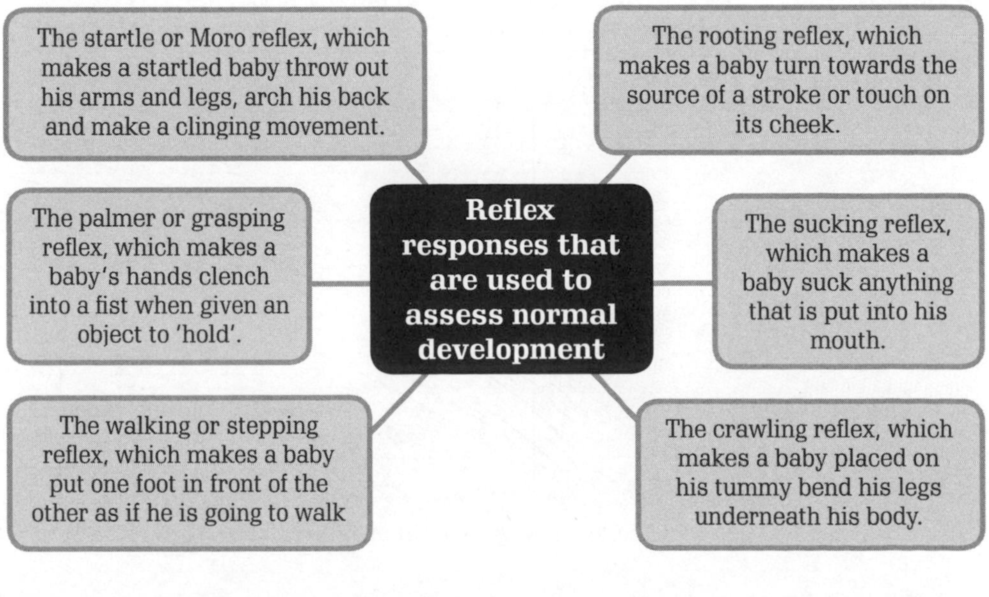

The startle or Moro reflex, which makes a startled baby throw out his arms and legs, arch his back and make a clinging movement.

The rooting reflex, which makes a baby turn towards the source of a stroke or touch on its cheek.

The palmer or grasping reflex, which makes a baby's hands clench into a fist when given an object to 'hold'.

Reflex responses that are used to assess normal development

The sucking reflex, which makes a baby suck anything that is put into his mouth.

The walking or stepping reflex, which makes a baby put one foot in front of the other as if he is going to walk

The crawling reflex, which makes a baby placed on his tummy bend his legs underneath his body.

Fig 4.5 Reflex responses

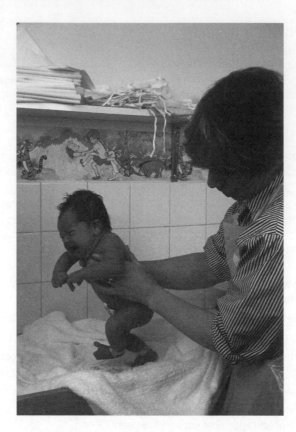

score between zero and two. The scores are summed: neonates who score between eight and ten are in good to excellent condition; those who score between five and seven are in fair condition and may require some help; those who score under five may be in poor condition and require specialist help.

The Guthrie test (heel-prick, blood spot) is used to screen neonates for the abnormal conditions phenylketonuria (PKU), sickle cell anaemia, cystic fibrosis and Medium Chain Acyl CoA Dehydrogenase Deficiency (MCADD).

Normal patterns of growth from the foetal stage through to adulthood have been established against which individuals can be compared. They illustrate the normal change in proportions of different parts of the growing body. For example, the head of the early foetus forms half of its body length while the adult's head is less than a quarter of body length. **Centile** charts provide ranges of measurements against which the height of individuals can be assessed. A measurement that falls between the range denoted by the 3rd and 97th centile usually demonstrates that growth in height is progressing normally.

Fig 4.6 Centile chart

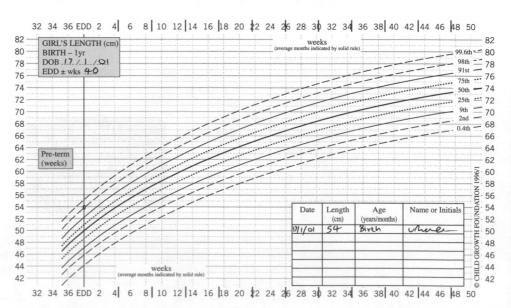

Some screening techniques are carried out at all life stages. For example, hearing tests enable hearing abnormalities to be identified, screening of the eyes checks for visual abnormalities such as **cataract** and **squint**, dental screening assesses the condition of the teeth and mouth and identifies the development of abnormal disorders such as cancer of the mouth, and measuring of Body Mass Index (BMI) determines whether an individual's weight is normal for their height. BMI is calculated by dividing an individual's weight in kilograms by the square of their height in metres. A BMI of:

- less than 18.5 indicates that a person is underweight
- 18.5 to 24.9 indicates that their weight is ideal
- 25 to 29.9 indicates that they are overweight
- 30 to 40 indicates that they are obese
- more than 40 indicates that they are very obese.

At the end of life, before a body can be removed and prepared for burial or cremation, a doctor has to complete a death certificate. To do this, he or she has to check for the normal signs of death, which include cessation of respiration and heart beat, pallor, loss of skin elasticity, a flattening of the body due to loss of muscle shape, and a reduction in body temperature.

Developmental milestones

These are important stages in an infant and child's development. The normal range for the timing of their achievement is very wide, but significant deviations from the norm generally indicate that development is not proceeding normally. For example, 90% of infants walk by the time they are 15 months; some of those who have not started to walk by 18 months may have an underlying problem such as muscular dystrophy.

See page 123 in this unit for more information about the timings of milestone development.

Life course

The life course is the course of developmental change through which an individual progresses between conception and death. These changes, or transitions, are often significant turning points in people's lives, and can be over in a short while, such as a wedding; take a day or more, as in giving birth; or span a number of years, such as the ageing process and the slow changes associated with puberty.

Developmental transitions change the way people feel and behave, and usually result in their being treated differently by others. For example, having a baby means a change in role from childlessness to parent, and is accompanied by new rights and responsibilities. Having a baby sibling changes a child's status within the family, such as from only child to older sister, which changes the way the child is treated and expected to behave.

Maturation

Maturation is the process of growth and development, and maturity is the state of being fully grown. Because the normal range for the rate of growth and development is very wide, it follows that different individuals reach maturity at different ages. Physical maturity is normally achieved by the end of adolescence or during early adulthood. Late maturing boys and girls are often smaller than their peers and may be less confident and less successful socially. Early maturation in boys is associated with high self-confidence and esteem and social and vocational success, and in girls with independence but also with premature sexual activity and poor academic performance. In both boys and girls early maturation can result in pressure to behave like adults because of the way they look.

Life expectancy

The number of years an individual can expect to live is called their life expectancy. This is calculated using **probability** statistics. According to the British Government's Office of National Statistics in November 2006:

- boys and girls born in the United Kingdom (UK) can expect to live, on average, to 76.6 years and 81.0 years of age respectively
- men aged 65 can expect to live a further 16.6 years and women a further 19.4 years (providing mortality rates remain the same for the rest of their lives).

Within the UK, life expectancy at age 65 varies by country. People living in England have the highest life expectancy (a further 16.8 years for men and 19.6 years for women) and people in Scotland have the lowest expectations (a further 15.5 years for men and 18.4 years for women). The equivalent figures for Wales and Northern Ireland are a little lower than those for England.

Development

Holistic development

You read earlier that, given appropriate conditions, human beings have the capacity for growth, to develop language skills and to develop physically, socially, emotionally and intellectually. These different aspects of growth and development do not proceed discretely; instead, growth and development has a holistic nature in which development in one area depends on and exerts an influence over development in another. For example, language development is dependent on the development of:

■ the physical structures needed to hear speech and to vocalise sounds, such as the tongue and **palate**. In the event of a disorder that prevents normal speech, such as a hearing impairment, language development depends on the development of the physical structures needed to communicate non-verbally, for example, in the form of pictures, symbols, writing and sign language.

■ the intellectual skills of thinking and understanding

■ the social and emotional need to engage with other people.

In turn, language skills enable an individual to develop socially, such as by developing relationships; to express emotions, for example, by articulating their needs; and to develop intellectually, for example, through discussion groups.

Physical development

The following table outlines some of the significant features of physical growth and development from conception through to the final stage of life.

Physical development through the life stages

Life stage	Age	Significant aspects of physical growth and development
Conception to pregnancy	1 to 2 weeks	The zygote travels along the fallopian tube to the uterus, dividing rapidly into two, four, eight cells, and so on, and eventually into a hollow ball of cells called an embryo. The embryo (blastocyst), in which the process of differentiation has commenced, implants into the thickened uterus lining (endometrium) between one and two weeks of age.
Pregnancy to birth	3 weeks	The embryo continues to divide, becoming pear-shaped with a rounded head end and a rudimentary spinal cord (notochord) along its back.
	4 weeks	The embryo has become C-shaped, with a distinct tail, rudimentary eyes, limb buds and an enlarged forebrain. It measures about 0.35 cm but weighs almost nothing.
	5 weeks	It is now about 0.5 cm long, still weighing very little, and has started to develop a heart, digestive organs and tract, a lung and a bladder.
	6 weeks	Limbs and sense organs are beginning to develop.
	8 weeks	All the major organs have formed, the heart has begun to beat, the tail has disappeared, the head and face are recognisable as being human and the limbs have become jointed with the addition of fingers and toes. The embryo is now known as a foetus, is about 3.5 cm long and its weight approaches 0.05 kg.
	12 weeks	Nerves and muscles are developing rapidly and the foetus can swallow, clench its fists, kick and make facial expressions. It weighs about 0.05 kg and is 9 to 10 cm long.

Life stage	Age	Significant aspects of physical growth and development
	20 weeks	The foetus is about 23 cm long and weighs up to 0.5 kg. Its skin is covered by very fine hair, the heart is beating rapidly, its movements can be felt and external sex organs have developed.
	30 to 40 weeks	This is the period when foetal development is completed and there is a marked increase in growth and strength. At birth, the neonate weighs about 3.5 kg and measures approximately 50 cm.
Infancy		Due to growth of the skeletal system, most infants grow rapidly during their first years, and by the age of three are between 95 and 100 cm tall, with boys, on average, being slightly taller than girls. Body proportions also change, the legs and trunk becoming longer in proportion to the head.
	0 to 6 months	Most infants are able to hold their head up steadily, sit with support, roll over in both directions, turn towards sounds and voices, and imitate sounds. Short-sightedness reduces and eyes begin to work together.
	6 to 12 months	Most infants are able to sit without support, crawl, stand alone for a few seconds, use a pincer grasp to pick things up, and pass objects from hand to hand.
	12 to 18 months	Most infants are able to walk, including backwards, point, ride toys and use pedals.
	18 to 24 months	Most infants are able to run, climb, kick and throw a ball underarm, use a spoon and fork, scribble with a crayon, build a small tower (about three bricks), remove clothing with help, and see as far as an adult.
	2 to 2½ years	Most infants are able to jump, and, with help, get dressed, undressed, wash and dry their hands and brush their teeth.
	By the 3rd birthday	Most infants are able to build a bigger tower (about six bricks), use scissors, stand on one leg and throw overarm.
Childhood		Body shape and proportion change during infancy and early childhood as the child develops a more adult-like body. Height and weight gain, primarily the result of bone and muscle growth, are less rapid in childhood than in infancy. Boys and girls tend to grow at the same rate until the age of about nine, boys being, on average, slightly taller and heavier than girls.
	4 to 6 years	Gross motor skills involving the use of larger muscles become more co-ordinated, allowing younger children to run, hop, skip and jump with confidence. Fine motor skills involving the use of the smaller muscles also develop, allowing younger children to handle small objects such as pencils with accuracy.
	6 to 9 years	Children continue to grow in size, strength and co-ordination. Their developing gross and fine motor skills allow them to become competent in activities such as swimming, tennis and football, and in activities that demand precision skills such as painting, model-making and playing a musical instrument.

Life stage	Age	Significant aspects of physical growth and development
Adolescence	10 to 18 years	Early adolescence is accompanied by a height spurt that tails off at about 16 years of age and normally ceases in late adolescence or early adulthood. Other physical changes are associated with puberty (the period of time during which sexual maturity is achieved). During puberty, changes in levels of growth and sex hormones cause growth of the sex organs: ovaries, fallopian tubes, uterus and vagina in females, and testicles, seminal ducts, prostate and penis in males. In addition, sex hormones promote development of the secondary sexual characteristics: ■ in females: deposition of fat, breast growth and broadening of the hips, giving the characteristic female shape; onset of menstruation and first ovulation; growth of pubic and axilla (armpit) hair; increased activity of the sweat glands. ■ in males: growth of muscles and broadening of the shoulders, giving the characteristic male shape; growth of the larynx, causing the voice to deepen (break); production of semen; growth of facial, body, pubic and axilla hair; increased activity of the sweat glands.
Adulthood	19 to 65 years	Most adults reach their full height in their late teens or early twenties, their peak strength in their mid- to late twenties and their maximum weight in their middle years. Hearing and vision are at their peak around the age of 20, as is reproductive capacity for women. Physical ageing starts in the mid-forties. Loss of muscle tone and flexibility lead to loss of strength and shape; loss of skin elasticity and strength leads to sagging skin, lines and wrinkles; the hair begins to thin and lose its colour; and body weight may increase, particularly in women. There is a decline in the functioning of body tissues and organs such as joints, the heart and the sense organs, and a slowing down in reaction time. Changes in hormone levels in a woman's late forties or early fifties cause ovulation and menstruation to cease. This is known as the menopause and is often accompanied by flushing and sweats due to changes in the ability of blood vessels to maintain body temperature. Other physical features associated with the menopause include headaches, insomnia, weight gain, growth of facial and body hair, and dry skin and hair. Many men experience menopausal changes in their middle life, for example, impotence, irritability, insomnia, a reduction in size of the testicles, a decrease in their sperm count and an enlargement of their prostate. However, sexual activity can play a role in the lives of both men and women through to old age.
Older adulthood	65+ years	Physical ageing continues and as time progresses, there is an increased risk of developing age-related degenerative diseases such as osteoporosis, macular degeneration and prostate cancer. However, the rate and effects of ageing vary from person to person.

case study
4.1

The Smith family

Jean and Ray Smith are in their late forties. They have four children, Samantha, aged 21, the twins David and Glenda, who are 11, and Julia, who is 7. They are in the process of adopting a 12-month old girl called Alison. Ray's mother, Betty, who is 67, lives with the family.

activity
INDIVIDUAL WORK

1 Which life stage is each individual progressing through?

2 What physical changes can each individual expect to experience in the near future?

Intellectual development

The development of thinking, learning, understanding, reasoning, problem-solving skills and memory begins in infancy and continues throughout life. Intellectual development in infants is initially through sensory awareness and later through physical exploration of their environment. Some important achievements include:

- by six months, recognising the faces of primary carers and distinguishing between bold colours
- by one year, understanding simple instructions such as the word 'no'
- by 18 months, having an interest in story books, pointing to a small number of body parts when asked, and knowing the correct way to use everyday objects such as a cup
- by two years, following simple instructions, naming a growing number of everyday objects and body parts, and recognising when something is wrong
- by three years, naming colours and people, knowing how a few simple everyday objects are used and understanding more complex instructions.

Pre-school children have an endless curiosity but a low attention span and so are easily distracted. By the age of four, many are able to distinguish between fact and fiction and are beginning to think about things beyond their own experience. As they reach middle childhood, they develop an understanding of concepts such as time and number and an ability to classify (sort) objects into groups according to, for example, their colour, size, shape and function. At six years, most children can focus their attention for up to thirty minutes and have developed memories of a number of significant facts and events.

Between the ages of seven and nine, children begin to be able to think logically and to reason. Their understanding is limited by their reliance on what they can actually observe, but their observational skills enable them to understand such concepts as length, area, weight and volume. Attention span, memory and skills of classification develop, as does an understanding of humour, other people's perspectives and the need for rules and standards of behaviour. One of the functions of school is to provide a setting which exploits children's ability to develop intellectually and prepare them for success as adults.

Fig 4.7 Intellectual development

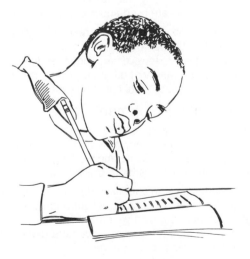

Adolescence is when young people start to be able to think analytically and in more abstract, theoretical terms, to explore and challenge ideas, beliefs, morals and conventions, to use **metaphors**, to formulate and test hypotheses, to solve problems and to plan for the future.

The intellect continues to develop throughout adulthood. Certain intellectual skills peak during early adulthood, for example, **short-term memory**, the ability to think and respond quickly, and the creation of original ideas and products. As the years progress, understanding increases, ways of thinking are refined, problem-solving skills evolve, and so on, through formal participation in learning and training programmes, and through experiences associated with, for example, life events and personal, social and occupational change.

At the time of writing (April 2007), lifelong learning continues to be promoted in order that people might enjoy, in their later years, the health and personal and social well-being associated with intellectual achievement. The expressions 'Use it or lose it' and 'You're never too old to learn' are based in fact: intellectual skills can be lost through disuse but regained by deliberate learning, regardless of age.

Exercising the brain in older adulthood can:

- improve intellectual agility, such as speed of response and the ability to stay focused and interested
- slow down the intellectual deterioration associated with ageing, such as memory loss
- provide an opportunity to maintain and develop social contacts.

However as people age their ability to process information by, for example, reasoning, thinking in abstract terms and solving problems, decreases. On the other hand, their vocabulary and social judgement, and their knowledge and understanding based on previous learning, socialisation and experience, improve.

See page 278 in Unit 8 for information about theories of intellectual development.

Language development

Language is a method of human communication based on a structured and conventional use of spoken and written words. Language development begins in infancy with crying. By two months, an infant has begun to coo; and by five or six months, can understand about three spoken words and produce a variety of different sounds such as 'la' and 'ba', which he strings together when he babbles.

Babbling has no connection with a particular language, for example, with English or Arabic, but by about six months, the infant starts to produce or imitate sounds contained in the language he hears. This develops into expressive jargon, which is a speech pattern that sounds like conversation but is meaningless in content. By the age of one, most infants understand about 100 spoken words and begin to use words they hear on a daily basis, such as the names given to people, toys and food; and simple expressions such as 'bye-bye'.

By eighteen months, most infants can understand more than 750 words, say in excess of 400, use a handful of words regularly and place emphasis on words to convey more meaning. By the age of two, most understand more than 1000 words, can say more than 500 and can use simple sentences, such as 'Nanna gone home'. By three, their sentence length has grown to in excess of four or five words, they can carry on conversations of two or three sentences, describe how two simple objects are used and are developing grammar.

Between the ages of two and six, vocabulary, sentence length and grammar increase and improve dramatically, and by the age of six, most children have mastered the essential features of their native language. However, an understanding of language and the ability to express oneself effectively in a variety of different situations continues to develop throughout life, supporting and promoting successful communication.

Social and emotional development

Social and emotional development are closely linked and sometimes described as socio-emotional development. Social development is to do with developing relationships, values, beliefs and behaviours necessary for living and working in society; emotional development is to do with the development of feelings, both towards others and about the self.

By the age of three months, most infants have developed the social skill of smiling at others, and positive and negative emotions such as delight and frustration. By nine months, they engage socially with everyone, but by a year, have formed a strong, trusting and affectionate attachment to or bond with their primary caregiver and demonstrate anxiety and distress when separated or in the presence of a stranger.

During their second year, infants develop strong emotions, including rage and anger, which are often expressed in the form of temper tantrums. They also begin to develop an identity or sense of self, including their sex, and can recognise their reflection in a mirror.

The process of primary socialisation occurs during the first few years and takes place within the home. The child takes on the values, beliefs and behaviours that the family respect and hold dear through a developing sense of self, observation of role models (members of the family for whom he has admiration), and parental discipline and reinforcement of socially acceptable conduct.

Fig 4.8 Primary socialisation

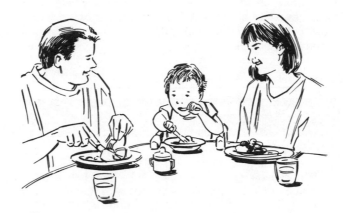

Prosocial behaviour and social play develop in early childhood. Prosocial behaviour develops as the young child becomes aware of other people's feelings, and teaches him to share and to care for and be helpful to others. Social play provides pleasure and teaches the young child to get along with others and to follow rules. As they grow older, children begin to develop relationships with their peers, which give them an opportunity to practise and refine their developing social skills and learn to deal with emotions caused by, for example, popularity and rejection.

Secondary socialisation starts in early to middle childhood and is due to exposure to society outside the home and the family, for example, at school, in the community and on television. It brings about the development of personal ways of thinking and behaving, which in turn help shape self-concept and build self-confidence and self-esteem. Secondary socialisation continues throughout life, causing people's values, beliefs and behaviours to change as they mature and grow older.

Link

See page 2 in Unit 7 for more information about socialisation.

Adolescence is the time for establishing a personal identity and set of values, beliefs and behaviours (although these change with time); developing autonomy, responsibility for self and emotional independence; becoming a group member and developing a sense of belonging; and forging mutual, intimate relationships.

Adults continue to grow and develop emotionally and socially. Identity changes as values, beliefs and roles are modified, new relationships built and new emotions experienced, for example, at work, within marriage and parenthood, and following divorce. In older adulthood, unless people have a mature sense of autonomy and independence and a reliable social and emotional support network, events such as retirement, ill health, bereavement and impending death can have disturbing and distressing effects on their socio-emotional well-being. Effects include loneliness, isolation, anger, depression and resignation to the fact that they have no further purpose.

remember

Physical, intellectual, language and socio-emotional growth and development progress at different rates for different people.

activity

INDIVIDUAL WORK

Look back at case study 4.1 on page 126 about the Smith family.

1   What intellectual changes can each individual expect to experience in the near future?

2   What socio-emotional changes can each individual expect to experience in the near future?

3   How would you expect Alison's language to develop over the next 12 months?

Change along the continuum of life

Even though there is a distinct difference between the neonate and someone in the final stages of their life, change along the continuum of life is not clearly visible, i.e. the adjacent features of the different aspects of growth and development are not obviously different from one another. However, changes do become obvious when they do not occur as expected, in cases of delayed development.

Delayed development

Delayed development is defined as the failure of a child to achieve specific developmental milestones at the age when it is expected that most children will have achieved them. The following table describes some of the disorders associated with delayed development, their potential causes and their effects.

Causes and effects of developmental delay

Developmental disorder	Potential causes	Effects of delayed development
Infantile autism: a **psychological** disorder which occurs in up to 10 births per 10,000 and which usually becomes apparent by the time a child is three years old. Signs include abnormal behaviour, such as a lack of imagination and an obsession with routine; emotional coldness; and an inability to develop relationships and use language to communicate.	It is thought that infantile autism may be inherited; it is also linked with Rett's syndrome, which is a developmental disorder of the nervous system. At one time, autism was linked with the MMR vaccine but no evidence has been found to support this suggestion.	Some children improve between four and six years of age, can attend ordinary schools and gain ordinary employment, but they continue to have abnormal behaviour and communication problems, and remain emotionally cold. Others can live at home but attend special schools. Their chances of gaining ordinary employment are very slim. Most are unable to lead an independent life and need residential care.
Speech delay: a delay in the development of normal speech. The normal range of vocabulary in infants and children is very wide but about 6% of children between three and four years of age show a significant delay in development.	Possible causes include deafness, infantile autism, cerebral palsy, degeneration of the central nervous system, **elective mutism** and social deprivation.	The effects of speech delay depend on the cause, but speech therapy is usually necessary.
Specific motor disorder: a condition where the child is able to carry out normal movements but is clumsy and lacks coordination.	Delayed development of motor control, i.e. nervous control of the skeletal (voluntary) muscles.	Children with this condition are poor at physical performance. There may be an emotional disorder for which they are referred to a psychiatrist.
Specific reading retardation: a serious delay in learning to read. The child's reading age is below that expected, given her age and IQ.	Specific reading retardation is not due to a poor education or low IQ but is linked with a delay in the development of speech and language.	A delay in learning to write and spell and poor self-confidence and self-esteem due to perceived failure.
Specific arithmetic disorders: serious delays in learning to use numbers.	There is no known single cause but, like specific reading retardation, specific arithmetic disorders are not explained by a low IQ.	Less of a handicap than specific reading retardation but there can be emotional problems in situations where arithmetic is used.

Developmental disorder	Potential causes	Effects of delayed development
Delayed puberty: lack of pubertal changes in a girl aged 13 or a boy aged 14 or where puberty fails to progress over a two year period.	There are a number of causes, including a delay in bone growth, hormone deficiencies, chromosomal abnormalities and anorexia nervosa.	Emotional problems and abnormal behaviour.

Website dedicated to helping new and expectant parents	www.babycentre.co.uk
Website for parents and midwives	www.midwivesonline.com
Website for parents and health visitors	www.healthvisitors.com
National Childbirth Trust	www.nct.org.uk
Health information	www.publichealthmatters.org
Home of official UK statistics	www.statistics.gov.uk
Online encyclopaedla of medicine	www.gpnotebook.co.uk
Up-to-date health information provided by GPs	www.patient.co.uk

activity
INDIVIDUAL WORK
4.1

P1

Write case studies for two imaginary people, one of whom has experienced some form of delayed development, which describe their growth and development from conception through to their final life stage. Your target readers should be level 3 learners preparing to work in a health or social care setting.

Professional Practice

When working with different individuals:

■ don't apply your personal definition of normal development and make judgements about an individual's skills and abilities. Remember that everyone grows and develops at a different rate.

■ if you have any concerns about an individual's development, for example, a child who you feel has not achieved the appropriate developmental milestones, talk to someone in a position of responsibility.

How life factors and events may influence the development of the individual

The nature-nurture debate

For centuries, people have debated why we develop as we do. More recently, the controversy has centred around two key principles: genetics (nature) and environment (nurture).

Interrelationship between genetic and environmental factors

Extreme views support the notion that either nature or nurture is the primary influence on development. However, just as development has a holistic nature in which development in one area depends on and exerts an influence over development in another, development can be better explained in terms of an interrelationship between genetic (nature) and environmental (nurture) factors. This interrelationship is not necessarily equally balanced. For example, the development of the physical structures needed to crawl is dependent more on biological programming than, for example, the space within the physical environment in which an infant can move. In addition, the balance of interrelationship changes over time. For example, physical maturation during adolescence is primarily dependent on biological programming whereas in adulthood, development is more significantly influenced by social and emotional experiences.

Fig 4.9 The nature–nurture debate

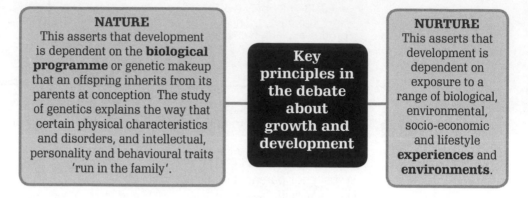

NATURE
This asserts that development is dependent on the **biological programme** or genetic makeup that an offspring inherits from its parents at conception The study of genetics explains the way that certain physical characteristics and disorders, and intellectual, personality and behavioural traits 'run in the family'.

Key principles in the debate about growth and development

NURTURE
This asserts that development is dependent on exposure to a range of biological, environmental, socio-economic and lifestyle **experiences** and **environments**.

The following section describes, in brief, the influence on development of a number of genetic, environmental and experiential life factors.

Life factors

Genetic factors

It is argued that our genetic makeup **predisposes** us to certain behaviours, disorders and diseases. For example, females are seen to be more predisposed than males to eating disorders such as anorexia nervosa, and males more predisposed than females to risk-taking behaviours such as committing criminal offences. Another suggestion is that such behaviours, disorders and diseases are explained by nurture, that is the different expectations that society (the social environment) has of men and women.

There are a number of disorders to which people are predisposed because their genetic makeup contains one or more of a large number of genes, which are inconsequential on their own but when acting together can have an effect. They include diabetes mellitus, hypertension, depression, MS, schizophrenia and Alzheimer's disease; and common congenital malformations such as hip dislocation, cleft lip, cleft palate, club foot and spina bifida. However, many disorders caused by the interaction of multiple genes are also affected by environmental factors, for example, a lack of folic acid in early pregnancy contributes to the development of spina bifida and smoking increases the risk of developing Alzheimer's.

The function of genes is to initiate the construction of proteins such as enzymes that are crucial for normal body functioning. Genes are packaged together in specific sequences to form chromosomes and each human body cell has 23 pairs of chromosomes, one of each pair inherited from the mother and the other from the father (sex cells – eggs and sperm - have 23 single chromosomes). Gene **mutations** and chromosomal abnormalities result in protein defects, which in turn cause a variety of genetic diseases, for example:

- phenylketonuria (PKU), in which a defect in the enzyme phenylalanine hydroxylase prevents the body from converting phenylalanine, which is found in most protein foods, into tyrosine. An accumulation of phenylalanine in the body tissues affects brain development, causing learning difficulties. PKU may be treated by a diet that is free from high-protein foods such as meat, cheese, eggs and milk, and which contains artificial, phenylalanine-free protein.

- cystic fibrosis, in which the protein responsible for transporting salts and water across cell membranes is defective. As a result, mucus in the lungs, intestines and pancreas becomes thick and sticky, causing coughs, chest infections, abnormal stools and poor weight gain. Treatment includes physiotherapy to clear mucus from the lungs, antibiotics to treat infections and drugs to reduce inflammation. A high-calorie diet is important for weight gain and maintenance of health. Gene therapy for cystic fibrosis is in the early stages of development.

- Down's syndrome, in which there is an extra part of chromosome 21 or there are three copies of chromosome 21 (instead of two). The additional genes that result cause proteins to be made that disturb normal growth. Down's syndrome is characterised by a variety of physical features, including low birth weight, differences in appearance, lower than average height, poor muscle tone, and delayed development, which results in poor health and learning difficulties. Treatment includes special educational programmes, physiotherapy, and occupational and speech therapy.

■ sickle-cell disease, in which the protein in red blood cells (haemoglobin) cannot carry oxygen in the normal way. As a result of deoxygenation, the protein becomes rod-like, which in turn causes the blood cells to become sickle-shaped and rigid. As a result, the cells are unable to pass through capillaries, which leads to anaemia. If the cells clump and block blood vessels, tissues can die, causing severe pain and ill health due to organ damage. Treatment includes oxygen, painkillers and blood transfusions.

Biological factors

As you read above, it is also argued that development is influenced by a range of biological, environmental, socio-economic and lifestyle experiences and environments. From conception to birth, the developing child is exposed to the internal environment of its mother. Two factors within this environment that exert a significant influence on the child's biological development are alcohol and infectious agents.

The first few weeks of life are described as a critical period of development. This is when an embryo is most susceptible to alcohol. If a woman drinks alcohol in early pregnancy, she puts her baby at risk of developing foetal alcohol syndrome (FAS), which is characterised by physical and intellectual developmental delay; a range of physiological disorders, in particular of the nervous system; and abnormalities of the face and skull. FAS is of current concern because of the trend for women's alcohol consumption to rise and because many continue to

Fig 4.10 Foetal alcohol syndrome

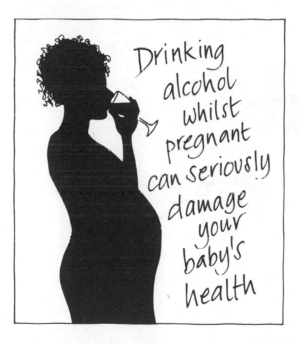

drink several weeks into pregnancy before they are aware of their condition.

Infectious agents that cause infectious diseases, such as bacteria and viruses, can pass from a mother to her unborn baby. Infectious diseases in pregnancy that affect development within the uterus include:

■ rubella

■ toxoplasmosis

■ hepatitis B

■ syphilis

■ HIV

■ listeriosis, which can be caught from eating unwashed fruit and vegetables and soft cheeses made from unpasteurised milk, and which can be life-threatening and lead to premature delivery

In addition if a pregnant woman has genital herpes and weeping ulcers on her cervix, vagina and **vulva**, normal delivery through the birth canal puts the baby at risk of infection that can lead to blindness.

Environmental factors

Pollution in the environment into which a child is born can affect its development in a number of ways. For example, infectious agents that enter the drinking water supply due to poor personal hygiene and inadequate public health sanitation measures, such as ineffective sewage disposal, cause a variety of diseases, including diarrhoea which remains an important cause of child mortality. Exposure to small amounts of lead in water, food and the air can damage the nervous system of infants and small children, impairing their intellectual development. Pollution from traffic fumes can affect lung development and function and damage various body systems. And noise pollution, such as loud background noise from aeroplanes, washing machines and television, has been linked with delayed intellectual development.

Access to leisure and recreational facilities is important for healthy growth and development throughout life. Facilities such as out-of-school clubs, hobby and interest groups, evening classes, and sports and social clubs give people an opportunity to develop:

- intellectual skills, such as learning and understanding, creativity, decision making and problem solving
- emotional and social skills, such as confidence, self-esteem, interaction, communication, team work, sharing and awareness of their personal, social and community responsibilities as individuals, group members and citizens
- physical skills, such as mobility, fitness and co-ordination.

Fig 4.11 The importance of access to leisure and recreational facilities

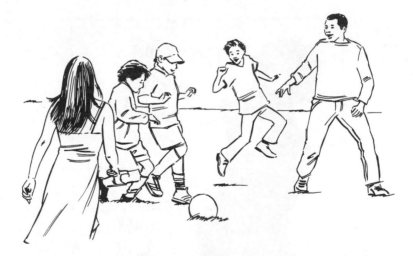

Access to health and social care services is important for monitoring growth and development through the different life stages, in particular of the foetus, infant and child, and of vulnerable people such as those who are elderly or who have a low socio-economic status. When access to health and social care services is limited or denied, for whatever reason, growth and development needs may not be identified and addressed, which results in health and social inequalities and disadvantage.

Access to employment and income is also important for growth and development. For example, employment provides an opportunity to develop personal skills such as responsibility, time-keeping, reliability and motivation, and to develop:

- intellectually, through learning, understanding and using a range of work-related skills
- socially, through building and maintaining work relationships, team work and co-operation
- emotionally, through a change in role and a growth in self-awareness, self-confidence and esteem.

Having an income promotes intellectual development through learning how to manage money responsibly and having the wherewithal to buy into an education. It promotes physical development through an opportunity to purchase nutritious food, decent housing in a secure and clean environment, and health care. Finally, it promotes socio-emotional development through social and financial independence and the ability to purchase goods that promote self-confidence and esteem.

Socio-economic factors

Socio-economic factors that affect growth and development include:

- family, friends, peer groups, teachers and media personalities who are involved in the socialisation process. Positive peer pressure and the influence of these people as role models spread attitudes, values, beliefs and cultural ways of living and behaving. By showing emotions such as love, companionship and support, they encourage positive emotional development in others. Any by providing each other with a variety of social roles, for example, daughter, friend and student, they promote the development of relationships and a sense of belonging.

- social class, which is defined by employment status, income, education and housing. Employment and income have positive consequences for development, as does an education that enables people to make choices that promote their own personal development, and housing that provides warmth and protection. A low socio-economic status, i.e. unemployment, poverty, an inadequate education and cold, damp, over-crowded, insecure, filthy living conditions flies in the face of human growth and development.

- gender. The state of being male or female has a marked influence on development. Biological differences impact on physical development, for example, the female hormone oestrogen helps to protect against heart disease and osteoporosis. **Cultural and social norms**, expectations, role models, and so on, influence the intellectual and socio-emotional development of boys and girls and the roles they play as adults at work and in the home.

 Link

See page 65 in Unit 2 for more information about the effects of bullying and discrimination on growth and development.

Lifestyle factors

Lifestyle encompasses factors such as nutrition and dietary choice, exercise, stress and substance abuse. The type and amount of food and drink that is consumed and levels of physical activity greatly affect physical growth and development, which can have knock-on effects on emotional and, consequently, social development. For example, a child who is reared on fast food and who has little if any exercise is likely to become obese, which will impact on his self-esteem and ability to develop relationships. Too much stress has a wealth of negative influences on physical and emotional health, putting development at risk; and substance abuse has been linked with developmental delay, particularly of the foetus.

case study 4.2   Sunhil and Georgina

Both Sunhil and Georgina are 11 years old. Sunhil lives with his mother and father who are qualified nurses and work full time. Georgina lives with her mum, who is a widow and unemployed. Both children live on the same busy housing estate, which is surrounded by heavy industry and a motorway network. They go to the same school although Sunhil is driven there while Georgina walks. Georgina and her friends are very interested in local leisure opportunities and pop culture but Sunhil's parents are strict about how he spends his spare time, preferring him to stay home and study.

activity
GROUP WORK

1   What life factors could influence each child's growth and development?
2   How might each factor influence their development?

Genetic Interest Group	www.gig.org.uk
NHS Direct	www.nhsdirect.nhs.uk
The National Childbirth Trust	www.nct.org.uk

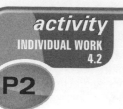

activity

INDIVIDUAL WORK
4.2

P2

Using the information in case study 4.2 and the results of your further reading, use the table below to show your understanding of the potential influences of five life factors on human development.

Influences of life factors on human development

Life factor	Potential influences on development
Genetic	
Biological	
Environmental	
Socio-economic	
Lifestyle	

activity

INDIVIDUAL WORK
4.3

M1

D1

Write an article entitled 'The nature–nurture debate' for your school or college magazine.

1 Using examples, discuss the nature–nurture debate in relation to five different life factors that influence development.

2 Sum up your article by evaluating the debate with regard to development of the individual.

Major life events

Life events are often significant turning points in people's lives. Some are predictable, such as starting school; others are unpredicted, such as being made redundant. This section aims to help you understand the influence that a number of life events can have on individual development.

Birth of a sibling

Most people have at least one sibling, and because sibling relationships are usually the longest lasting relationships people experience, their potential for influence is huge. The birth of a sibling can be confusing and upsetting for a young child, who has to deal with a range of new, negative emotions such as jealousy, suspicion and distrust, and novel social situations in which she has to adjust to a different role. However, realisation that the sibling is here to stay is usually accompanied by positive socio-emotional and intellectual changes, such as the development of affection, concern and a new relationship in which the child has an opportunity to build on her language skills and to learn, for example, to be supportive, responsible and to deal with and resolve conflict.

Starting school

Starting school or nursery can be as perplexing and distressing for young children as the birth of a younger brother or sister. Unless they have been adequately prepared for the big event, they may feel anxious, abandoned and distressed, lonely and alone in the company of so many. However, with support, reassurance and encouragement, positive outcomes include an opportunity for children to:

- make their own friends
- adjust to other people's ways of doing things
- develop a new identity and sense of belonging within a social group
- progress their independence
- build on their prosocial skills and start to play alongside and, later, with others
- further their language skills
- increase their intellectual skills.

Leaving home

Leaving home usually happens towards the end of adolescence or in early adulthood and is associated with aspects of socio-emotional development such as an adjustment to identity; the building and maintenance of supportive and enduring friendships and sexual relationships; and the development of autonomy and responsibility for self and **significant others**. It is also associated with the development of the intellectual skills needed for, for example, financial competence and, in the event of moving into one's own home, home management.

Moving house

Moving house at any age can be daunting. However, it offers opportunities, such as socio-emotional development through the evolution of an increasingly complex identity; the cultivation of new social contacts; membership of new groups; and the taking on of new roles; and intellectual development through learning about official transactions associated with moving house, local politics, geography and history and developing an understanding of the cultural backgrounds of people living within the new neighbourhood.

Marriage

While there has been a general decrease since the early 1970s in the number of people getting married, people do still choose to marry or get re-married. A marriage to which both partners are committed and in which there is trust, equality and mutual love and respect has a strengthening effect on their relationship, and the care, support and encouragement they give each other promotes positive personal development such as improved self-esteem and self-confidence, trustworthiness and dependability. It also provides an opportunity to grow intellectually, through, for example, the development of conflict resolution skills.

Parenthood

Bringing up children is a huge responsibility but a great personal and social achievement. Parenthood goes hand-in-hand with learning parenting skills, how to manage change and make decisions, how to deal with conflict such as challenging behaviour, how meet a child's need for love, safety and security, and so on. It also requires development of a less self-centred identity, a new role, new relationships, added responsibilities and the need for self-sacrifice.

Fig 4.12 The magic of parenthood!

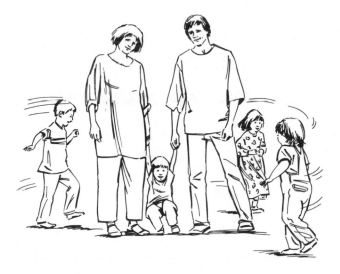

Divorce

Divorce can be traumatic, destroying confidence, self-esteem and trust in others, which can, in turn, hinder the development of new relationships. On the other hand, divorce can be liberating, offering an opportunity for the divorcee to regain their independence, rebuild their confidence and self-esteem, learn new skills and develop new relationships. The vast majority of children cope well when their parents divorce but more children from broken homes have serious social or emotional problems than children from families that stay together.

Employment

Link

Refer back to page 133 to remind yourself about the influence of employment on development. See page 145 for more information about the influence of retirement from work.

Redundancy, or losing one's job prior to retirement, implies that workers are no longer needed or useful. Withdrawal of their role can hold back socio-emotional development as confidence and self-esteem are lost, relationships curtailed, and loneliness and depression take effect. In addition, a check is put on intellectual development as workplace learning opportunities cease. However being made redundant can promote development, for example, it frees up time to develop a new career, take up new interests and re-kindle old and establish new relationships.

Serious injury

The consequences of serious injury can change a person's identity and present them with new roles to play. While many people rise to the challenge that their disability or changed health status presents, the effect of serious injury on others can mean a loss of confidence, self-esteem and independence; difficulty in adjusting to a new lifestyle; problems developing new and maintaining existing relationships; and difficulty accessing services that promote socio-emotional development, such as leisure facilities, and intellectual development, such as employment.

Abuse

Abuse can be physical, sexual, emotional or financial. It can happen at home and in the institutions in which people live and work; and very often, the perpetrators are those one would least expect to be abusers, for example, friends, family and carers. Abuse of whatever form is traumatic and can cause lasting socio-emotional damage, for example, loss of confidence and self-esteem, anxiety, fear, depression, difficulty expressing feelings and building relationships, withdrawal, loneliness, social isolation and a loss of a sense of belonging. Some people who have experienced abuse become abusers themselves.

> Everyone is influenced by their own individual set of personal experiences and life factors. For this reason, everyone is different and will continue to develop in their own unique way.

remember

i

| Home of official UK statistics | www.statistics.gov.uk |
| A website dedicated to offering support, information, and friendship to everyone raising children | www.raisingkids.co.uk |

---

activity

INDIVIDUAL WORK 4.4

P3

M2

Talk to three or four people about predicted and unpredicted events they have experienced during their life times.

1   Use your findings to write anonymous case studies, two of predicted events and two of unpredicted events.

2   Describe and explain the influence of life events on individual development.

Physical changes and psychological perspectives in relation to ageing

Theories of ageing

As you know, ageing is brought about by biological and psychological changes that:

- reduce life expectancy
- reduce the ability to use physical, intellectual, emotional and social skills
- reduce social and emotional well-being and quality of life
- increase vulnerability to physical and mental ill health and disability, social isolation, and so on.

Psychological changes

Disengagement theory

The disengagement theory, proposed by Cumming and Henry in 1961, suggests that older people make a positive effort to withdraw from life as a response to their lessening physical, intellectual, emotional and social skills and abilities, diminishing interests and expectations of how they should behave. It suggests that they willingly retire from work; willingly withdraw from relationships and disengage from roles, preferring to pursue passive, solitary activities; and willingly give up their traditional, normal ways of behaving, becoming less and less friendly and companionable and sometimes hostile in their interactions.

Although the disengagement theory was put forward in the early 1960s, society still seems to facilitate older people's withdrawal from life and shape their perception of how they should behave by offering them incentives to disengage.

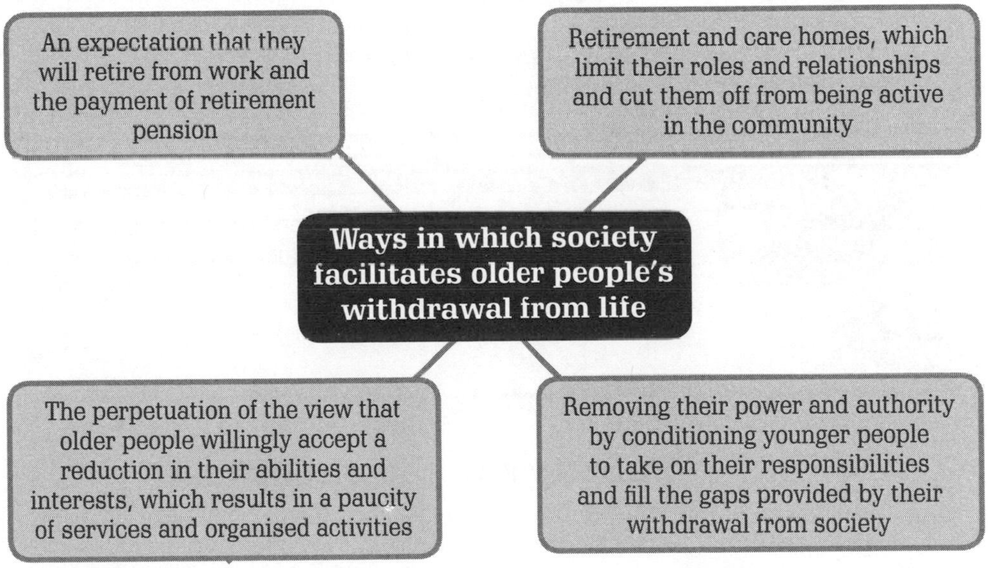

Fig 4.13 Ways in which society facilitates older people's withdrawal from life

An expectation that they will retire from work and the payment of retirement pension

Retirement and care homes, which limit their roles and relationships and cut them off from being active in the community

Ways in which society facilitates older people's withdrawal from life

The perpetuation of the view that older people willingly accept a reduction in their abilities and interests, which results in a paucity of services and organised activities

Removing their power and authority by conditioning younger people to take on their responsibilities and fill the gaps provided by their withdrawal from society

Activity theory

The activity theory, proposed in 1972 by Lemon, Bengtson & Peterson, has a more optimistic view of ageing than the disengagement theory. It suggests that older people age more successfully when they maintain their roles and relationships, keep busy with a full round of daily activities and preserve a positive attitude to life. Further, the more social contacts, activities and positive attitudes an older person has, the better their quality of life.

To maintain their physical, intellectual, emotional and social skills, well-being and quality of life, people need support, and opportunities for support come from having roles and relationships. However, as people become older, events such as retirement and bereavement diminish their social networks and limit their social contacts. By engaging in new and alternative activities that promote and add to their relationships and that give them fulfilment and a sense of achievement, older people continue to receive the support they need.

The 'busy ethic' that underlies the activity theory works for people who like to live a structured life, who enjoy good health and who have the means to pursue a full schedule of activities. However, activity is still seen as the key to successful ageing although the definition of beneficial activity varies from person to person. For example, some older people obtain meaningful support from taking part in informal activities with family and friends, whereas others derive support from formal activities such as volunteering, or solitary activities such as reading.

The social creation of dependency theory

This theory suggests that discriminating social policies, such as age-restricted retirement policies and opportunities to participate in the community, and poverty caused by low pension and income levels, cause older people to become dependent on society.

The effect of these social policies is to single out and isolate older people. As a result, they feel stigmatised and stand out as being vulnerable and helpless, signalling a stereotypical image of being useless and inadequate. They then become the focus of negative attitudes, which in turn cause them to act in the way they think they are expected to, for example to become increasingly dependent on family, friends and social care services.

activity
INDIVIDUAL WORK 4.5

P4

M3

Complete the following table to show your understanding of two different theories of ageing.

Theories of aging

Theories of ageing	Similarities (M3 part)	Differences (M3 part)
Theory 1 Name: Description:		
Theory 2 Name: Description:		

activity
GROUP WORK 4.6

D2

In your group, research local health and social care provision for people who are elderly and evaluate how it is influenced by different theories of ageing.

Puberty and the menopause

Although puberty and the menopause are not generally linked with the ageing process, they are hormone-controlled changes that are predicted to take place as life progresses.

Puberty

Puberty occurs during adolescence and is the period during which an individual reaches sexual maturity. It lasts between two and four years and is accompanied by both physical and psychological changes. Three significant physical changes that are stimulated and controlled by sex hormones during puberty are the growth spurt, when girls and boys suddenly grow taller, the change in body shape and the development of the reproductive system, i.e. the growth and development of the sex organs and secondary sex characteristics.

Refer back to page 125 to remind yourself about physical development at puberty.

Physical changes are stimulated and controlled by a dramatic increase in the amount of sex hormones secreted into the bloodstream:

■ androgens, for example, testosterone, are produced in the testes (testicles) and control the development and functioning of the male sex organs and the development of male secondary sex characteristics. Normal females have small amounts of androgens.

- oestrogens, for example, oestradiol, are produced in the ovaries and control the development and functioning of the female sex organs and the development of female secondary sex characteristics. Normal males have small amount of oestrogens.

Change in body shape is principally due in girls to a laying down of body fat around the hips and breasts, and in boys to a growth in muscle mass. While muscle growth and, as a result, an increase in strength and stamina occur in both sexes, differences in muscle shape and composition in adolescent boys and girls can be partly accounted for by differences in participation in hard physical sports.

Probably the most important and memorable physical change for girls during puberty is their first menstruation (menarche), which normally occurs between the ages of 11 and 15. Menstruation in the first phase of the **menstrual cycle**, which has four distinct phases:

- Phase 1: menstruation (about five days) when the broken down endometrium (uterus lining) is shed from the body in a flow of blood known as a period.

- Phase 2: the repair phase (about eleven days) when the endometrium thickens in preparation for the implantation of a fertilised egg cell (zygote).

- Phase 3: the receptive phase (about five days) when the endometrium is sufficiently prepared to receive a zygote. Implantation of a zygote into the endometrium indicates the beginning of pregnancy.

- Phase 4: the pre-menstrual phase (about seven days) when, in the event that a zygote does not implant, the endometrium begins to break down.

At birth, a female has about one million immature eggs in her ovaries. On day one of her menstrual cycle, follicle stimulating hormone (FSH) from the pituitary gland at the base of the brain stimulates several eggs to start maturing, each one surrounded by a layer of cells called a follicle. The developing follicle produces oestrogen, which causes the endometrium to thicken (repair phase). On day 14 or thereabouts, luteinising hormone (LH), also from the pituitary, stimulates **ovulation**, the follicle surrounding the fully grown egg cell ruptures, releasing it into the fallopian tube where muscle movements and tiny hair-like cilia waft it toward the uterus. In the meantime, FSH and LH cause the follicle, which remains in the ovary, to develop into the corpus luteum, which produces progesterone, the hormone that prepares the uterus for and helps maintain pregnancy in the event that the egg cell is fertilised.

Fig 4.14 Hormonal control of the menstrual cycle

Hormonal action	FSH from the pituitary gland stimulates development of egg cells, and the developing follicles produce oestrogen, which causes the endometrium to thicken.													On about day 14, LH from the pituitary stimulates ovulation. FSH and LH cause the ruptured follicle to develop into the corpus luteum, which produces progesterone that prepares the uterus for a fertilised egg.														
Day	1	2	3	4	5	6	7	8	9	10	11	12	13	14	15	16	17	18	19	20	21	22	23	24	25	26	27	28
Phase	1 Menstruation					2 Repair phase											3 Receptive phase					4 Pre-menstrual phase						

Menopause

The menopause, like puberty, is under the control of hormones. Female menopause normally occurs during a woman's late forties or early fifties and is signalled by menstruation becoming more irregular and more infrequent until it eventually ceases altogether. This is due to the fact that the ovaries cease to produce mature egg cells at regular intervals, thus levels of oestrogen decline. It is this lack of oestrogen that is responsible for many of the unpleasant physical symptoms associated with the menopause that you read about earlier.

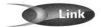

Refer back to page 125 to remind yourself about physical development at menopause.

The female menopause is over relatively quickly; male menopause, on the other hand, occurs over quite a long period of time. It too involves a decline in the production of hormones but while women lose their ability to produce children, men continue to be able to father children well into their old age. This is because hormone levels diminish very slowly and the effect is to reduce rather than terminate their sperm count. However, like women, they can experience unpleasant physical menopausal symptoms, some of which you read about earlier.

Hormonal changes during puberty and the menopause can also have psychological effects:

■ pre-menstrual syndrome (PMS) is thought to be caused by an increased sensitivity to progesterone, one effect of which is to reduce production of the mood-controlling hormone serotonin. This helps explain the depression, irritability, anxiety and aggression that many women experience in the days leading up to their menstrual period.

■ emotional changes such as mood swings and a change in sexual interest are brought about by the rapid decline in levels of oestrogen that cause the female menopause. But because levels of testosterone fall far more gradually over many years, it is thought that the male menopause has more of a psychological than hormonal cause, for example, the recognition by men that the years are taking their toll and that their role and appearance are not what they used to be.

Physical changes

Body systems decline with age, and there are a number of physiological disorders that are specifically linked with advancing years.

Cardiovascular system

The cardiovascular system consists of the heart, blood vessels and the blood. The functions of the cardiovascular system are to maintain the body's supply of oxygen and to transport materials such as nutrients, hormones and antibodies to parts of the body where they are needed and waste products such as carbon dioxide and urea away from body cells to where they can be eliminated.

Several conditions may occur within the cardiovascular system as a person ages:

■ Cholesterol is a fatty substance made by the body but also consumed in animal foods such as meat, fish, eggs and dairy products. It is carried in the blood. If blood cholesterol levels become too high, some of the cholesterol is deposited as a thick, fatty sludge (atheroma) on the inside walls of blood vessels. Over time, atheroma deposits, known as plaques, build up, causing the condition atherosclerosis in which blood vessels are narrowed and blood flow decreased. As a result, the circulation is unable to maintain a supply of oxygen to the body, causing conditions such as breathlessness, weakness and **cyanosis**.

■ Atherosclerosis of the coronary arteries, which deliver oxygenated blood to the heart, causes coronary heart disease (CHD). Angina, which is a symptom of CHD, occurs when there is a temporary reduction in blood flow within the coronary arteries. It causes pain but no damage; however, it does warn of an increased risk of a heart attack. A heart attack (myocardial infarction) happens when blood flow to part of the heart is fully blocked, causing that part of the heart to die. This blockage can be caused by blood clots forming over atheroma (coronary thrombosis) or when the coronary arteries go into spasm. Heart attacks can cause permanent damage to the heart and can be fatal.

Respiratory system

The respiratory system consists of the nose, the respiratory tract (larynx, trachea and bronchi) which connects the nose with the lungs, the lungs (bronchioles and alveoli), blood vessels that circulate around the alveoli, pleural membranes that surround the lungs, the ribs, intercostal muscles that run between the ribs, and the diaphragm. The functions of the respiratory system are to maintain the body's supply of oxygen and to eliminate the waste product carbon dioxide.

A number of physiological disorders affect the respiratory system:

■ The respiratory tract of people with asthma is very sensitive and when irritated, for example, by allergens, becomes swollen and narrow, its muscles tighten and there is usually an increase in the production of mucus. As a result, the chest feels tight, it becomes hard to get enough breath and the person coughs and wheezes.

■ In emphysema, the walls of the alveoli break down, creating much larger air sacs and reducing the elasticity of the lungs. The larger the air sacs, the smaller the total surface area available for **gaseous exchange**. As the area for gaseous exchange reduces, so does the amount of oxygen that can diffuse into the blood from the lungs and the amount of carbon dioxide that can diffuse into the lungs from the blood. As a result, blood becomes oxygen-poor and carbon dioxide-rich, which results in shortness of breath and a reduced amount of oxygen reaching all the body cells. It is often linked with years of smoking.

■ Chronic obstructive pulmonary disease (COPD) is the name for a collection of respiratory disorders including chronic bronchitis (inflammation of the respiratory tract) and emphysema, all of which can occur together. It is one of the most common respiratory diseases and occurs as a result of permanent damage to the lungs, and is, like emphysema, linked with years of smoking. The main symptoms are persistent, productive coughing, recurring chest infections and shortness of breath and wheezing, which reduces oxygen supply to the heart, causing heart failure.

Fig 4.15 Ill health in old age

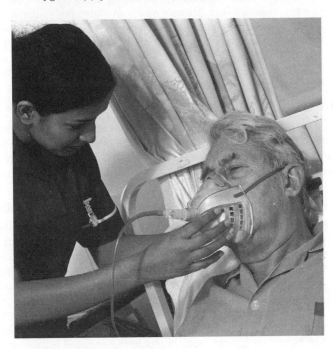

The nervous system

The nervous system consists of the central nervous system (CNS – brain and spinal cord); sensory cells in sense organs, which receive information about stimuli in the environment; nervous tissue, which carries information in the form of electrical impulses and which is made from bundles of sensory neurones (nerve cells that link sensory cells with the CNS) and motor neurones (that link the CNS to effector cells); and effector cells in muscles and glands, which effect or bring about a response to the stimulus. Its main function is to receive information about the environment so that the body can respond appropriately.

Degeneration of sense organs may lead to a number of conditions:

■ Macular degeneration results in the loss of central, detailed vision, making it difficult to see straight ahead, for example, to watch television, drive and recognise people; and to see detail, for example, the printed word. In addition, vision can become distorted, making it difficult to make judgements about height and distance; the eyes can become sensitive to light; and lights and colours may appear that do not actually exist. Eventually, central vision is replaced by a black spot.

■ Conductive hearing loss is interference with transmission of sound from the outer ear to the inner ear, caused by, for example, middle ear infections, wax and fluid blockages, injury to the eardrum and rheumatoid arthritis.

■ Sensorineural hearing loss is caused by a problem with the inner ear or with the nervous tissue connecting the inner ear to the brain, for example, age-related hearing loss; injury to the ear due to loud noise; inner ear and auditory nerve infections, such as mumps and rubella; and disorders such as Meniere's disease, meningitis, MS, brain tumour and stroke.

Degeneration of nervous tissue may lead to a number of conditions:

■ Multiple sclerosis (MS) occurs when there is a scarring or loss of the myelin sheath that surrounds neurones (demyelination). The myelin sheath has an insulating function and when it is lost or damaged, electrical messages cannot travel normally from the brain to different parts of the body, resulting in, for example, blurred vision, unsteady walking and poor coordination. There is evidence to suggest that some people are predisposed to MS, that it is caused by a virus and that it is an **autoimmune disorder**, where antibodies attack and destroy the myelin sheath.

- Motor neurone disease (MND) is a highly debilitating disease that damages and kills the motor neurones in the brain and spinal cord. Evidence suggests that the neurones are killed or damaged by an overproduction of the **neurotransmitter** glutamate.

- Alzheimer's disease is a form of dementia, a word which originates from the Latin word *demens*, meaning 'out of one's mind'. In Alzheimer's, clumps and bundles (called plaques and tangles) of certain proteins accumulate inside and outside of the brain cells, gradually destroying the connections between them that are essential for normal mental activity. It results in a gradual deterioration of brain function leading to cognitive changes such as loss of memory, confusion, disorientation and changes in behaviour. Age and lifestyle are the greatest risk factors for Alzheimer's disease, but it is also inherited.

Musculo-skeletal system

The musculo-skeletal system consists of muscles that are attached to bones; bones and joints of the skeleton, cartilage; which is the flexible tissue lining the bones in a joint and that enables smooth movement; tendons which attach muscles to bone; and ligaments which attach bones to bones. The function of the musculo-skeletal system is to enable movement and mobility and to support and protect the body.

Degeneration of the musculo-skeletal system may lead to a number of conditions:

- Arthritis is the general term for several painful conditions of the joints that limit movement and cause a decline in mobility. The most common form is osteoarthritis, which is where cartilage gradually wastes away, causing bones to rub together, most frequently in the hands, knees, hips and spine. Rheumatoid arthritis is an autoimmune disease in which the immune system attacks the lining of the joints, causing inflammation, pain and swelling. Other forms of arthritis include spondylitis, which is inflammation of the joints in the backbone; gout, in which crystals of uric acid collect in the joints, causing pain and inflammation; and lupus, another autoimmune disease in which symptoms include aches and pains in the joints. Arthritis is often associated with older people, but can also affect children.

- Muscle thinning, atrophy or wasting is caused by a shrinkage of muscle fibres (muscle cells) and a decrease in their number. It is often associated with physical inactivity but can be caused by a number of physiological disorders.

- Osteoporosis, also known as brittle bone disease, occurs when more bone cells are lost than replaced, which causes bones to become thinner and weaker. It happens more commonly in old age, when the body is less able to replace worn-out bone, and in post-menopausal women. Like painful joint conditions, it causes a decline in mobility.

Skin

The skin has a number of important functions. For example, it protects the body by producing oil which makes it waterproof, and melanin which protects against UV rays in sunlight; and, because it contains sensory cells that are stimulated by temperature, pain and touch, it protects against environmental hazards. It is hairy, has a rich blood supply and produces sweat, each of which contribute toward body temperature regulation; and it produces vitamin D.

The skin has two layers. The epidermis, the uppermost layer contains the cells that produce melanin. New epidermal cells are produced in the basal (bottom) cell layer of the epidermis. They gradually rise to the outer layer, the stratum corneum, from where they are shed. The dermis, which is below the epidermis, contains blood and lymph vessels, sensory cells, and glands that produce sweat and oil. It also contains the proteins collagen and elastin, which give the skin strength and elasticity respectively. Below the skin is a layer of fatty tissue, which gives the skin its structure.

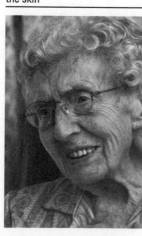

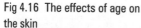

Fig 4.16 The effects of age on the skin

The speed at which skin ages is partly influenced by genes and partly due to exposure to factors such as the sun, tobacco smoke, pollution, stress, a poor diet, lack of water in the diet and lack of sleep. Signs of an ageing skin include:

- thinning, wrinkling and crêping as the rate of cell production slows down. Older skin is often described as being 'papery'.

- sagging, drooping and a loss of elasticity as production of collagen and elastin slows down and the skin yields to the forces of gravity

- age or liver spots caused by an increase in activity of the cells that produce melanin, particularly in areas that have been exposed to the sun such as the back of the hands

- dryness, because ageing skin has fewer oil glands. As a result, the skin can become rough and itchy.

Illnesses resulting from ageing

Illnesses that are more likely to occur as a result of ageing include:

- Dementia, for example, Alzheimer's disease, the signs of which include progressive memory loss, confusion, disorientation and unpredictable changes in behaviour. One in 1000 people aged between 40 and 65 have dementia, rising to one in 50 between the ages of 65 and 70, one in 20 between 70 and 80 and one in five at age 80 plus. One third of people over 95 have dementia.

- age-related macular degeneration (ARMD), which is the most common form of macular degeneration and its incidence also increases with age: almost 15% of 75 year olds are affected, in particular females.

- hearing loss due to progressive damage to and loss of **hair cells** in the **cochlea**. By the age of 40, most people have lost some of their hearing; by 80, most people have significant hearing loss, particularly of high frequency sounds such as children's and female voices.

- prostate cancer, which is an enlargement of the prostate gland caused by a tumour, and which, if left untreated, may spread to other parts of the body. It is rarely found in men under 45 but its incidence increases with age and nearly three out of four men in their 80s have tiny specks of prostate cancer.

Psychological changes

Developmental changes or transitions that characterise growing older are often significant turning points in people's lives. As you know, they can have physical effects; they can also change the way people feel and behave. You read earlier about some of the emotional changes associated with different life stages. This section focuses on the psychological effects associated with ageing, that is those experienced as an individual passes through older adulthood.

The disengagement theory of ageing suggests that older people make a positive effort to withdraw from society, and the activity theory suggests that successful ageing is dependent on maintaining social contacts and earlier levels of activity. However, older people are likely to find it difficult to adjust if they are not willing to withdraw but instead are cut off prematurely, for example, because of forced retirement, loss of role, requirement to live in residential care or if declining mobility and income prevents them remaining active or maintaining relationships. Cutting older people off from society, removing their authority, changing their identity and having their lifestyle curtailed can be demoralising and reduce their confidence and self-esteem, resulting in frustration, depression, loneliness and social isolation.

The effects of physical decline can have severe psychological effects:

- Progressive sight loss, ill health and immobility reduce confidence and self-esteem and bring worry and uncertainty about the future, for example, about carrying out everyday living activities, staying safe, getting out and about, remaining independent, maintaining relationships and taking part in social activities

- Progressive hearing loss impacts on relationships, because listening requires a great deal of physically and emotionally draining concentration, and speaking can be difficult if there are problems in hearing one's own voice. As a result, communication becomes strained, confidence and self-esteem are lost, and people become isolated and lonely.

- Changes in ability and physical appearance can affect some older people's confidence and self-esteem.

See page 145 in this unit for more information about ageism and how it affects older people's perceived image of themselves.

At the time of writing (April 2007), there are about 700,000 people in the UK with dementia-type conditions such as Alzheimer's disease. The impact of Alzheimer's can be far reaching, for the individual concerned and their carers. For example, progressive memory loss causes frustration and anxiety; confusion and disorientation cause alarm and agitation. And frustration, anxiety, agitation and alarm can, in turn, lead to unpredictable changes in behaviour. Changes in behaviour, particularly to behaviour that is socially unacceptable such as loss of inhibition, rudeness, paranoia and violence can lead to social isolation, loneliness and depression.

You read earlier about Kubler-Ross' (1969) five-stage process of dying, which proposes that the emotions experienced by people when they are dying include denial, anger, pleading, sorrow, depression and, finally, acceptance. Dying people may also experience a number of fears.

Link

Refer back to page 119 to remind yourself about Kubler-Ross' five-stage process.

Fig 4.17 Fears associated with dying

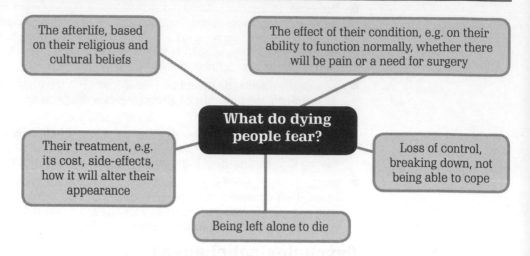

Negative perspectives

Adjusting to growing older is greatly influenced by changes in employment, employability, roles and relationships; by societal and personal attitudes; and by financial concerns. For many people, these events and experiences have a negative connotation.

Effects of retirement

Retirement from work, for example, can be summed up as 'loss': loss of personal identity, purpose, value, relationships, financial comfort and security, daily activity, contact with and knowledge of the world outside of the home and family, confidence, self-esteem, and so on. It presents a challenge to adjust, but if viewed with a negative attitude or if it is forced or accompanied by ill health, disability or financial constraints, adjustment can be difficult.

Role changes

The course of developmental changes through which an individual progresses between conception and death present opportunities for a variety of social roles. However, many older people can find it difficult to come to terms with role changes if, because of negative attitudes, advancing years, ill health and disability, they perceive that the roles left for them to play have limited usefulness, value and influence.

Loss of a partner

Loss of a partner is distressing at any age but can be overwhelming for an older person and the single greatest loss they ever suffer. In addition to coping with emotional reactions to the loss of a companion, friend or loved one, new roles and tasks have to be learnt, for example, making meals and maintaining the car; and lifestyle has to be adapted, for example, to living alone and being independent. Many older people, because of grief, loneliness, ill health, disability, lack of support or an inability to communicate their feelings, are unable to recover from their loss and re-establish their lives. Their distress, despair and depression accompany them to the end of their lives.

Loss of peers

Loss of peers or friends can be equally distressing. For most people, friends are very important. They are chosen on the basis of shared interests and compatibility, and they provide an opportunity to give and receive affection, emotional and social support, security and intellectual stimulation. Death is anticipated as the years advance but witnessing the loss of friends can leave a large gap in an older person's life, provoke fears of dying and confirm their imminent demise.

Ageism

Many people, including some older people themselves, have a negative attitude to ageing. Ageism is a form of discrimination and happens when people are treated unfairly because of their age.

Fig 4.18 Ageism

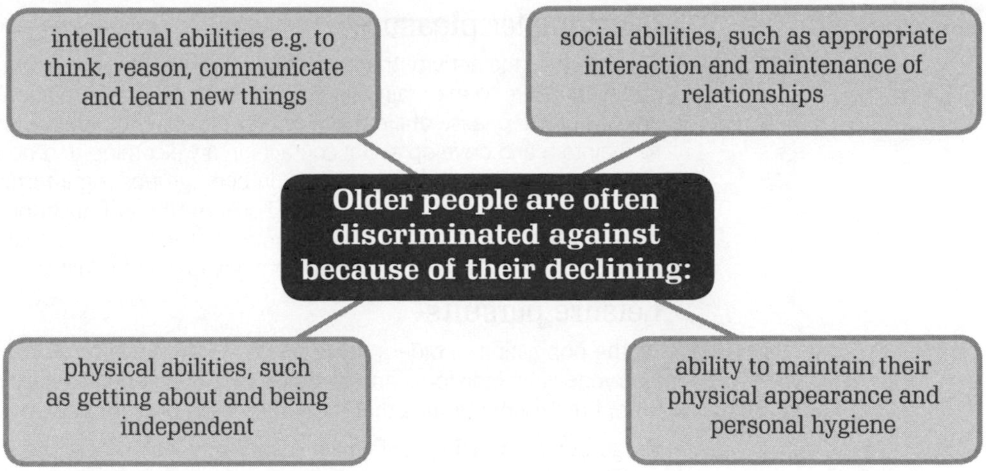

intellectual abilities e.g. to think, reason, communicate and learn new things	social abilities, such as appropriate interaction and maintenance of relationships

Older people are often discriminated against because of their declining:

physical abilities, such as getting about and being independent	ability to maintain their physical appearance and personal hygiene

Ageism can have tragic effects on older people. Bullying and exploitation can cause a loss of confidence and self-esteem and a fear of others, which lead to isolation, loneliness and vulnerability. In addition and as the social creation of dependency theory of ageing suggests, discrimination singles out older people and presents them as weak and helpless, useless and inadequate. Some older people embrace this negative image and behave in the way they think they are expected to. As a result, they become increasingly dependent on family, friends, social care services, and so on.

Financial concerns

Because of the growth in the elderly population and because people are living longer, pensions are likely to decrease and many older people can expect to experience financial concerns. This could affect their ability to pay for basic needs such as nutritious food; fuel for cooking, warmth and hot water; telephone bills; housing and general maintenance; transport; health and personal care.

Positive perspectives

Effects of retirement

While retirement has negative associations for some, others, especially those who are able to choose when and whether or not to retire, who enjoy relatively good health, who are financially comfortable and who welcome personal and social change, see it as an opportunity to:

- extricate themselves from a dissatisfying job role and achieve satisfaction and fulfilment in a new role, such as carer or voluntary worker
- spend time nurturing existing and building new relationships
- try out new activities and join the activities of friends and relatives who have already retired
- devote time and energy to achieving new goals, developing a hobby or second career, and so on
- spend time relaxing, examining their thoughts and feelings, dwelling on happy memories and personal achievements, and preparing for their future.

Role changes

Like all life stages, late adulthood brings role changes that, if welcomed and embraced, reassure older people that they remain valued and from which they gain pleasure and satisfaction. The experiences and wisdom of older friends, parents and grandparents, and their freedom to spend time as they choose, enable them to give, for example, emotional support, advice and child care, and to carry out household services such as shopping, cleaning and repairs until such time that they need care and support themselves. Acknowledging that role change is inevitable and preparing for on-going change helps make it acceptable and enjoyable.

Learning for pleasure

According to the activity theory of ageing, older people who have a positive attitude to life and who aspire to maintain and develop their roles and relationships, whether retired or not, enjoy a better quality of life. Learning for pleasure in older adulthood provides an opportunity to maintain and develop social contacts in a welcoming and non-threatening setting. It takes place at quiz nights at the local pub, in book groups, on internet learning programmes, through the media, at classes run by Local Authority Education Departments, and so on. It does not have to be formal or result in a qualification, it can simply be to develop an existing interest or learn something new in an enjoyable and relaxing way.

Leisure pursuits

As the population of older people grows, so do the leisure services provided for them. Everyone is an individual and has their own preferences regarding how to spend their leisure time, but leisure pursuits that meet the needs of older people include:

- gardening, walking, swimming, dancing, yoga and playing golf, that improve and maintain fitness
- arts and crafts, writing and playing musical instruments, that improve and maintain dexterity
- reading, discussion groups, cooking, visits to museums, art galleries and sports events, theatre trips, use of computers and reminiscence therapy, that develop and maintain intellectual agility, imagination, problem-solving skills, memory and so on
- taking part in drama and role play, researching family history, and arts and crafts, that improve confidence and self-esteem
- games and quizzes that get people together, promote communication, friendships and encourage mutual support, care and understanding.

Cultural variations

Although in general attitudes throughout the world to ageing are very positive, different cultures have different values and these values affect perceptions of older people and the care they are given. In individualistic societies, such as the United States and the UK, independence is important from the beginning of life and the general expectation is that people should remain independent well into their old age. Most people strive to be independent but an expectation to remain so in older adulthood can cause problems. For example, older people often hesitate to ask their family for help because they fear they will become a burden. Residential homes, as opposed to the family, provide more and more older people with care, and communal living is expected to become more common as older people's children grow old themselves and become unable to care for them in ways that are appropriate to their needs.

In collective societies, where the notion of family is strong and interdependence is stressed, attitudes and caring strategies are different. For example, in India, older people are respected for their wisdom and authority. Although they strive to remain active and live independently for as long as possible, it is expected that they will become dependent on the family. Similarly, in Islamic societies, age commands authority and the status and therefore confidence and self-esteem of older people increases with their age. Care homes for older people in collective societies are rare as it is assumed that families, particularly sons, will look after their elderly relatives.

activity
INDIVIDUAL WORK 4.7

P5

You have been asked by a local carers' organisation to give a presentation that describes the physical and psychological changes caused by the ageing process to a group of people who care for older people. Produce a series of slides to use in your presentation and two information sheets entitled 'The physical changes caused by the ageing process' and 'The psychological changes caused by the ageing process' that the carers can take away to read.

National Osteoporosis Society	www.nos.org.uk
BUPA	www.bupa.co.uk
NHS Direct	www.nhsdirect.nhs.uk
The Alzheimer's Society	www.alzheimers.org.uk
Royal National Institute for the Blind	www.rnib.org.uk
Royal National Institute for the Deaf	www.rnid.org.uk
The Prostate Cancer Charity	www.prostate-cancer.org.uk
National Statistics Online	www.statistics.gov.uk
BBC website	www.bbc.co.uk
Government public services website	www.direct.gov.uk

Progress Check

1 Name the different life stages.

2 Distinguish between the terms growth and development.

3 Define *holistic development*, *developmental norms*, *life course*, *maturation* and *life expectancy*.

4 Describe physical development through the life stages.

5 Describe intellectual development through the life stages.

6 Describe emotional development through the life stages.

7 Describe social development through the life stages.

8 Describe language development through the life stages.

9 Use examples to explain the nature-nurture debate in relation to human development.

10 Describe the influence of one genetic, one biological, one environmental, one socio-economic and one lifestyle factor on human development.

11 Explain the influence of two predictable and two unpredictable major life events on human development.

12 Describe two theories of ageing and how they can influence care services for older people.

13 Describe the physical and psychological changes that accompany ageing.

14 Describe positive and negative perspectives on ageing.

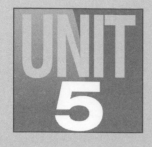

Fundamentals of anatomy and physiology for health and social care

This unit covers:

- The organisation of the human body
- The functioning of the body systems associated with energy metabolism
- How homeostatic mechanisms operate in the maintenance of an internal environment
- Interpreting data obtained from monitoring routine variations in the functioning of healthy body systems

Health and social care workers need to have an understanding of the anatomy and physiology of the human body, how body systems work and routine variations in this functioning in order to undertake their role in monitoring and promoting service users' health and well-being. They need to understand how the body produces energy and maintains an internal equilibrium to enable body systems to work effectively. They need to understand the importance of monitoring body function through observation and non-invasive measurement of the respiratory and cardiovascular systems as well as body temperature and how to interpret this data to determine an individual's health and well-being.

grading criteria

To achieve a **Pass** grade the evidence must show that the learner is able to:	To achieve a **Merit** grade the evidence must show that, in addition to the pass criteria, the learner is able to:	To achieve a **Distinction** grade the evidence must show that, in addition to the pass and merit criteria, the learner is able to:
P1 describe the functions of the main cell components _Pg 152_		
P2 describe the structure of the main tissues of the body and their role in the functioning of two named body organs _Pg 156_		
P3 describe the gross structure and main functions of all major body systems _Pg 163_		

To achieve a **Pass** grade the evidence must show that the learner is able to:	To achieve a **Merit** grade the evidence must show that, in addition to the pass criteria, the learner is able to:	To achieve a **Distinction** grade the evidence must show that, in addition to the pass and merit criteria, the learner is able to:
P4 describe the role of energy in the body and the physiology of three named body systems in relation to energy metabolism Pg 165	**M1** explain the physiology of three named body systems in relation to energy metabolism Pg 165	**D1** use examples to explain how body systems interrelate with each other Pg 163
P5 describe the concept of **homeostasis** and the homeostatic mechanisms that regulate heart rate, breathing rate, body temperature and blood glucose levels Pg 184	**M2** explain the probable homeostatic responses to changes in the internal environment during exercise Pg 188	**D2** explain the importance of homeostasis in maintaining the healthy functioning of the body Pg 184
P6 measure body temperature, heart rate and breathing rate before and after a standard period of exercise, interpret the data and comment on its validity Pg 188	**M3** analyse data obtained to show how homeostatic mechanisms control the internal environment during exercise Pg 188	

The organisation of the human body

The starting point in understanding the **anatomy** and **physiology** of the human body is to consider the body's basic organisation.

Organisation

The body is organised into cells, tissues, organs and systems.

BBC Science	www.bbc.co.uk/science
BBC Health	www.bbc.co.uk/heath

Cells

Fig 5.1 Parts of a cell

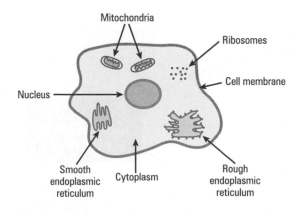

A cell is the basic, **microscopic** structural and functional part of all living **organisms**. It is the smallest structure capable of performing all the activities vital to life. All cells are made up from a cell membrane, nucleus, organelles and cytoplasm.

Cell membrane

This is the flexible yet tough outer surface of the cell. It separates the cell's inner contents from the external environment. It is a selective barrier and regulates the flow of materials in and out of the cell. This selectivity helps to create and maintain the best environment for normal cell activities to take place. The cell membrane is also important in communication among cells and between cells and their external environment.

Nucleus

This is the part of the cell that controls how the cell works. It is spherical or oval in shape and is the most prominent part of the cell. It contains the **chromosomes** each of which consists of a single **molecule** of **DNA** associated with several proteins. A chromosome contains thousands of **genes** that control most aspects of cellular structure and function.

Organelles

Within the cytoplasm there are a number of specialised parts called **organelles**.

Mitochondria

These are known as the powerhouse of the cell because they play a central part in the production of the chemical adenosine (or ATP). Adenosine is important in transferring energy from chemical reactions to fuel cellular activities.

Endoplasmic reticulum (ER)

This is a membranous network of flattened sacs or tubules. Rough endoplasmic reticulum has **ribosomes** attached and is involved in making and transferring proteins within the cell organelles and through the cell membrane. Smooth endoplasmic reticulum has no ribosomes and is involved in making fatty acids and steroids. It also removes the toxicity of drugs and stores and releases calcium from muscle cells.

Golgi apparatus (or complex)

A group of four to six flattened membranous sacs stacked on one another with expanded areas at their end giving a cup-like shape. Their function is to sort, package and deliver proteins and lipids to, for example, the cell membrane and lysomes. Most cells have several Golgi complexes.

Lysomes

Sacs enclosed by a membrane and filled with fluid that form from the Golgi complex. They contain powerful digestive **enzymes** which can breakdown other molecules.

Cytoplasm

This is a jelly-like fluid (cytosol) which contains all the organelles that enable a cell to function.

Fig 5.2 Cells in the human body

The human body contains many different types of cells with different functions.

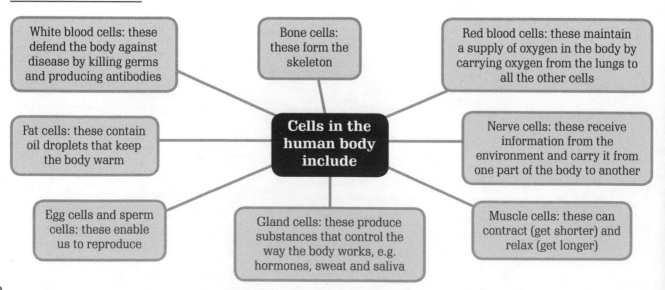

White blood cells: these defend the body against disease by killing germs and producing antibodies

Bone cells: these form the skeleton

Red blood cells: these maintain a supply of oxygen in the body by carrying oxygen from the lungs to all the other cells

Fat cells: these contain oil droplets that keep the body warm

Nerve cells: these receive information from the environment and carry it from one part of the body to another

Cells in the human body include

Egg cells and sperm cells: these enable us to reproduce

Gland cells: these produce substances that control the way the body works, e.g. hormones, sweat and saliva

Muscle cells: these can contract (get shorter) and relax (get longer)

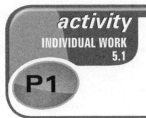

Describe the functions of each of the main cell components. [activity ends]

Tissues

A tissue is made up of cells that have the same function. There are four basic types of tissue in the human body contributing to homeostasis by providing diverse functions including protection, support, communication among cells and resistance to disease. The four main tissue types are epithelial, connective, muscle and nervous.

Epithelial tissue

This type of tissue covers the body's surfaces and lines hollow organs, body cavities and ducts. It also forms glands.

Simple epithelial tissue

Simple epithelial tissue is a single layer of cells. These cells are involved in the movement of substances as well as the production, release and absorption of substances. To achieve this, simple epithelial tissue contains cells of different shapes.

- Cuboidal cells may have microvilli (microscopic finger-like projections that increase surface area) and are responsible for secretion or absorption. In the body, these cells are found, for example, on the surface of the ovary, lining kidney tubules and in smaller ducts (passages or tubes) of many glands such as the thyroid and pancreas.

- Columnar cells may have cilia (microscopic hairs) or microvilli often specialised for secretion or absorption. In the body, these cells are found, for example, lining the digestive tract.

- Squamous cells are flat to allow rapid movement of substances through them. In the body, these cells are found, for example, lining the heart, blood vessels and the air sacs in the lungs.

- Ciliated cells are cuboidal cells with cilia or hairs which assist the movement of substances and secretions along the tissue. In the body, these cells are found, for example, in the upper respiratory tract where it assists the movement of mucus and in the Fallopian tubes where it assists the movement of the egg cell (ovum) towards the womb (uterus).

Compound epithelial tissue

This consists of two or more layers of cells that protect the underlying tissues in parts of the body where there is considerable wear and tear. The cells may be simple, formed from one of the cells types already described, or they may be keratinised. **Keratin** is a tough fibrous protein that helps to protect the skin and underlying tissues from heat, microbes that may cause infections and disease and chemicals. Compound epithelial tissue can be found, for example, lining the urinary tract (bladder, ureters and urethra) and keratinised cells form the outer layer of the skin.

Fig 5.3 Cell types

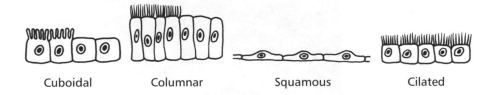

| Cuboidal | Columnar | Squamous | Cilated |

Connective tissue

This is one of the most plentiful and widely distributed tissues in the body. It consists of two elements: cells and matrix. The matrix fills the spaces between the cells and consists of protein-based fibres usually secreted by the connective tissue cells. It may be flexible or hard and firm. In its various forms, connective tissue binds together, supports and strengthens other body tissues. It provides protection and insulation to the internal organs of the body and compartmentalises (separates) structures such as the muscles of the skeleton. Connective tissues generally have a plentiful blood supply and nerve endings.

There are five types of connective tissue: blood, cartilage, bone, areolar and adipose.

Blood

Blood is a fluid connective tissue and it functions as the major transport system within the body. Blood is made up of a number of different types of blood cells:

- red blood cells (erythrocytes)
- white blood cells (leukocytes)
- platelets (thrombocytes)
- plasma (the matrix)

Fig 5.4 Blood cells

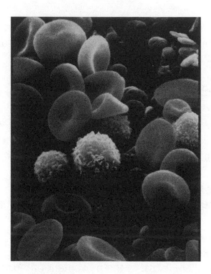

Cartilage

This is different from other types of connective tissue as it has no blood or nerve supply. It is a closely packed network of collagen fibres and elastic fibres embedded into a gel-like substance. Its density makes it able to withstand more stress than the loose connective tissues and so it can be found where bones meet, such as in the knee joint and between the spinal vertebra. It acts as a shock absorber. It is also found in other flexible parts of the body, such as the external ear.

Fig 5.5 Outer ear

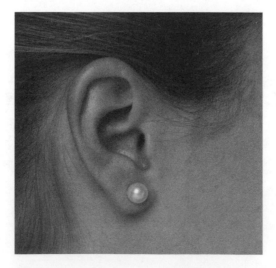

Bone

Bone is part of the skeletal system. Bone connective tissue is mainly made up of collagen fibres (cells) and calcium (matrix). Bone is either compact or spongy depending on how the cells and matrix are organised. The hardness of bones is due the density of calcium within the bone matrix, while bone strength derives from the collagen fibres. A bone is made up of several types of connective tissue working together. Each individual bone is therefore an organ as well as connective tissue.

Areolar tissue

This is a loose connective tissue. Unlike other types, it lines joint cavities such as hip joints. It is made up of three types of fibres: collagen, elastic and reticular. Along with adipose tissue it forms the layer of tissue that attaches the skin to the underlying tissues and organs.

Adipose tissue

This is also a loose connective tissue with specialised fat (energy) storage cells. Adipose tissue is also a good insulator and reduces heat loss through the skin as well as protecting major body organs.

Individuals who are malnourished lose adipose tissue and this can make it difficult for them to maintain their body temperature. Babies and young children have more of a particular type of adipose tissue not present in adults which generates heat and, in newborn babies, helps to maintain body temperature.

Muscle tissue

The main function of muscle tissue is to change chemical energy into mechanical energy in order to produce force, perform work and produce movement. Muscle tissues also stabilise the body's position, regulate organ volume, generate heat and push fluids through the various body systems.

There are three types of muscle tissue: striated, non-striated and cardiac.

Striated muscle tissue

This is made up of long cylinder-shaped striated fibres. They are referred to as being striated due to the alternating dark and light bands of fibres which give a striped appearance under a microscope. These muscle tissues are usually found attached to bones and are often referred to as skeletal muscle. These are voluntary muscles, which means we can choose to contract or relax them.

Non-striated muscle tissue

This is also known as smooth muscle. It is found in the walls of hollow internal structures of the body such as blood vessels, airways to the lungs, the stomach and intestines. Non-striated muscle fibres are small, thin in the middle and tapered at each end. They constrict in a wave-like motion to move substances through the vessels, for example to break down and move food through the intestines. The contraction or relaxation of these muscles is involuntary, and so not under conscious control. Sometimes the smooth muscle fibres contract together which creates a strong action, such as the contractions of the uterus during childbirth labour. At other times they act individually, for example in the movement of the iris of the eye.

Fig 5.6 Muscle types

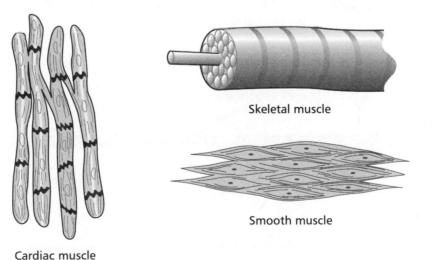

Skeletal muscle

Smooth muscle

Cardiac muscle

Cardiac muscle

This is a specialised muscle which forms most of the heart wall. It is striated and involuntary in action. The function of this muscle is to pump blood to all parts of the body from the heart.

Nervous tissue

Nervous tissue can be found in the central nervous system i.e. the brain and spinal cord and in the peripheral nervous system; the part that lies outside the brain and spinal cord.

Nervous tissue consists of two types of cells: neurones and neuroglia.

Neurons

These are also known as nerve cells. They are sensitive to various stimuli (factors which create a response or reaction, such as light, heat or pain). Neurons change stimuli into nerve impulses and send these impulses to other neurons, to muscle tissue or to glands, in order for the body to respond. Most neurons consist of three parts, a cell body, dendrites and axons. Dendrites are short tree-like cell processes which receive the nerve impulse. An axon is a single, thin, often very long cylinder shaped process which transmits or conducts the nerve impulse towards another neuron or other tissue.

Neurolgia

These do not generate or conduct nerve impulses. Their function is to act as the 'glue' that hold the nervous tissue together. Neuroglia are smaller than neurons and can multiply and divide to fill the spaces if neurons are damaged. There are six different types of neuroglia. Four are only found in the central nervous system and the other two in the peripheral nervous system. Some provide nutrients to neurons and help to form the barrier between the blood and the brain. Two types of neuroglia are responsible for producing the insulating myelin sheath that covers the axon to increase the nerve impulse conductivity (speed of message transmission).

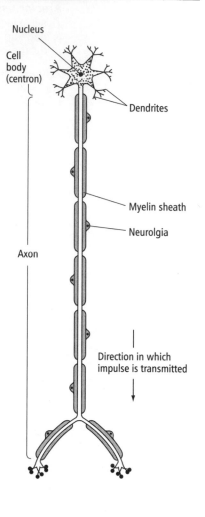

Fig 5.7 Neuron and neurolgia

- Nucleus
- Cell body (centron)
- Dendrites
- Myelin sheath
- Neurolgia
- Axon
- Direction in which impulse is transmitted

Link

See page 159 for more information about the central nervous system and the peripheral nervous system.

Body organs

A body organ is a part of the body made up of two or more types of tissue and which has one or more particular functions.

---

activity

INDIVIDUAL WORK
5.2

P2

1 Describe the structure of the main body tissues.

2 Identify two body organs and describe the role of different body tissues in how each organ functions.

Fig 5.8 Locations of main body organs

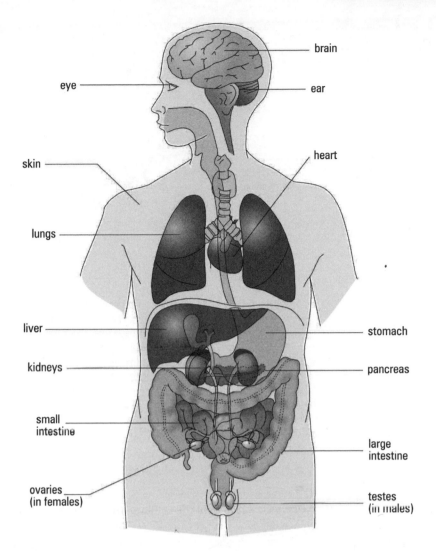

Systems

A body system is a group of two of more body organs working together to perform a particular function. All body systems interact to ensure the body functions effectively and efficiently. The digestive system provides energy for the muscles to work and for bones to move in response to stimulation from the nervous system which in turn is responding to external stimuli. All three systems rely on the respiratory and cardiovascular systems to provide the oxygen and nutrients to the organs, tissues and cells to fuel these responses. The skin, renal and the respiratory systems ensure that efficiency is maintained by eliminating toxic waste from the body while the lymphatic and immune systems keep the body free from infection. The endocrine system ensures that the body maintains its internal balance. The reproductive system relies on all the other systems for health reproduction.

Skin

The skin is the largest organ in the body and is made up of many different cells and tissues.

The main functions of the skin are:

- to regulate body temperature
- to act as a reservoir for blood
- to provide protection for the inner structures from the external environment
- to receive information through the form of sensations about the external environment, i.e. through touch, pressure, vibration, pain and temperature
- to produce sweat which helps the body get rid of waste products
- to absorb vitamins, such as A, D, E and K, as well as certain drugs and gases, such as oxygen and carbon dioxide
- to manufacture vitamin D.

Fig 5.9 Cross-section of the skin

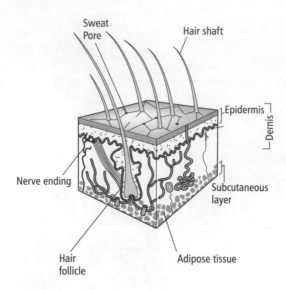

Most drugs are absorbed into the body through the digestive system or by injection. However, some drugs can be absorbed through the skin by using an adhesive skin patch. This enables the drug to be released into the body at a controlled rate over a period of time as it passes through the epidermis of the skin and into the blood vessels of the dermis. This method is commonly used to administer hormone replacement therapy for women during the menopause; to give small doses of nicotine to people who want to stop smoking and glycerintrinitrate to prevent angina (chest pain associated with heart disease).

Cardiovascular system

The cardiovascular system is made up of:

- heart
- blood vessels
- blood.

The main function of the cardiovascular system is to supply oxygen and transport materials throughout the body in order to maintain life.

Fig 5.10 Cardiovascular system

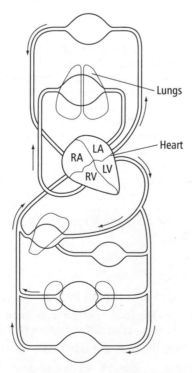

Respiratory system

This system is made up of:

- nose, through which oxygen-rich air is inhaled and carbon dioxide-rich air is exhaled (breathing)
- larynx, trachea and bronchi, which are all air tubes that connect the nose with the lungs
- two lungs, which are made up of bronchioles and alveoli
- blood vessels, which circulate around the alveoli
- muscles of the thoracic (chest) cavity which aid breathing.

Fig 5.11 Respiratory system

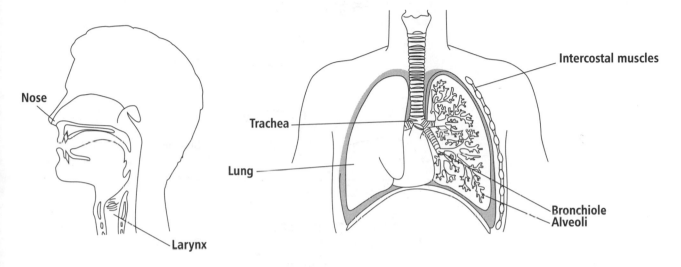

The function of the respiratory system is supply the body with oxygen and rid it of waste carbon dioxide.

Digestive system

Two groups of organs make up the digestive system: the gastrointestinal tract and the accessory organs.

Gastrointestinal tract

The gastrointestinal tract, or alimentary canal, is a continuous tube that extends from the mouth to the anus. The organs of the gastrointestinal tract are:

- mouth
- most of the pharynx
- oesophagus
- stomach
- ileum (small intestine)
- colon (large intestine).

Accessory organs

The accessory organs are:

- teeth
- tongue
- salivary glands
- pancreas
- liver
- gallbladder.

Apart from the teeth and the tongue the other accessory digestive organs do not come into direct contact with food, instead they produce or store secretions that then flow into the gastrointestinal tract through ducts (small tubes) to aid the chemical breakdown of food.

Fig 5.12 Digestive system

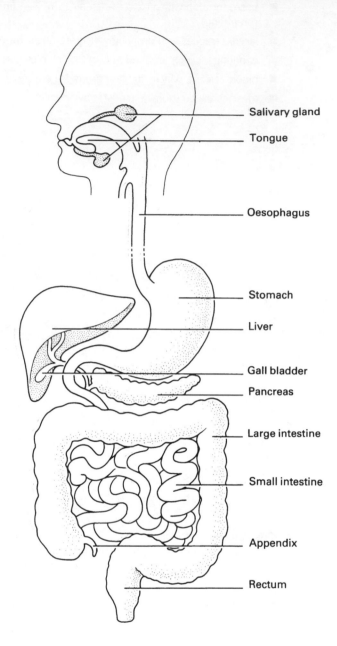

- Salivary gland
- Tongue
- Oesophagus
- Stomach
- Liver
- Gall bladder
- Pancreas
- Large intestine
- Small intestine
- Appendix
- Rectum

The main functions of the digestive system are the digestion of food, the absorption of nutrients from food and the elimination of waste products.

Renal system

The renal system consists of:

■ two kidneys

■ two ureters, which enable urine to pass into the urinary bladder

■ urethra, which enables urine to pass out of the body.

The function of the renal system is to excrete waste products from the body. The kidneys purify the blood and act as a filtration system ensuring that nutrients are retained and only excess salt, water and waste products such as urea are filtered out to make urine which the passes into the bladder before being eliminated from the body.

Fig 5.13 Renal system

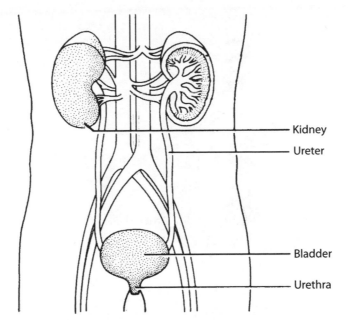

- Kidney
- Ureter
- Bladder
- Urethra

Nervous system

The nervous system is divided into two parts: the central nervous system (CNS) and the peripheral nervous system (PNS).

Central nervous system (CNS)

The CNS consists of:

- brain
- spinal cord

Peripheral nervous system (PNS)

The PNS consists of:

- sense organs, which receive information about the environment both outside the body (the skin, eyes, ears, nose and tongue) and inside the body (within the ears, muscles and organs that sense, for example, the body's position and heartbeat)

- sensory nerves, which carry information from the sense organs to the CNS

- relay nerves in the CNS, whose purpose is to form a link between sensory and motor nerves

- motor nerves, which carry information from the CNS to effectors

- effectors, which are muscles and glands which respond to information coming from the CNS, i.e. when information is received a muscle contracts and a gland produces a secretion, such as a hormone or saliva.

The function of the nervous system is to receive information about the environment so that the body can respond appropriately. The nervous system also coordinates and controls skeletal muscles to ensure our movements are smooth and we maintain our balance.

Fig 5.14 Nervous system

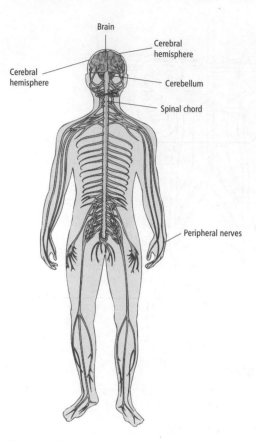

- Brain
- Cerebral hemisphere
- Cerebral hemisphere
- Cerebellum
- Spinal chord
- Peripheral nerves

Endocrine system

The endocrine system is made up of a number of glands that produce hormones which act on the body to control and coordinate the way the body works.

Fig 5.15 Endocrine system

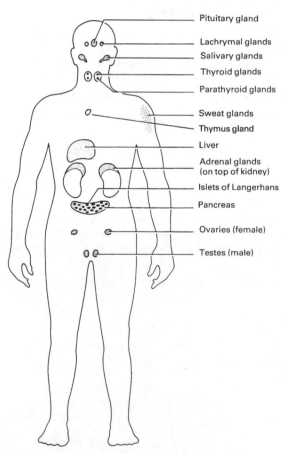

- Pituitary gland
- Lachrymal glands
- Salivary glands
- Thyroid glands
- Parathyroid glands
- Sweat glands
- Thymus gland
- Liver
- Adrenal glands (on top of kidney)
- Islets of Langerhans
- Pancreas
- Ovaries (female)
- Testes (male)

Reproductive system

Refer back to page 156 to remind yourself about the position of the reproductive organs.

The female reproductive system
The female reproductive system is made up of:

- two ovaries whose function is to produce and store egg cells and produce female hormones
- two fallopian tubes which carry eggs away from the ovary to the uterus
- uterus, a strong muscle which protects and feeds the unborn baby (foetus) as it develops and then contracts during childbirth to push the baby out down the birth canal so the baby is born
- vagina.

The male reproductive system
The male reproductive system is made up of:

- two testicles whose function is to produce and store sperm cells and produce the male hormones
- vas deferens (sperm tubes) which carry sperm away from the testicles to the penis
- prostate gland and a seminal vesicle which produces a fluid that mixes with sperm to form semen
- penis which places sperm in the female vagina during sexual intercourse.

The function of both the female and male reproductive systems is reproduction through the fusion of the ovum and sperm cell to create first an embryo, which develops into a foetus and finally a baby.

The lymphatic and immune systems

These systems are responsible for resisting damage or disease to the body. We are born with some resistance e.g. babies have some resistance to infections at birth, while specific resistance results from coming into contact with a particular substance that may cause damage or disease, such as a bacteria. These two systems are closely related and work together with other body systems to keep the body healthy.

Fig 5.16 Lymphatic and immune systems

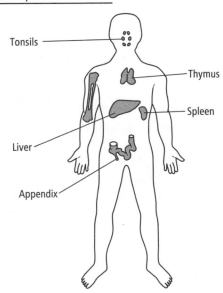

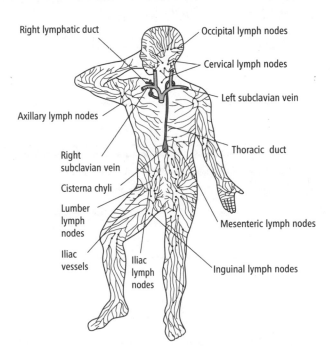

The lymphatic and immune systems consist of:

- lymphatic vessels, which form the second transport system of the body that carry a fluid known as lymph around the body
- lymph
- structures and organs containing lymphatic tissue, such as the spleen, thymus, tonsils and appendix
- red bone marrow, where stem cells develop into various types of blood cells including lymphocytes which work to counteract the effects of infection on the body tissues.

The three primary functions of the lymphatic and immune systems are:

- draining excess fluid from the spaces between body tissues and returning it to the blood
- transporting dietary fats (lipids) and the lipid-soluble vitamins A, D, E and K which are absorbed by the gastrointestinal tract via lymphatic vessels to the blood
- carrying out immune responses.

The immune response starts when lymphocytes and **macrophages** recognise foreign matter within the body. The lymphatic system starts specific responses to particular cells, microbes (micro-organisms), toxins and abnormal cells to protect the body from disease or damage. The lymphocytes and macrophages respond either by destroying the intruders (causing them to break or by releasing a cell-killing substance) or by producing cells called antibodies which then cause destruction to the specific invader.

Musculo-skeletal system

This system is made up of the bones of the skeleton and the muscles attached to those bones. The calcium within bones makes them hard and gives bones their rigidity which enables them to support the body. Muscles are made up of thousands of individual cells that are able to contract and relax. When muscle cells contract, the muscles get shorter and fatter and this action moves the bone the muscle is attached to. The continued muscle contraction holds the bone in position. When the muscle cells relax, the muscle lengthens and this allows the bone to return to its original position.

Link

Refer back to page 154 to remind yourself about bones and muscles.

---

activity
INDIVIDUAL WORK
5.3

P3

1 Draw labelled diagrams which show the gross structure of all major body systems.
2 Describe the main functions of all major body systems.

---

activity
INDIVIDUAL WORK
5.4

D1

Explain how the following different body systems interrelate with each other:
1 Circulatory and respiratory systems
2 Reproductive and endocrine systems.

The functioning of body systems associated with energy metabolism

 See in Unit 21, in BTEC National Health and Social Care Book 2, for more information about energy metabolism.

Energy laws

Energy is the capacity for matter and radiation to do work. Potential energy is energy associated with matter due to its position, such as the energy stored in a battery or in a person before they move. Kinetic energy is energy associated with matter in motion. When the battery is used to run something such as a clock or when the person moves, the potential energy is converted into kinetic energy.

Conservation of energy

Although energy can be neither created nor destroyed, it may be converted from one form to another. For example, the food we eat contains potential energy in the form of chemicals. Some of this will be converted into various forms of kinetic energy, such as mechanical energy to enable us to walk.

Transformation of energy

The process by which energy changes its form is called the transformation of energy. For example, energy from the sun is used by plants in photosynthesis. It is then stored as chemical energy. Plants are eaten by animals. Animals use some of the energy produced from eating the plants as kinetic energy to enable them to move and function. Eventually, the animal dies and decomposes. Over millions of years, the nutrients released from the animal's body become fossil fuels and they can then be burnt to produce energy in the form of heat and light.

Forms of energy

There are a number of different types of energy.

Fig 5.17 Types of energy

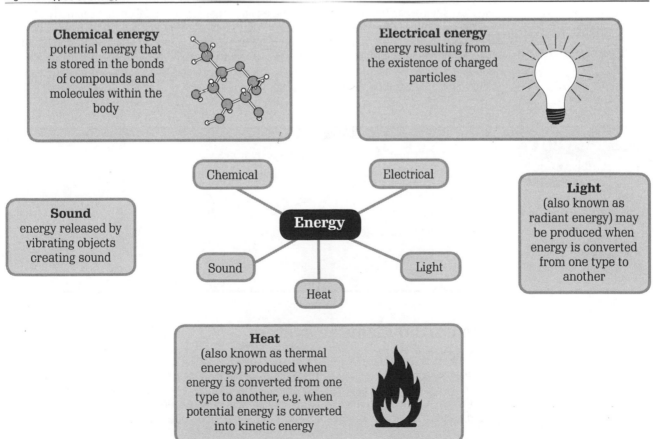

Energy metabolism

Energy is essential for body function. Some actions create energy, while others use energy. Metabolism is the process by which the energy produced and used up by all the chemical reactions that occur in the body is balanced.

Catabolism

Catabolic reactions are those chemical reactions that break down complex organic molecules into simpler ones. These reactions release the chemical energy which is stored in organic molecules. An example of an important catabolic reaction is the breakdown of fats stored in the body into glucose so that it can be used as an energy source (this is known as Krebs cycle).

Anabolism

Anabolic reactions are **synthesis** actions: chemical reactions that combine simple molecules to form the body's complex structural and functional components. Anabolism requires a supply of energy to facilitate the process. Energy produced as a result of catabolic reactions drives anabolic reactions.

Anabolism is about 'building up' cells. Some of the body's anabolic reactions are:

- tissue growth
- tissue repair
- when amino acids join at each stages of protein synthesis, e.g. forming dipeptides
- process of small sugar molecules joining to make dissacharides
- when glycerol reacts with fatty acids to form lipids
- storing nutrients in fatty tissues

Activities involved in supplying energy to the body

The digestive, cardiovascular and respiratory systems are all essential in ensuring that energy is released through metabolic reactions. The body is unable to produce enough energy through cellular respiration, the chemical reactions in the cytoplasm that breakdown glucose in the absence of oxygen, and so requires a continuous supply of oxygen in order to perform efficiently. The digestive system produces enzymes that break down carbohydrate so that glucose is released. The respiratory system ensures that oxygen is taken into the body and distributed to the lungs where it is passed to the red blood cells for transportation around the body. The cardiovascular system then plays its part by circulating the oxygen-rich blood around the body so that oxygen can be exchanged at a cellular level to facilitate catabolic and anabolic reactions and release energy. The circulatory and respiratory systems are also involved in the excretion of carbon dioxide.

activity
INDIVIDUAL WORK
5.5

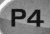

1   Describe the role of energy in how the body works.
2   Describe and explain how energy is metabolised in the:
   - digestive system
   - respiratory system
   - cardiovascular system.

The cardiovascular system

The heart

The heart is about 10 cm long and roughly cone-shaped. It is a hollow, muscular organ that lies in the centre of the chest between the lungs a little more to the left than the right. The heart is a powerful pump made up of four chambers. The two upper chambers, atria, receive blood and the two lower chambers, ventricles, pump blood out of the heart.

Fig 5.18 Structure and
cross-section of the heart

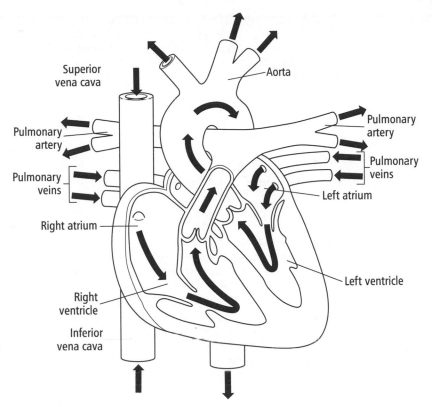

Superior
vena cava

Aorta

Pulmonary
artery

Pulmonary
artery

Pulmonary
veins

Pulmonary
veins

Left atrium

Right atrium

Left ventricle

Right
ventricle

Inferior
vena cava

* Diagram to practise

The main function of the heart is to pump blood around the body. This ensures that all body cells receive a plentiful supply of oxygen through the circulation of blood, a supply of nutrients, hormones and antibodies to enable the body to function normally, and that waste products produced by the body cells are removed so they and their harmful effects can be eliminated from the body.

The cardiac cycle

All the events that make up one heartbeat are called a cardiac cycle. On average, one cardiac cycle will take approximately 0.8 of a second, and thus the usual number of cardiac cycles per minute is between 60 and 80.

The cardiac cycles consists of the following actions:

■ Atrial systole, the contraction of the atria (upper chambers of the heart), which lasts on average 0.1 second

■ Ventricular systole, the contraction of the ventricles (lower chambers of the heart),which lasts on average 0.3 second

■ Complete cardiac diastole, the relaxation of both the atria and ventricles, which lasts on average 0.4 second.

The heart has its own system of stimulating the myocardium (heart muscle) to contract in a sequence to empty and fill the heart chambers and so pass blood through the heart. There are small groups of specialised neuromuscular cells in the myocardium which initiate and conduct impulses of contraction over the heart muscle.

■ The Sinuatrial node (SA node) is a small mass of specialised cells in the wall of the right atrium. It is often referred to as the 'pacemaker' as it initiates impulses of contraction more rapidly that other groups of neuromuscular cells.

■ Atrioventricular node (AV node) is a small mass of neuromuscular tissue situated in the wall of the atrial septum near the atrioventricular valves. It is normally stimulated by the impulse of the contraction that sweeps over the atrial myocardium.

■ Atrioventricular bundle is a mass of specialised fibres that come originally from the AV node. The AV bundle crosses the fibrous ring that separated the atria from the ventricles. At the upper end, it divides into two and this enables the impulses to pass from the AV node to the bottom or apex of the heart from which the impulse then sweeps upwards pumping blood into the pulmonary artery and the aorta.

An electrocardiogram (ECG) is a tracing that demonstrates the electrical activity of the heart during the cardiac cycle. ECGs are examined for changes to the normal wave pattern (PQRST) as the position and type of changes provide valuable information about how the heart is performing, showing how healthy it is or if damage has occurred the extent and position of the damage.

Fig 5.19 Electrocardiogram showing one cardiac cycle

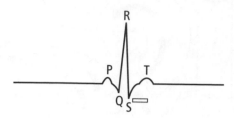

Deoxygenated blood from the body pours into the right atrium via the superior and inferior vena cavae (veins) at the same time as the four pulmonary veins pour oxygenated blood into the left atrium. The valves between the atria and ventricles are open and blood flows through into the ventricles. The SA node emits an impulse of contraction which stimulates the muscles (myocardium) of both atria to contract (the P wave on the electrocardiogram). This empties the atria and fills the ventricles with blood. When the wave of contraction reaches the AV node, it is stimulated to emit an impulse of contraction which spreads to the ventricular muscles via the AV bundle and its fibres. This wave of contraction sweeps upwards from the apex of the heart and pushes blood into the pulmonary artery and the aorta (the QRS wave on the electrocardiogram). After the ventricles have contracted there is complete cardiac diastole or resting phase (the T wave on the electrocardiogram). The valves of the heart and great blood vessels open and close as the pressure within the heart chambers change and this ensures that blood flows only in one direction.

Heart rate

The heart rate is the rate at which the heart is working and is usually described as a number of beats per minute. At rest, a newborn baby's normal heart rate is fast at around 120 beats per minute. This gradually decreases as the baby grows and the heart develops. An adult's normal heart rate at rest will be around 60 to 80 beats per minute. The heart rate indicates how hard the heart is working. If you ran up a flight of stairs or were anxious, your heart rate would increase as your body works harder and requires more energy to cope with the demands being made on it.

The heart rate is usually measured by taking the person's pulse. The pulse is the wave of distension and elongation felt in an artery wall as a result of blood being forced out of the heart and into the aorta. As the aorta distends, a wave passes along the walls of the arteries and this wave can be felt by pressing the artery next to a bone.

See page 184, to find out how to locate and measure pulse rate.

Stroke volume

The amount of blood pumped out of the heart by each ventricular contraction is called the stroke volume. This represents the difference between the amount of blood left in the ventricle during the relaxation or diastole and the amount of blood left in the ventricle at the end of contraction or ventricular systole. The end diastolic volume (EDV) is usually about 120 ml and the left ventricular EDV is usually about 5 ml, so the stroke volume is therefore 120 ml – 50 ml = 70 ml. A change to these volumes will alter the stroke volume and an increase in the stroke volume increases the systolic pressure more than the diastolic pressure.

Cardiac output is the quantity of blood being ejected by the left ventricle every minute and is expressed in litres per minute. To calculate cardiac output, multiply stroke volume by heart rate. For example, if stroke volume is 70 ml per beat and heart rate is 80 beats per minute, cardiac output is 70 × 80 = 5600 ml per minute or 5.6 litres per minute.

As the average adult has five litres of blood. This means that this entire volume passes through the heart every minute. The cardiac output increases as physical fitness increases or if the person is performing physically strenuous work.

Blood pressure

This is the force which blood exerts on the walls of the blood vessels. The delay in blood flow through the arteriolar and capillary systems means that blood pressure is higher in arteries than in veins. Arterial blood pressure results from the flow of blood out of the ventricles into an already full aorta. When the left ventricle contracts and pushes blood into the aorta, the pressure that results is called the systolic blood pressure. In adults, this is usually around 120 mmHg (millimetres of mercury). When the heart is resting (complete cardiac diastole), the pressure within the arteries falls and this is called the diastolic blood pressure. In adults, this is usually around 80 mmHg. Like the pulse rate, the blood pressure can vary as a result of different factors. For example, the time of day, position, i.e. standing or lying down, age, gender and physical activity and fitness, as well as emotional state. Blood pressure increases with age and is higher in women than in men. Blood pressure is measured using a sphygmomanometer and is an important part of any routine health screening test.

Blood vessels

The circulatory system is the network of blood vessels called arteries, arterioles, capillaries, venules, and veins throughout the body that transport the blood to and from the heart.

Arteries

Arteries usually carry the oxygenated blood away from the heart to all the body cells. The exception to this is the pulmonary arteries in the adult as these carry deoxygenated blood from the heart to the lungs. Elastic arteries are large vessels, such as the aorta that can be up to 25 mm in diameter. These vessels need to be able to stretch to accommodate the increases in blood volume and pressure that occur when the ventricles contract and to recoil when they relax. Muscular arteries are the distributing arteries and are medium sized vessels (1 to 4 mm in diameter). They have a greater capacity to regulate blood flow through contraction or dilation than the larger arteries whose capacity for this is limited. Arterioles are the smallest arteries that deliver blood to the capillary vessels within tissues.

Venous system

The venous system is the collection system as its function is to transport the deoxygenated blood towards the heart. Capillaries are smaller vessels between cells which take blood from arteries to the veins. The pressure in capillaries is medium and their walls are thin to allow the oxygen and nutrients to pass through them into the cells and waste products from the cells to pass into the capillaries. Capillaries merge to form venules and these become larger in diameter as they become closer to connecting with the larger veins. Veins carry deoxygenated blood and have very thin inflexible walls. As a consequence, the pressure within veins is low. At any time, about two-thirds of the total blood volume is found in the venous system.

Pulmonary and systemic circulation

Fig 5.20 Pulmonary and systemic circulation

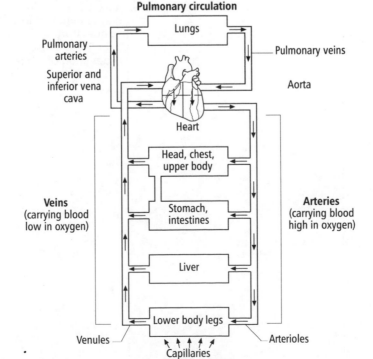

167

Blood continuously circulates around the body. Pulmonary circulation consists of the circulation of blood from the right ventricle of the heart to the lungs and back to the left atrium. The pulmonary arteries carry deoxygenated blood to the lungs. In the lungs, carbon dioxide is excreted and oxygen is absorbed. The oxygenated blood is returned to the left atrium of the heart by the pulmonary veins. During atrial systole, the oxygenated blood passes into the left ventricle and then into the aorta.

Systemic circulation is the general circulation throughout the body. Blood is pumped out of the left ventricle of the heart and distributed around the body via the branches of the aorta which supply every part of the body, for example, femoral arteries supply blood to the legs. Blood is returned to the heart via veins and the superior and inferior vena cavae (the major veins of the body).

Structure and function of blood

As described earlier in this unit, blood is the major transport system within the body. Blood is made up of a straw-coloured transparent fluid, plasma, within which there are different types of blood cells. Plasma constitutes about 55% and the cells 45% of blood volume.

Blood structure and function

Constituent	Composition	Function
Red blood cells (erythrocytes) Fig 5.21 Red blood cell 	■ Develop in red bone marrow ■ Contain a complex protein called haemoglobin which has an affinity for oxygen. This enables the cells to transport oxygen through the body efficiently ■ Life span of a red blood cell is 120 days	Transport oxygen and carbon dioxide from cells to the lungs for excretion
White blood cells (leukocytes) Fig 5.22 Neutrophils Fig 5.23 Eosinophils Fig 5.24 Basophils Fig 5.25 Monocytes Fig 5.26 Lymphocytes 	■ Develop in red bone marrow. ■ Largest of blood cells ■ There are several different types: granulocytes (neutrophils, eosinophils and basophils) and non-granular leukocytes (monocytes and lymphocytes)	To protect against foreign material, e.g. germs that may enter the body. Kill invading substances by ingesting them or by secreting substances to protect the body, e.g. histamine. They surround the foreign or waste material and isolate it to limit cell damage. Both types of non granular leukocytes produce interleukin 1 which acts on the hypothalamus causing the rise in temperature which occurs with microbial infections. It also encourages further production of white cells that fight infection.

Constituent	Composition	Function
Platelets (thrombocytes) Fig 5.27 Platelets	■ Very small discs with no nucleus ■ Come from the cytoplasm of cells in red bone marrow ■ Contain a variety of substances, e.g. platelet fibrinogen ■ Life span of usually 8 to 11 days	Important in the blood clotting process as the platelet's surface becomes sticky and sticks to the blood vessel wall around the damaged area to form a plug. They also stimulate constriction to reduce further blood flow and then initiate blood clot formation.
Plasma (the matrix)	■ 90 to 92% water ■ Dissolved substances are plasma proteins, e.g. albumen, globulin, fibrinogen, blood clotting factors, mineral salts, e.g. sodium chloride, iron, calcium, nutrients from food, e.g. glucose, amino acids from fats and vitamins, organic waste, e.g. urea, creatinine, hormones, antibodies, gases, i.e. oxygen, carbon dioxide, nitrogen	The means by which substances and blood cells are transported.

The respiratory system

The respiratory system is made up of a number of parts all of which have a part to play in respiration.

Refer back to page 158 for a diagram of the respiratory system.

Nose

The nose is lined with ciliated columnar epithelium which has a good blood supply. The membrane also has special goblet cells that secrete mucous and is often referred to as a mucous membrane. Air enters the respiratory system through the nose and mouth. When air is breathed in, it is warmed as it passes over the inner surface and is also moistened when it comes into contact with the mucus. The nose also acts as a filter to ensure we do not inhale dust and other impurities including germs. The cilia of the mucous membrane waft the air towards the throat and the next part of the journey. Nerve endings in the nose give us our sense of smell when they send messages via the olfactory nerves to the brain.

Refer back to page 152 to remind yourself about the structure of epithelial tissue.

Pharynx
Lying behind the nose, mouth and larynx this is a hollow tube approximately 12 to 14 cm in length which is wider at its upper end. The pharynx is involved in both the digestive and respiratory systems with food passing through the oral and laryngeal parts and air passing through the nasal and oral parts. The pharynx is also lined by mucous membrane. At the nasal end, it is continuous with the lining of the nose, having ciliated columnar epithelium. In the oral (mouth) and laryngeal parts, it is stratified squamous epithelium as this is continuous with the mouth and oesophagus. There is a layer of fibrous tissue and muscle tissue including several constrictor muscles. These involuntary muscles play an important part in swallowing ensuring the upper end of the oesophagus is closed when swallowing. Air is also warmed and moistened as it passes through the pharynx in the same way as when it passes through the nose.

Larynx
This is also referred to as the 'voice box'. The size of the larynx changes during puberty becoming larger and more prominent in males (the Adam's apple) and leading to a deeper voice tone. The larynx is made of five irregularly shaped cartilages held together by ligaments. It plays an important part in the production of voice and sounds. In relation to respiration, it provides a passageway for air to flow between the pharynx and the trachea.

As air passes through the larynx, it is further warmed, moistened and filtered. During swallowing, the larynx moves upwards so that it becomes closed, thereby preventing food from entering it and going into the respiratory passages.

Trachea

This is the windpipe and is continuous with the larynx. It is made up of 16 to 20 C-shaped rings of cartilages situated one above the other. The open part is at the back of the trachea which is covered by connective and involuntary muscle tissue. Three layers of tissue cover the trachea. The outer tissues are elastic and fibrous. The middle layer is cartilage, bands of smooth muscle winding around the trachea. The inner layer consists of ciliated columnar epithelium. This arrangement of tissues allows the trachea to extend when needed (i.e. when swallowing) but not collapse and obstruct the airway. Ciliated epithelial tissue plays an important part throughout the respiratory tract as its action moves potentially harmful impurities away from the lungs and out to the surface where it can be excreted either through coughing or sneezing.

Bronchial tree

This is formed when the trachea divides into two bronchi (singular bronchus), each leading into a lung. They are made of the same tissues as the trachea. The bronchi subdivide into progressively smaller branches called bronchioles. The bronchioles divide into alveoli and alveolar sacs. Oxygen and carbon dioxide exchange occurs across the capillary walls of the alveolar sacs.

Lungs

The lungs are a pair of cone-shaped organs in the thoracic cavity (chest). They are separated by the heart and other structures in the middle of the chest. Each lung is divided into lobes and has a bronchus or muscular air tube. They are surrounded by two membranes, the pleural membranes, which enclose and protect each lung and the other parts of the thoracic cavity. There is a small amount of fluid between the pleural membranes which acts as a lubricant to reduce friction between them as they slide over one another during breathing. The fluid also enables the membranes to stick together creating surface tension.

> **remember**
>
> The respiratory system maintains the body's supply of oxygen and eliminates the waste product carbon dioxide.

Respiratory muscles

These consist of:

- 11 pairs of intercostal muscles that lie in the space between the 12 pairs of ribs
- diaphragm, a large dome-shaped muscular structure which separates the thoracic and abdominal cavities

When we breathe in (inhalation), the intercostal muscles and the diaphragm contract, causing the ribs to rise and the diaphragm to flatten, which increases the space in the chest cavity. The pressure in the chest, alveoli and air passages decreases and air is drawn into the lungs thereby expanding them. This is an active process as it results from muscle contraction. The blood circulating around the alveoli absorbs oxygen from the inhaled air and the oxygen is pumped around the body to maintain the body's oxygen supply. At the same time, carbon dioxide passes from the blood into the alveoli.

When we breathe out (exhalation), the process is reversed as the intercostal muscles and diaphragm relax. The chest cavity decreases in size ensuring that carbon dioxide is pushed out of the lungs and eliminated from the body. This is a passive process. There is a pause before the next breath in occurs.

When we are resting, the diaphragm alone contracts, but the lungs are still adequately ventilated.

Gaseous exchange

Oxygen and carbon dioxide are exchanged in the blood within the capillary network that surrounds the alveoli and the air in the alveoli. To understand how this works, it is important to understand how gases react:

- Gas molecules are always moving.
- Gases tend to diffuse (move) from higher concentrations to lower concentrations.
- Gases will always fill whatever contains them (i.e. they do not leave any space) and if they are not contained they will escape.

Inhaled air will contain the normal levels of gases present in the air, i.e. 21% oxygen, 0.04% carbon dioxide, 78% nitrogen and rare gases and a variable amount of water vapour. Exhaled air will contain 16% oxygen, 4% carbon dioxide, 78% nitrogen and rare gases and be saturated with water vapour.

During respiration, the lungs always contain some air. When air reaches the alveoli, it is saturated with water vapour and because of the amount of air moving in and out of the lungs the concentration of gases in the alveoli remains fairly constant. Taken together, the partial pressures (which are proportionate to their concentrations) exerted on the alveoli walls by the different gases is the same as the atmospheric pressure 760 mmHg.

Partial pressures of gases in mmHg

Gas	Alveolar air	Deoxygenated blood	Oxygenated blood
Oxygen	100	40	100
Carbon dioxide	40	44	40
Nitrogen & other gases	573	573	573
Water vapour	47		
Total	760	657	713

As you can see from the above table, the partial pressure of oxygen in the alveoli is higher than that in the deoxygenated blood in the capillaries of the pulmonary arteries. Therefore, as gases diffuse from higher to lower concentrations, this accounts for the movement of oxygen from the alveoli to the blood and the movement of carbon dioxide from the deoxygenated blood to the alveoli. The partial pressure of each gas in the blood when it leaves the lungs via the pulmonary veins is the same as in the alveolar air. Blood moves slowly enough through the capillaries to allow the exchange of gases and for oxygen to be taken up by the red blood cells ready to be transported around the body.

Fig 5.28 Gaseous exchange

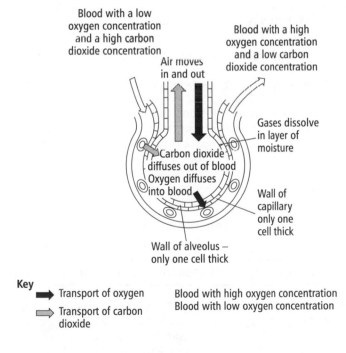

Section through alveolus showing gas exchange

Blood with a low oxygen concentration and a high carbon dioxide concentration

Blood with a high oxygen concentration and a low carbon dioxide concentration

Air moves in and out

Gases dissolve in layer of moisture

Carbon dioxide diffuses out of blood
Oxygen diffuses into blood

Wall of capillary only one cell thick

Wall of alveolus — only one cell thick

Key
→ Transport of oxygen
⇒ Transport of carbon dioxide

Blood with high oxygen concentration
Blood with low oxygen concentration

Digestive system

The main part of the digestive system is the alimentary canal, a long tube through which food passes and which starts at the mouth and ends at the anus. The remaining parts of the digestive system are the accessory organs, i.e. the salivary glands, pancreas, liver and biliary tract. Each part is linked both anatomically and physiologically as the process of digestion and absorption is dependent on the previous stage or stages.

Alimentary canal

The tissues of the alimentary canal are consistent from the oesophagus onwards with modifications dependent on role and function in the digestive and absorption processes. There are four layers:

- The outer layer is loose connective tissue and in the abdomen is covered by a serous membrane known as the peritoneum
- The muscle layer has two layers of smooth, involuntary muscle.
- The submucous layer contains the sympathetic and parasympathetic nerve endings from the autonomic nervous system.
- A mucous membrane lining provides protection and secretions, and maximises absorption.

Oesophagus

This is the first part of the alimentary canal and is about 25 cm long and 2 cm in diameter. It lies in front of the vertebral column and behind the trachea and heart. It is continuous with the pharynx and passes through the muscle fibres of the diaphragm then curves upwards (to prevent food regurgitation from the stomach) to join with the stomach. At each end of the oesophagus, there is s sphincter muscle. At the upper end, this sphincter prevents air passing into the oesophagus when breathing in, and stops food and liquid from the oesophagus from being inhaled. At the lower end, the sphincter prevents the acidic contents of the stomach from being regurgitated into the oesophagus.

The oesophagus is responsible for passing food into the stomach. The presence of food in the pharynx stimulates the involuntary smooth muscle contractions called peristalsis which push food downwards in a wave-like action. Peristalsis only occurs in the oesophagus after food is swallowed.

> **remember**
> The mucus secretions in the oesophagus aid the passage of food downwards to the stomach.

Stomach

This is the J-shaped muscular organ that has mucosal folds (rugae) that enable it to change shape and size depending on its contents and respiratory phase.

Refer back to page 159 to see the location of the stomach.

Like the oesophagus, the stomach has sphincter muscles, which are normally contracted, at each end (cardiac at the upper end and pyloric at the lower end). These ensure the stomach's acidic contents do not escape. Gastric glands in the lining of the stomach secrete two to three litres of gastric juice each day. This converts the food entering the stomach into semi-liquid chyme and produces an enzyme called protease which is responsible for beginning the breakdown of proteins. Gastric juice is acidic and the stomach is covered by a layer of cells that ensures the gastric juices do not breakdown the stomach wall. A number of digestive enzymes are produced in the stomach to break down food before it passes into the intestines where the absorption of nutrients takes place. The alimentary canal continues into the duodenum.

Duodenum

This is first and shortest part of the small intestine. It is C-shaped and about 25 cm long extending from the pyloric sphincter.

Refer back to page 159 to see the location of the duodenum.

The duodenum is divided into four parts with the pancreatic and bile ducts emptying the second (descending) part of the duodenum via a circular ring of involuntary muscle called the sphincter of Oddi. In the duodenal sub mucosa are glands called Brunner's glands. These secrete alkaline mucus which, along with pancreatic and bile salts, neutralise the acid chyme as it enters the duodenum from the stomach. This creates a slightly alkaline environment which assists the activation of pancreatic enzymes to ensure they work effectively in the intestines.

Extending from the duodenum is the jejunum which is about 2 m long. Both are concerned with the digestion and absorption of nutrients from food.

Ileum

The final part of the small intestine is the ileum which is about 3 m in length.

Refer back to page 159 to see the location of the ileum.

This is the main area where nutrients from food are absorbed. The lining of the ileum has circular folds called plicae with finger-like villi projecting from them. These increase the surface area of the ileum and so increase the digestion of the chyme and the absorption of nutrients as it passes through. At the base of the villi are glands that secrete intestinal juices which assist the digestive process. The ileum joins the colon at the ileo-caecal valve.

Colon

The colon is wider in diameter (about 6.5 cm) than the small intestine and about 1.5 m in length. The colon forms an arch around the small intestine. It is divided into the caecum, ascending colon, transverse colon and descending colon, sigmoid colon and the rectum. The rectum is about 16 to 20 cm long with the last 2 to 3 cm becoming the anal canal with the anus opening to the exterior of the body.

Refer back to page 159 to see the location of the colon.

The colon is made up of longitudinal muscle fibres. The arrangement of these fibres is different as they are not arranged as a continuous smooth layer but are collected in three bands, called taeniae coli, situated at regular intervals around the colon. These muscle fibres are shorter than the actual length of the colon and so this gives the colon its characteristic 'pouched' appearance. Sphincter muscles at the anus control excretion. The mucous membrane lining of the colon up to the rectum contains simple goblet cells that secrete mucus which helps to lubricate any **faeces** (waste) and ease its elimination from the body. The main purpose of the colon is to store indigestible food until it can be eliminated from the body as well as absorb most of the remaining water, mineral salts such as sodium and some vitamins. Bacteria in the colon also produce small quantities of vitamin K, B complex and folic acid as well as fermenting any remaining carbohydrates. This fermentation process produces gases (carbon dioxide, hydrogen and methane) and these contribute to flatulence. The amount of flatulence produced varies according to the type of food eaten. For example, onions, beans and some cabbage can increase the rate of fermentation and so increase flatulence. Bacteria in the colon also complete the breakdown of any remaining fatty acids or proteins and convert the pigment bilirubin into urobilinogen (which gives urine its characteristic colour) and stercobilirubin (which gives faeces its characteristic colour).

Liver

This is the largest gland in the body weighing 1 to 2.3 kg.

Refer back to page 159 to see the location of the liver.

The liver lies on the right side of the abdomen. It is covered in part by the peritoneum and folds of peritoneum form supportive ligaments to attach the liver to the lower surface of the diaphragm. The liver has four lobes, two at the front and two at the back. The right front lobe is larger than the wedge-shaped left front lobe. The liver is a very active organ and has many functions.

The liver produces a substance called bile. This is made up of water, mucus, a pigment called bilirubin, salts and cholesterol. Bile flows from the liver via the common bile duct into the duodenum entering through the sphincter of Oddi. Bile helps to emulsify (evenly disperse) fats to aid their digestion. The gall bladder is a reservoir for bile. It also adds mucus to the bile and concentres it by absorbing water in the bile. Fat, the acidity of chyme and a hormone produced by the duodenum all act to stimulate the gall bladder to contract and expel bile.

Pancreas

The pancreas is a pale grey gland, tapering in shape with its broad head lying in the loop of the duodenum and its thinner tail lying in front of the left kidney. It is 12 to 15 cm long, 2.5 cm thick and weighs about 60 grams.

Refer back to page 159 to see the location of the pancreas.

Fig 5.29 Functions of the liver

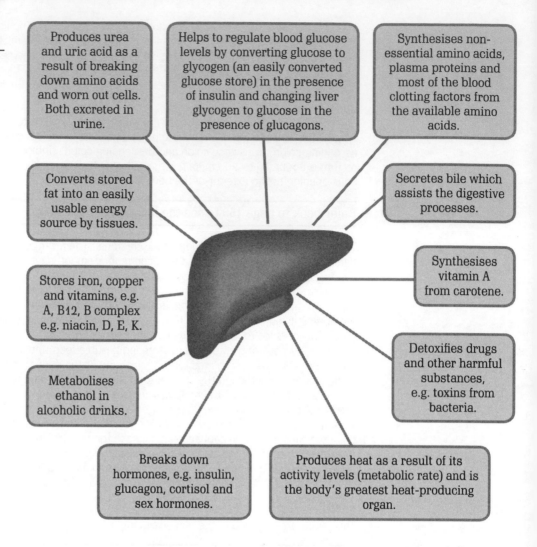

Produces urea and uric acid as a result of breaking down amino acids and worn out cells. Both excreted in urine.

Helps to regulate blood glucose levels by converting glucose to glycogen (an easily converted glucose store) in the presence of insulin and changing liver glycogen to glucose in the presence of glucagons.

Synthesises non-essential amino acids, plasma proteins and most of the blood clotting factors from the available amino acids.

Converts stored fat into an easily usable energy source by tissues.

Secretes bile which assists the digestive processes.

Synthesises vitamin A from carotene.

Stores iron, copper and vitamins, e.g. A, B12, B complex e.g. niacin, D, E, K.

Detoxifies drugs and other harmful substances, e.g. toxins from bacteria.

Metabolises ethanol in alcoholic drinks.

Breaks down hormones, e.g. insulin, glucagon, cortisol and sex hormones.

Produces heat as a result of its activity levels (metabolic rate) and is the body's greatest heat-producing organ.

The pancreas's role in the digestive process is an exocrine function, one which produces a product (pancreatic juice) through a duct. The cells involved in this function are lobules made up of small alveoli with secretory cells within their walls. Small ducts drain each lobule and these combine to form the pancreatic duct that runs the length of the gland joining the common bile duct to form the ampulla just before opening into the midpoint of the duodenum. Pancreatic juice is strongly alkaline (pH 8) and contains the enzymes amylase, peptidase and lipase that digest carbohydrates, proteins and fats. When the acidic stomach contents enter the duodenum, they mix with the pancreatic juice and bile and the pH is raised to between 6 and 8 thus enabling the pancreatic juice to work effectively.

The pancreas's other role in the production of the hormone insulin. This is an endocrine function, one which releases its product directly into the blood.

Salivary glands

There are three pairs of salivary glands which pour their secretions into the mouth to begin the process of food digestion.

■ Submandibular glands are positioned under the angle of the jaw opening onto the floor of the mouth.

■ Sublingual glands are positioned under the mucous membrane of the floor of the mouth and in front of the submandibular glands.

■ Parotid glands are positioned on each side of the face just below the ear opening into the back of the mouth near the molar teeth.

The salivary glands are surrounded by a fibrous capsule and consist of a number of lobules made up of small alveoli lined with secretory cells. Saliva is secreted by the salivary glands and this is made up of mineral salts, an enzyme, salivary amylase (ptyalin), lysozomes, immunoglobulins and blood clotting factors. The salivary glands produce the first of the digestive enzymes, salivary amylase which begins the breakdown of cooked starches changing them from polysaccharides to disaccharide maltose. The pH in the mouth depends on the rate of salivary flow: the more rapid the flow the higher the pH (alkalinity). The optimum pH for salivary amylase is slightly acid pH6.8.

The role of the digestive system in the breakdown and absorption of food materials

To summarise the digestive process, digestion begins at the mouth when food materials are ingested. The teeth begin the physical breakdown of food and the tongue assists with chewing and swallowing. The digestive process continues as the food bolus (the round mass of chewed food) passes into the oesophagus and as a result of peristalsis is pushed down the oesophagus and into the stomach. As food passes through the gastrointestinal tract (stomach and intestines), it is broken down by digestive enzymes that are present in each section of the tract. The stomach contains pepsin, an enzyme that starts the breakdown of proteins. Glands in the stomach wall produce acid which kill any germs ingested with the food and which also creates the correct environment for pepsin to work effectively. The food is partly digested when it leaves the stomach and goes into the duodenum and then into the ileum (small intestine). Muscles in the stomach and ileum churn the food and this action ensures that food and enzymes are mixed thoroughly and food molecules become dissolved. Digestive enzymes are also produced by the pancreas and ileum and they all cause a catalytic reaction (one which makes the reaction work faster) in the chemical digestion of food substances. A few substances such as cholesterol, glucose, water and vitamins can be digested without a chemical reaction. Nutrients, water, salts and vitamins are absorbed as the broken down food materials pass through the intestines before waste products and undigested food is egested (excreted) through the anus.

Role of enzymes in digestion

Enzymes play a crucial role in the breakdown and digestion of food materials. There are three main groups of enzymes:

- Amylases act upon carbohydrates.
- Proteases act upon proteins.
- Lipases that act upon fats.

The following table summarises the main enzymes, their site of secretion, their role in digestion and their product.

Role of enzymes in digestion

Enzyme	Site of secretion	Role in digestion	Product
Salivary amylase (ptyalin)	Mouth	Begins breakdown of cooked starches	Polysaccharides to disaccharide – maltose
Pepsinogen – converts to pepsin	Stomach	Breaks down proteins	Polypeptides
Pancreatic amylase	Pancreas	Acts in the small intestine to breakdown starches	Disaccharides (maltose)
Enterokinase	Small intestine	Activates trypsinogen	Trypsin
Trypsinogen converts to trypsin	Pancreas	Trypsin acts on large protein molecules (polypeptides) breaking them down into smaller protein molecules. Also acts on chymotrypsinogen	Peptides Chymotrypsin
Chymotrypsinogen converts to chymotrypsin	Pancreas	Chymotrypsin acts on polypeptides	Peptides
Carboxypeptidases and aminopeptidases	Pancreas	Act on peptides to break them down into smaller peptides	Oligopeptides
Lipase	Pancreas	Acts on large glycerol molecules (e.g. triglycerol) to detach fatty acids and glycerol	Diglycerides, monoglycerides, fatty acids and glycerol
Nucleases	Pancreas	Essential to enable the body to use the nuclear components of cells of ingested food. Acts on nucleic acids (**RNA**) to break them down	Nucleotides

Enzyme	Site of secretion	Role in digestion	Product
Disaccharidases (maltase, sucrase and lactase)	Small intestine	Acts on disaccharides (maltose, sucrose and lactose) to break them down into small molecules	Glucose, fructose and galactose
Peptidases	Small intestine	Acts on oligopeptides to break them down	Amino acids
Nucleotidases and Nucleosidases	Small intestine	Acts on nucleotides to produce nucleosides. Nucleosidase then works on nucleosides	Nucleosides, phosphoric acid, sugars, purines and pyrimidines (RNA and DNA derivatives)

Major products of digestion

The process of food breakdown to enable nutrients to be utilised in the body produces energy and heat. Metabolism is used to describe the series of interrelated chemical interactions that make up this process.

Refer back to page 164 for more information about metabolism.

Peptides and amino acids

Peptides and amino acids are the basic units of protein that are essential for health. They are involved in the building and repair of body tissues. Amino acids are transferred into the blood capillaries of the villi of the small intestine and then circulated to the liver where they are further broken down so their components can be utilised by body tissues and cells. If the intake of proteins is in excess of the body's requirements for building and repair function or immediate energy, the amino acids will be broken down in the liver. The nitrogenous part of the amino acid will be converted by the process of deamination into urea which is then excreted by the kidney in the urine. The remainder will be stored as fat, for example under the skin, around the kidneys and in the abdomen.

Sugars

When carbohydrates are metabolised, the glucose that makes them up is absorbed into the blood capillaries of the villi and mircovilli of the small intestine and then circulated to the liver where it is synthesised. Some glucose will be used to provide energy to fuel body activities, while some will remain circulating in the blood to maintain the blood glucose level. In the liver and muscles, the action of insulin will convert some glucose into glycogen so it can be stored for later use. The action of other hormones, such as adrenaline, thyroxine and glucagons, reverse this process changing glycogen to glucose when needed. Any excess carbohydrate is converted into fat and stored as fat. All cells require energy to function and, although some energy can be produced without oxygen being present (anaerobic process), most of the body's energy requirements are met through the aerobic oxidation (adding oxygen) of carbohydrate and fat.

The process of carbohydrate oxidation requires a good oxygen supply and this produces energy, carbon dioxide and water. Energy from anaerobic processes is not as efficient in releasing all the energy from the glucose molecules as aerobic oxidation, although it can be maintained for a short time (for example, the energy for the flight or fight response that the outpouring of adrenaline produces). As the energy conversion is inefficient, it produces a by-product, lactic acid, which if it accumulates in the muscles can cause pain and discomfort following an unusual level or intensity of exercise.

Fatty acids and glycerol

The fatty acids and glycerol produced when fat is metabolised circulate in the blood and provides energy for organs and glands to undertake their functions. In the liver, some fatty acids and glycerol provide heat and energy while others are reorganised and recombined to form other fatty compounds. Excess fatty acids are taken up by fat cells and changed to natural fat and stored ready for reconversion when required for energy. The end products of fat metabolism are energy, heat, carbon dioxide and water.

When fats are oxidised, ketone bodies and ketone acid is produced and excreted in the urine and in expired air as acetone. Excessive amounts of keto acids in the body are toxic to brain cells.

Absorption of food

Nutrients resulting from the breakdown of food materials are absorbed mainly in the small and large intestines. The ileum absorbs about 90% of nutrients and is well adapted for this absorption process with its large surface area, created by its length and the presence of folds, plicae and finger-like projections of villi and microvilli. It also has a thin absorbent epithelium and extensive blood and lymphatic supplies, all of which contribute to the ease with which nutrients are absorbed. Nutrients are absorbed into the blood through the processes of facilitated diffusion (carried by another substance) and passive diffusion (movement from high concentrations to low concentrations).

The finger-like projections or villi, have walls made up of columnar epithelial cells (enterocytes) with tiny microvilli on their free border. They are interspersed with mucus-secreting goblet cells. The enterocytes have a network of blood and lymph capillaries (lacteals). The lacteals absorb fat giving them their milky appearance. Absorption and some final nutrient digestion take place in the enterocytes before entering the blood and lymph capillaries.

Fig 5.30 Cross-section of ileum villi

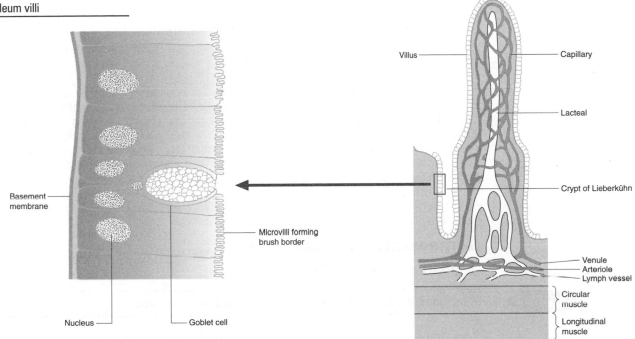

How homeostatic mechanisms operate in the maintenance of an internal environment

 Link

See Unit 13, in BTEC National Health and Social Care Book 2, for more information about homeostatic mechanisms.

Homeostasis

Homeostasis is the term used to describe the state of equilibrium (balance) that exists in the internal environment of the human body to enable systems to function at their optimum (most efficient) level. Homeostasis involves monitoring 'normal' levels (i.e. levels that occur in around 95% of the population), and instigating action to regulate if change is identified.

Homeostasis maintains:

- body temperature, normally 37°C and regulated by the nervous and endocrine systems
- water potential, regulated by the endocrine system and kidney
- blood pH, normally 7.35 to7.45 and regulated by the nervous and endocrine systems

■ oxygen and carbon dioxide concentrations, regulated by the nervous and respiratory systems

■ blood glucose, regulated by endocrine system.

Internal environment

Even small changes in the body's internal environment can considerably disrupt normal functioning and be detrimental to an individual's well-being. However, it is important to remember that this adaptive mechanism is also of benefit to humans as it enables them to cope with different circumstances, such as when exercising or during pregnancy.

During pregnancy, the levels of oestrogen and progesterone in a woman's body are considerably higher than they are when she is not pregnant. The variations in hormone levels are necessary to maintain pregnancy and ensure the development of the unborn baby. During this time, the variations in homeostatic range are considered to be normal given the changed inner environment of the body.

To ensure efficient body functioning however, homeostasis needs to be carefully monitored. For example, if blood glucose levels or temperature is either too high or too low this can be fatal. Homeostasis works through a process called negative feedback.

Negative feedback as a regulatory mechanism

If the inner environment becomes unbalanced, i.e. there is a change to the norm in any of the areas regulated by homeostasis, this triggers the body to act to restore the balance as quickly as possible before there is an impact on body function. For example, if there is a drop below a normal level of a substance within the body, the body takes action to increase the level to bring it back to the norm. Sometimes only one homeostatic control mechanism is required to redress the balance, such as when blood glucose levels rise beyond normal limits the hormone insulin is released to remove glucose from the circulating blood. However, if the situation cannot be redressed quickly the effects on the body's internal environment mean that other normal ranges are affected, for example not only a raised blood glucose level but also a change in blood pH (acidosis). In these circumstances, more than one control is needed to bring about equilibrium. So, continuing the previous example, chemical buffers will try and neutralize the acidic environment, respiratory rate will increase to try and excrete more carbon dioxide and the kidneys will excrete more acidic urine.

Homeostatic mechanisms

Regulation of heart rate

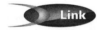

Refer back to page 167 to remind yourself about heart rate.

The heart has internal receptors that along with the sinoatrial node (SA node) are responsible for initiating and conducting the electrical messages through the heart that regulate heart rate. It is the SA node that controls heart rate although other factors such as hormones, autonomic nervous system and chemical imbalances in body tissues can also have an impact.

Blood pressure is the force or pressure that the blood exerts on the blood vessel walls. The cardiovascular, nervous, endocrine and renal systems work together to regulate heart rate and blood pressure.

The medulla oblongata in the brainstem has two cardiac centres controlling autonomic nerve activity to the heart. The cardiac accelerator centre controls sympathetic nerve activity and the cardiac inhibitory centre controls parasympathetic nerve activity. Neurons from both centres innervate (stimulate) nerve cells in the heart wall and these stimulate the SA and AV nodes as well as heart muscle. Sympathetic stimulation raises the heart rate, for example in exercise or stress, and parasympathetic stimulation lowers the rate. In normal conditions, both the sympathetic and parasympathetic systems are active in order to maintain the heart rate at the optimum level. A number of factors will affect the heart rate.

remember
The heart rate and blood pressure are interlinked as the one affects the other.

■ Changes in blood volume, for example a decrease due to haemorrhaging (excessive bleeding), reduce the pressure being exerted on blood vessel walls and so the blood pressure falls. This stimulates the sympathetic nervous system which in turn stimulates the adrenal glands. The adrenal glands secrete noradrenaline and adrenaline which cause vasoconstriction (tightening) in peripheral blood vessels and increase the force of heart muscle contraction. These changes increase the blood pressure and the heart rate. The secretion of these hormones in other circumstances, such as the 'flight or fight response', cause increased heart rate to ensure sufficient oxygen is being pumped to the lungs to meet the increased oxygen demands of the muscles.

- If the parasympathetic neurons are activated, for example in severe depression, the affect of acetylcholine decreases the heart rate and when activated to a maximum it can cause the heart rate to decrease to 20 to 30 bpm. Maximum activation of the sympathetic neurons can mean the heart rate reaches 200 bpm.

- Over-secretion of the hormone thyroxine when, for example, the thyroid gland is enlarged, causes an increase in heart rate. This change takes place over a longer period of time than the effects of adrenaline and noradrenaline.

- Chemical imbalances in the body tissues, in particular the relative concentrations of potassium, calcium and sodium, also stimulate changes to the heart rate. For example, higher (or lower) than normal levels of potassium result in increased (or decreased) cardiac stimulation and this raises (or lowers) the heart rate.

- Changes in blood pressure stimulate a response by the renal system to either increase or decrease circulating blood volume and concentration.

- A raised body temperature also affects heart rate as the SA and AV nodes of the heart are activated more frequently. If the body is exposed to cold for a period of time and there is a drop in temperature, then this decreases the heart rate.

Regulation of breathing rate

The control of breathing is partly voluntary but mainly involuntary as it is essential that we keep doing it and not forget if we are to stay alive! We exert voluntary control when undertaking activities such as singing, speaking, during exercise and swimming underwater.

Voluntary control is overridden by involuntary responses from the nerve cells in respiratory centre in the brain stem (medulla oblongata) which stimulate the stretch receptors in the lung, intercostal muscles and diaphragm to stretch and so inspiration (breathing in) takes place.

Nerve cells in another part of the brain (the pneumotaxic centre in the pons varolii) are responsible for stimulating expiration (breathing out).

Respiratory chemoreceptors are found in the brainstem and these monitor acidity levels of the cerebrospinal fluid and the base respiratory rate. It is the peripheral chemoreceptors in the blood vessel walls, especially the aorta arch and where the common carotid arteries divide, that are responsible for continuously monitor levels of oxygen, carbon dioxide and acidity in the blood. Changes to oxygen or carbon dioxide levels (and resultant increase in acidity) stimulate these receptors to send impulses to the respiratory centres of the brain to increased breathing rate to try and reinstate homeostasis. Changes in carbon dioxide levels appear to have a greater stimulating effect on respiratory rate.

During exercise, the breathing becomes deeper and faster as the muscles of the body require more oxygen and to excrete the resultant higher levels of carbon dioxide. The increase in respiratory rate is in part due to the action of the sympathetic nervous system which stimulates the production of adrenaline and this relaxes and dilates the bronchioles in the lungs to increase the volume of air entering the lungs to maximise the potential take up of oxygen from arterial blood. The parasympathetic nervous system acts on the airways to decrease the diameter and in so doing decrease the respiratory rate.

Regulation of body temperature

Production of heat by the body

Heat is produced by the body as a result of metabolic reactions within the body. The optimum core temperature (i.e. the temperature of the brain and organs) for efficient metabolism in humans is a fairly constant 37°C. Homeostatic controls are needed to maintain the balance of heat production by metabolism and heat loss from the body through the skin and respiration. If there is a variation in temperature, the cardiovascular, endocrine and nervous systems all work together to reinstate the equilibrium. The receptors that detect changes to the body's core temperature are located in the hypothalamus, in the brain. The skin also has temperature receptors.

Loss of heat from the body

Heat is lost through four main processes: radiation, conduction, convection and evaporation.

- Radiation: Any physical body with a temperature above absolute zero (0°K) will radiate energy in the form of waves. The body temperature of humans radiates energy in the form of infrared waves and can only be detected using specialised equipment. Most heat is either gained or lost from the body by radiation is the way. The amount of loss or gain is determined by the difference between skin temperature and the external environment.

■ Conduction: This is the direct transfer of energy between molecules that connect with one another physically. Conduction results when molecules connect within the skin as well as when air or an object, such as a heat pad or ice cube, connects with the skin externally. The rate at which heat transfers between molecules depends on the difference in temperatures between the two.

■ Convection: This is the circulation of air or water around the skin. The rate at which heat is transferred relates to the level of difference between the temperatures of the skin

Fig 5.31 Body temperature flowchart (low temperature)

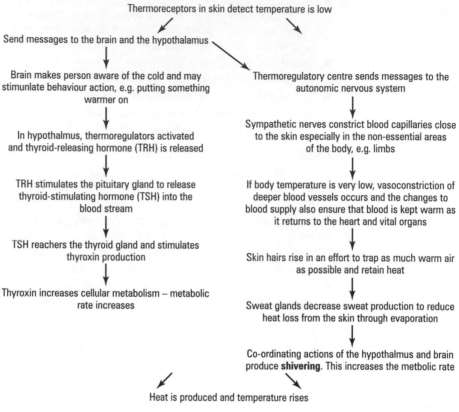

Fig 5.32 Body temperature flowchart (high temperature)

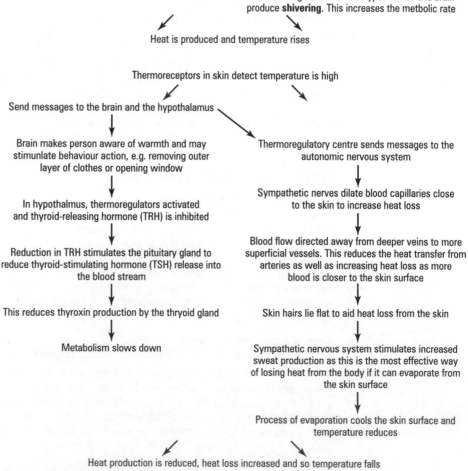

and the external environment: the greater the difference, the quicker the transfer. The circulation of air or water around the skin creates a new environment and this can either speed up or slow down the process of heat transfer. Convection is not in itself a means of heat transfer instead it facilitates the process of conduction.

■ Evaporation: This is the process by which a liquid changes to a vapour, and requires energy. The evaporation of sweat from the skin or the loss of water from the mouth and respiratory tract as part of respiration are the body's mechanisms for losing heat energy.

The hypothalamus and the autonomic nervous system

The hypothalamus is part of the endocrine system and controls involuntary functions including daily metabolic rhythm and body temperature. Within the hypothalamus, there is a thermoregulatory (temperature-regulating) centre which monitors blood temperature and takes action if there is a variation beyond normal ranges.

Temperature change stimulates the thermoreceptors in both the hypothalamus (internal changes) and the skin (external changes). To effect temperature regulation the hypothalamus has both heat gain and heat loss centres. When the thermoreceptors detect that the body temperature is lower than the optimum 37°C, the heat gain centre inhibits the activity of the heat loss centre and sends impulses to the skin, hair erector muscles, sweat glands and elsewhere to decrease heat loss and increase heat production.

Shivering is cased by involuntary muscle contractions or twitching and is the normal physiological response by the body at it attempts to increase heat production and warm the body. This action is accompanied by the hair erector muscles contracting and raising the hair on the skin in an attempt to trap warm air circulating around it and retain the heat within the body.

When the thermoreceptors detect a higher body temperature then it is the heat gain centre activity that is inhibited by the heat loss centre. The hair erector muscles relax and so flatten the hair on to the skin which aids heat loss when the body temperature is too high. The sweat glands only produce sweat when the body needs to lose heat. The sweat evaporates from the skin surface which assists in cooling the skin and aiding heat loss.

Internally, the arterioles supplying the blood capillaries widen (vasodilation) when the body needs to lose heat and becomes narrower (vasoconstriction) when the body needs to retain heat.

The skin is the largest organ in the body and in an adult this extends to about 1.8 m². This is where most body heat is lost. The body's surface area influences heat loss in cool environments while body volume influences heat generation through metabolism. The ratio of surface area to body volume affects body temperature. The limbs have the greatest surface area to body volume ratio and so the limbs generally are much cooler than the chest and abdomen. The surface area to body volume ratio is important to consider especially for babies whose temperature regulatory mechanisms are underdeveloped and where there is a relatively large surface area to body volume ratio. This means that babies are inclined to lose more heat than they can generate and so need to be cared for in an environment that has a more consistent temperature as they are less able to cope with temperature changes.

case study 5.1   Body temperature

Older people also find it more difficult to maintain their body temperature due to the effects of aging, such as the reduced capacity to shiver, slower metabolic rate and fewer sweat glands in the body. This makes them vulnerable to the effects of temperature extremes. Each winter a significant number of older people die as a result of hypothermia (body temperature below 35.5°C).

During the French heat wave between 4th and 13th August 2003, the majority of the 15,000 extra deaths that occurred were of people over 65 years old as a result of hyperthermia (body temperature above 40.6°C) and associated factors such as dehydration, respiratory problems, related to the prolonged high temperatures (between 35 to 40°C when the seasonal normal was 25°C). During the same period in England and Wales, it was estimated that over 2,000 more deaths occurred than normal.

activity
INDIVIDUAL WORK

1   Explain, using examples, what action could be taken to prevent deaths from hypothermia in winter.

2   What could be done to prevent deaths from hyperthermia during a prolonged period of higher than normal temperatures?

Regulation of blood glucose levels

Refer back to page 176 to remind yourself about the role of glucose in the body.

Glucose is an important energy source for the body and consequently levels of glucose circulating around the body in the blood need to be maintained at a fairly constant level to ensure the body functions effectively and efficiently. However, there are times when glucose levels change considerably due to the normal activities of daily living. For example, blood glucose levels rise after eating (the extent depends on what is eaten) and fall after exercise or if there has been a long period without eating, for example first thing in the morning. To try and minimise the extent of the swings in the blood glucose levels, the pancreas produces two hormones which work in opposition to one another. These hormones are insulin, which acts to reduce the blood glucose level, and glucagon, which acts to increase the blood glucose level. The level of blood glucose is monitored by the pancreas and the appropriate hormone is released to increase or decrease the blood glucose level.

Blood glucose levels

Blood glucose levels too HIGH	Blood glucose levels too LOW
Receptors in the pancreas send messages to the brain to indicate a feeling of satiety (fullness) which then stimulates the individual to stop eating	Receptors in the pancreas send messages to the brain to indicate a feeling of hunger which stimulates the individual to eat
Stimulates β cells in the pancreas to release insulin	Stimulates α cells in the pancreas to release glucagon
Reduces level of glucose in blood plasma	Increases level of glucose in blood plasma
Utilises excess glucose by increasing respiration rate	Reduces respiratory rate to slow down the rate that glucose is used
Removes glucose from blood plasma by increasing glucose absorption by the liver and body tissues	Reduces glucose absorption by the liver and other body tissues and stimulates the liver to convert amino acids into glucose
Converts glucose into glycogen so that it can be stored	Releases glycogen from liver and muscles where it is stored and converts it back into glucose (glycogenolysis); promotes the conversion of fatty acids into glucose (gluconeogenisis)
Blood glucose level falls	Blood glucose level rises
Blood glucose level returns to within normal limits (between 4 to 7 mmol/l)	

case study 5.2 — Diabetes mellitus

Diabetes mellitus is a condition where the blood glucose levels are higher than normal limits. There are two main types of diabetes.

- Type 1 diabetes is the least common type of diabetes occurring in 5 to 15% of all diabetics. It usually develops before the age of 40 years and is due to the body's inability to produce insulin. This is treated by regular insulin injections (two to four per day) and diet management.

- Type 2 diabetes occurs in 85 to 95% of all diabetics and usually occurs after 40 years of age. In this type, the body still produces some insulin but it is either not enough or it is not effective in controlling blood glucose levels. Type 2 diabetes is linked to being overweight. However people of South Asian and African-Caribbean origin may develop Type 2 diabetes after the age of 25 years. More recently, Type 2 diabetes has been diagnosed in children. This is usually treated with lifestyle changes such as healthier diet, increased exercise and weight loss. In addition, the person may be given medication or insulin treatment. The main aim of treatment is to regulate blood glucose levels, blood pressure and cholesterol to within normal limits and so reduce the potential risks to well-being. This is substantially supported by a healthy lifestyle.

In the UK there are currently over two million people with diabetes and it is estimated that as many as 750,000 are unaware they have the condition. In 1999, the government launched a National Service Framework for Diabetes setting out 12 standards to improve prevention, identification, care and long term management of diabetes.

In the short term, a faulty blood glucose control can cause life threatening situations, for example, if the blood glucose level either rises to excess levels (hyperglycemia) or falls too low (hypoglycemia) for normal body functioning. A person with diabetes is taught the early warning signs of these situations and what action to take to prevent the situation deteriorating. However, sometimes this is too late or insufficient to prevent either the need for emergency treatment or, in some cases, death.

High levels of glucose circulating in the blood stream are damaging to the blood vessels. There is an increased risk of fatty deposits on the blood vessel walls (arteriosclerosis) which narrows the lumen (opening) and constricts blood flow. Thus the complications that can arise as a result of uncontrolled diabetes are serious and widespread. For example, people with diabetes are more at risk of developing vascular disease, heart disease and stroke, problems with eyesight (retinopathy), kidney disease, neuropathy (poor conduction of nerve impulses) and skin problems.

---

activity
GROUP WORK

Discuss the following questions:

1   What constitutes a healthy diet?

2   How can individuals reduce their risk of developing diabetes?

Diabetes UK - Measure up	www.diabetes.org.uk/measureup
Department of Health	www.dh.gov.uk
Diabetes UK	www.diabetes.org.uk

---

activity
GROUP WORK
5.6

P5

1   Describe what is meant by homeostasis.

2   Draw a diagram which describes the homeostatic mechanisms that regulate:

- heart rate
- breathing rate
- body temperature
- blood glucose levels.

---

activity
INDIVIDUAL WORK
5.7

D2

Explain why maintaining homeostasis is vital if the body is to function effectively and remain healthy.

Interpreting data obtained from monitoring routine variations in the functioning of healthy body systems

Measurements

Taking physiological measurements in order to monitor and record body functions is an important part of health and to a lesser extent social care work, as these measurement establish a baseline and help to identify changes in homeostasis. These relatively non-invasive procedures provide vital information about an individual's well-being and are quick and easy to perform. When recorded over a period of time, they also give clear information about patterns of change and the effectiveness or otherwise of various medical and nursing interventions, such as reduction of anxiety, oxygen therapy or medication.

Before undertaking any measurements, it is important to ensure that you have all the equipment you require, that you are competent in its use and it is ready, clean and safe to use. You must also ensure that your hands and any equipment used are cleaned effectively before and after working with each individual. You must also check that you have the individual's current records and are aware of any specific instructions regarding that individual and the manner of taking the physiological measurements, such as safe practice before and after activity measurements. Before beginning, ensure the individual is comfortable. For example make sure they are not in pain and do not need to use the toilet, as these factors can raise the pulse and respiratory rates. Make sure too that you can clearly observe the individual.

Pulse rate

The radial pulse can be located by placing two fingers (1st and 2nd) on the inner part of the forearm just below where the wrist bends and just down from the base of the thumb. To feel the pulse, gently press down using three fingers (not your thumb as this has a pulse) and slightly inwards towards the bone until you can feel a rhythmic beat. The pulse rate tells us how fast the heart is beating (measured as beats per minute) while the rhythm tells the regularity of heart activity.

The strength and the firmness of pressure required to locate the pulse tells us about heart function, cardiac output and blood pressure. If the pulse is faint, this indicates the blood pressure is low, such as when person is shocked or injured. An irregular pulse may indicate underlying problems and requires investigation. The pulse rate can vary for a number of reasons. For example, it will change depending on the person's position, i.e. lying or standing, temperature, age, gender, physical activity, physical fitness and emotional state.

The pulse can be located in other areas of the human body and each pulse point is named after the artery associated with it. These other pulse points may be used if the radial pulse is weak, for example if the individual has collapsed and requires resuscitation. In babies and children under two years of age it is usually more accurate to measure the apical pulse using a stethoscope, as the pulse rate can be affected by crying, feeding and movement. The apical pulse is also used if the individual has an irregular heart beat.

Fig 5.33 Taking a radial pulse

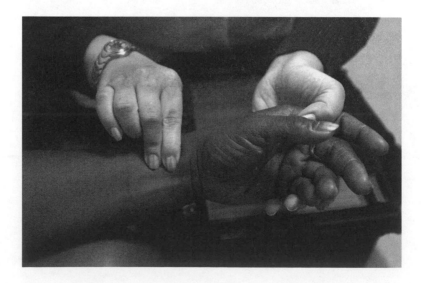

Fig 5.34 Pulse points in the
human body

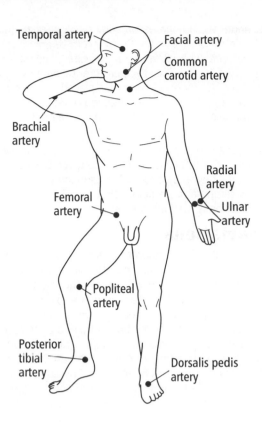

Breathing rate

The rate at which a complete respiratory cycle occurs in a 60-second period is known as the breathing rate. A respiratory cycle is one breath in (inspiration) and one breath out (expiration). The respiratory rate is affected by a number of factors, including activity, emotional state (calm, frightened or anxious), humidity (the level of moisture in the air), lung capacity and function, age and physical fitness. Altitude (height above sea level) affects the oxygen concentration in the air, with lower oxygen concentration occurring at higher altitudes, so respiration rate increases at higher altitudes in an attempt to meet the body's oxygen requirements.

To measure breathing rate, it is best to position yourself where you can clearly see the individual's chest movements. If it is difficult to see chest movements, you could either put your hand on the individual's chest and count the number of rises and falls or place your face close to their mouth and nose and count the number of breaths you can feel on your cheek. Observe and, using a watch with a second hand, count the number of complete cycles in a 60-second period.

Normal ranges of pulse and respiration rates

Age	Pulse rate (beats per minute)	Respiration rate (breaths per minute)
Newborn	120–140	40
Babies and children up to 5 years	1–5 yrs 105–110	40
Children up to 10 years	90–110	25
10 years old to adult	60–80	16

Variations in the pulse rate of 20 beats per minute would be considered significant if all other factors had been considered, for example, exercise or fitness level.

Temperature

The core temperature of an individual (i.e. the temperature of the brain and organs) is being measured and this can be access through the mouth, ear or anus or in the armpit. The recorded temperature may vary slightly depending on where the temperature reading is taken. A temperature of 37˚C should be measured by an oral reading, taken by placing a thermometer under the tongue, or an aural reading, taken in the ear using an electrical thermometer with a thermistor at the tip to record temperature change. For accurate readings place the thermistor close to the eardrum. A rectal temperature is usually slightly higher at around 37.5°C. An axilla temperature, taken under the armpit, will be slightly lower at around 36.5°C. Thermometer strips placed on the forehead provide an approximate measurement and are a quick and easy method of determining if the individual is too hot or too cold. These are useful for checking a child's temperature but not as accurate as using a thermometer.

In young children, the core temperature is slightly higher between 37.5°C and 38°C. Hypothermia is identifies as being when the body temperature is 35.5°C or lower. Hyperthermia (fever or pyrexia) is identified as being when the body temperature is 39°C or above. If the body temperature is below 25°C or if it reaches about 42°C then the person will die as a result of body systems collapsing.

Normal variations

There are normal variations in relation to pulse, temperature and respiratory rate dependent on the level of activity being undertaken or the situation. For example, if an individual is frightened, the outpouring of adrenaline creates the 'fight or flight' response which raises the heart and respiratory rate as well as the temperature. An individual's level of general fitness will also have and impact on measurements. The greater the level of physical fitness, the higher the level of physical activity before there are increases in heart and respiratory rate and temperature rise and associated sweating. It is important therefore to undertake physiological measurements at rest to establish a baseline when trying to determine the body's capacity to cope with stress of any kind. Physiological measurements taken during exercise or stress as well as the time taken by the body to recover from exercise or stress and return to the baseline (resting values) indicate the body's capacity to cope and fitness level. One standard exercise test is the Harvard step test used to establish fitness levels.

To do this, using a step 45 cm high, the individual steps up and down once every two seconds for five minutes (total 150 steps).

- One minute after completing the test take pulse rate (pulse 1)
- Two minutes after completing the test take pulse rate (pulse 2)
- Three minutes after completing the test take pulse rate (pulse 3)

To calculate the level of fitness, use the following equation:

Level of fitness = 30000 ÷ pulse 1 + pulse 2 + pulse 3

The higher the score, the better the level of the individual's fitness. This is useful when measuring the effectiveness of a fitness training programme.

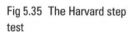

Fig 5.35 The Harvard step test

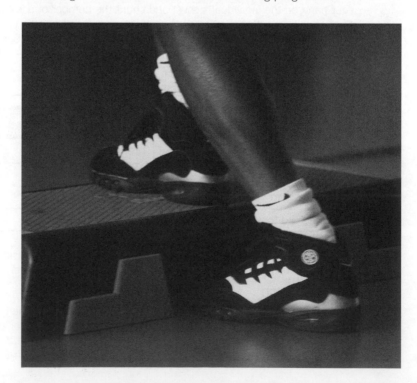

Data presentation and interpretation

Information collected as a result of taking physiological measurements must be recorded accurately and interpreted so that decisions can be made about appropriate responses and actions. Information is generally recorded on graphs or charts and supporting explanations or the data collected recorded in the individual's care, nursing or medical notes.

Graphs and charts

Graphs and charts usually record only quantitative (numerical) data although sometimes qualitative information may also be recorded, such as whether the pulse was taken at rest or following exercise. Graphs and charts are a good means for recording numerical data as it is easer to see patterns, trends, improvements and declines and link these to interventions, such as giving analgesia or increasing oxygen levels.

Fig 5.36 Temperature, pulse and respiratory rate chart

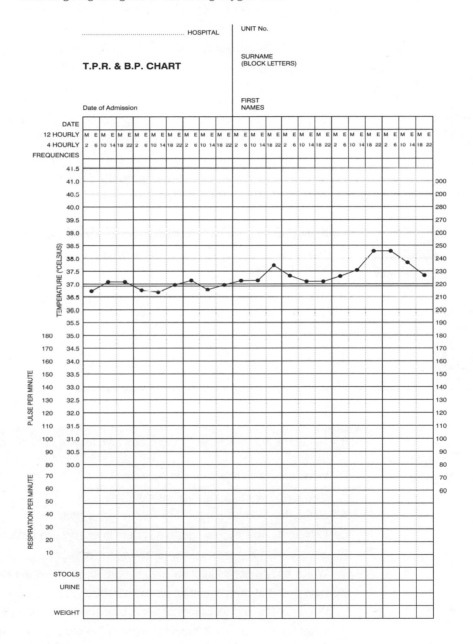

Supporting explanations of collated data

Numerical data alone can be misleading and not reveal the whole picture and so it is important to include an explanation to support collated data. This could be information relating to what the individual was doing at the time, for example how they coped with an activity such as an exercise stress test, their level of comfort or distress while undertaking the test, your observations of skin colour, sweating, and so on. If an individual is unwell and has a fever, other observations may also be relevant, such as skin colour and elasticity, and cognitive state (confused or alert). In relation to respiration, it is important that information about the effort taken to breathe, skin colour around the nose and mouth and the type of breathing (i.e. mouth or diaphragmatic breathing only, shallow breaths) is also recorded. When measuring the pulse rate, the regularity and strength of the pulse are important factors to be considered. If the physiological measurements and supporting explanations are taken together these help to provide a comprehensive picture of the individual's well-being.

activity
GROUP WORK 5.8

P6

1   Working in pairs, measure each other's body temperature, heart and breathing rate.
2   Take it in turns to undertake five minutes of active exercise, such as the Harvard step test.
3   Measure body temperature, heart and breathing rates at intervals of one minute, two minutes and three minutes following exercise completion.
4   Record the data collected on a chart or graph.
5   Discuss the data and comment on its validity.

activity
INDIVIDUAL WORK 5.9

M2

M3

1   Explain how the body makes internal changes to ensure that homeostasis is maintained during exercise.
2   Analyse the data obtained from activity 5.8. In your analysis, show how homeostatic mechanisms control the internal environment during exercise.

Progress Check

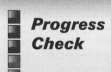

1   Name the four main body tissues and give an example of where each may be found.
2   What are the five main forms of energy?
3   How does the body produce energy?
4   Name the different parts of the respiratory system.
5   Explain the role of the digestive system in energy production.
6   Explain what is meant by the term *homeostasis*.
7   Which body systems interact to maintain homeostasis during exercise?
8   How does the body maintain its temperature?
9   What are the normal ranges of heart rate and how would you measure it?
10 What factors can affect the reliability of physiological measurements?

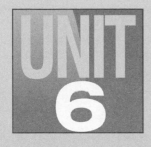

Personal and professional development in health and social care

This unit covers:

- The learning process
- Planning for, monitoring and reflecting on own development
- Service provision in the health or social care sectors

This unit enables the learner to bring together their learning from all the other units and place it in the vocational context of the qualification. It will enable the learner to make links between their study of theory and the practice of their vocational work experience.

Learners will explore the concepts of learning and relate these to their own preferred learning style. They will also explore factors that affect learning, including their own learning, the different ways in which learning can take place and how learning from individual experiences can be used to enhance the quality of knowledge, skills and practice.

Learners will consider their own knowledge, skills, practice, values and beliefs in relation to working in health and social care. They will draw up a personal development plan for the programme based on their personal abilities, learning and development needs, goals and career aspirations. They will monitor and review their progress at regular intervals through the programme and make appropriate adjustments as circumstances change. They will draw on a range of information sources to assess their personal and professional development including their vocational work experience, formal study, employment or voluntary activities.

They will also consider health and social care service provision and the fundamentals of research methodology.

grading criteria	To achieve a **Pass** grade the evidence must show that the learner is able to:	To achieve a **Merit** grade the evidence must show that, in addition to the pass criteria, the learner is able to:	To achieve a **Distinction** grade the evidence must show that, in addition to the pass and merit criteria, the learner is able to:
	P1 explain key influences on personal learning processes of individuals Pg 198	**M1** analyse the impact of key influences on personal learning processes on own learning Pg 198	**D1** evaluate how personal learning and development may benefit others Pg 207
	P2 describe own knowledge, skills, practice, values, beliefs and career aspirations at start of programme Pg 213		

grading criteria

To achieve a **Pass** grade the evidence must show that the learner is able to:	To achieve a **Merit** grade the evidence must show that, in addition to the pass criteria, the learner is able to:	To achieve a **Distinction** grade the evidence must show that, in addition to the pass and merit criteria, the learner is able to:
P3 produce and monitor an action plan for self-development and the achievement of own personal goals Pg 216		
P4 describe own progress against action plan over the duration of the programme Pg 223	**M2** explain how the action plan has helped support own development over the duration of the programme Pg 223	**D2** evaluate own development over the duration of the programme Pg 224
P5 produce and reflect on own personal and professional development portfolio Pg 225	**M3** reflect on own experiences and use three examples to explain links between theory and practice Pg 225	
P6 describe one local health or social care service provider and identify its place in national provision Pg 229		
P7 describe the roles, responsibilities and career pathways of three health or social care workers Pg 235		

The learning process

The way that individuals learn as adults have been found to be different to the way children learn. Adults have a wealth of experience to contribute to their learning as well as individual preferences and barriers to learning.

Theories of learning

Adult learning is different from childhood learning for a number of main reasons. Firstly, adults, being used to independence, are more inclined to be self-directing in their learning. Secondly, personal experience plays a large part in learning, as new ideas are checked against experience before being either rejected or, if accepted, grafted onto exiting knowledge frameworks. Thirdly, the purpose for learning is different for adults and is often associated with either a work role or social role. Learning becomes a chosen activity as the individual determines for themselves what they need to know rather than being given little choice. Lastly, the type of learning changes as adults mature and is often related to problem-solving or undertaking specific projects or tasks and so the individual can see the relevance to their life and the benefits that can result.

David Kolb produced his work on experiential learning in 1984 which expressed his belief that adults learned through discovery and experience. Kolb's work was based in the intellectual traditions and experiential work of Piaget, Lewin, Dewey and others. Kolb's experiential learning cycle provides a holistic model where experience plays a central role in the learning process. It is consistent with what is known about human growth, learning and development and is multi-linear. Peter Honey and Alan Mumford developed a theory concerning the preferred learning styles of individual based on four learning types. It remains the most widely used learning theory.

Kolb's experiential learning cycle

Kolb believes that learning is a four stage cycle: experiencing, reflecting, thinking and acting. For learning to be a complete, an individual must complete each aspect. An individual will experience something which leads to observations and reflections on the experience. Their reflections are then absorbed and translated into abstract models, theories, concepts and ideas, in an effort to make sense of what they have learned in relation to what they already know. The final stage of the learning cycle is when the learning is applied to practice and actively tested out to see if it works or the practice can be changed or adapted as a result. The application of learning to practice will lead to a different concrete experience and so the cycle continues. Kolb identified four learning styles to describe individual learning preferences which combined two of the stages of the learning cycle.

Kolb considers that all individuals have a preferred learning style and various factors influence this. Kolb identified three stages of an individual's development and suggests that their ability to utilise all four learning styles will develop as they mature. Kolb identified the three development stages as:

■ acquisition (birth to adolescence) and the development of basic abilities and cognitive structures

■ specialisation (school, early adult work and experience) as learning style becomes specialised dependent on social, educational or organisational specialisation, for example, e.g. theoretical or practical learning

■ integration (adult to older adult) as own style develops through work and personal life.

Kolb believes that individuals have to make two decisions regarding learning. The first is how to approach a task or how to 'grasp experience'. Is their preference to watch or to do? The second decision is their emotional response to the experience or how they will then 'transform experience'. Is their preference to feel or to think? The resultant decision determines their preferred learning style. If individuals are able to use all learning styles, they can get the most out of every potential learning situation. If they have strong preference for one style, this may limit this ability and hinder learning. Different learning opportunities relate to different learning styles.

Experiential based learning systems, inc.   www.learningfromexperience.com
This website lists a range of study skills sites

Fig 6.1 An experiential learning cycle based on Kolb

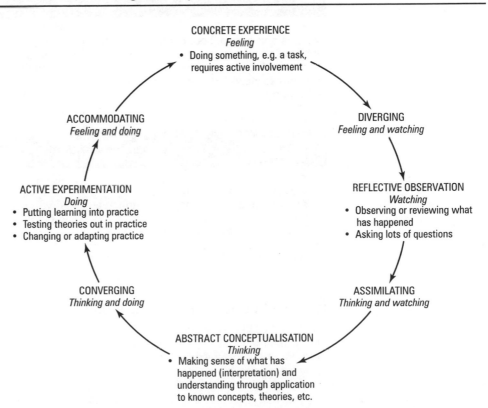

Honey and Mumford

Peter Honey and Alan Mumford built on Kolb's model and developed a model with four distinct learning styles: activist, theorist, pragmatist and reflector. Honey and Mumford identify that individuals develop a preference and, in order to get the most out of learning, individuals should understand their own learning style and identify learning opportunities appropriate to their preference. To help individuals identify their learning style, Honey and Mumford developed a learning styles questionnaire which is made up of numerous statements (the number depends on which version of the questionnaire is being used) which the individual is asked to agree or disagree with without too much analysis with each statement. The agreed statements are indicated on a score sheet and a pattern emerges which indicates the preferred learning style.

Honey & Mumford learning styles

Activists Links with Kolb: concrete experience, accommodating learning style	
Likes ■ Doing and experiencing ■ Give them a role-play or a game and they are into it before you have even finished giving them the instructions. ■ Eager participants in discussion	Dislikes ■ Sitting around for too long ■ Too much theorising ■ Anything that looks like slacking of the pace ■ Working alone ■ Reading
Reflectors **Links with Kolb: reflective observation, diverging learning style**	
Likes ■ Above all, time: to think, to watch, to ponder ■ Want to see how others do things first ■ Reading ■ Need some solitude to absorb ideas	Dislikes ■ Being hurried ■ Having to do things without preparation ■ Going first ■ Games and role plays where the intention is not crystal clear ■ Crammed timetable ■ Having to spend too much time with other people
Theorists **Links with Kolb: abstract conceptualisation, assimilating learning style**	
Likes ■ Ideas and abstract concepts ■ Knowing where something fits in with a general framework ■ Being stretched with new notions ■ Reading ■ Lectures ■ Analysis and logic	Dislikes ■ Ambiguity ■ Open-endedness ■ Anything that seems frivolous ■ Not being able to question and be sceptical ■ Timetables that lack structure.
Pragmatists **Links with Kolb: active experimentation, converging learning style**	
Likes ■ Activity that answers the question 'What does this mean for me in the 'real world?' ■ Opportunities to problem-solve ■ Concrete application ■ Useful tools and techniques	Dislikes ■ Anything that looks woolly or abstract ■ Anything that seems too far in the future to have meaning now

Race's experiential learning model

A third model of adult learning is emerging which, although it has some similarities, suggests that there are four process that interact with one another rather than progress through a cycle. Professor Phil Race's 2005 experiential learning model is circular which he describes as being like ripples in a pond.

Fig 6.2 Race's experiential
learning model

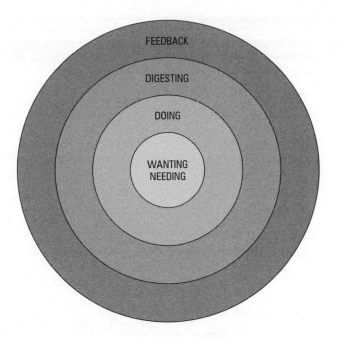

Race believes that effective conscious learning must start from the desire or motivation to
want to learn, and/or ownership of a need to learn. Effective experiential learning requires
the individual to be doing something and then practising it. Although practice does
sometimes make perfect, unthinking practice does not automatically lead to learning, so for
learning to be effective it requires the individual to digest what has happened, and to think
and reflect. A good way to reflect on something is to ask questions such as 'how did that
go?' 'what worked well or not so well?' Finally, essential to effective learning is feedback,
both intrinsic (the individual's own thoughts) and extrinsic (comments and information
from others). Knowing how you are progressing is essential for motivation, enjoyment and
confidence, all of which feed into one another.

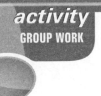

activity
GROUP WORK

1   Individually, use the learning styles learning styles inventory and assessment sheet
    below.
2   As a group, discuss your findings.

Influences on learning

By the time an individual reaches adulthood, they will have experienced many different
learning opportunities from those of early childhood through formal school education as well
as social learning through the processes of **socialisation**.

See page 110 in Unit 2 for more information about socialisation.
See page 278 in Unit 8 for more information on psychological perspectives.

Previous learning and experiences

Previous learning and experiences both play a major role in influencing attitudes towards
learning as an adult. Some individuals' learning experiences may have been positive
ones. For example, where they accessed a range of positive and encouraging learning
opportunities they found sufficiently challenging and stimulating. This would have
maintained their interest as well as enabled them to achieve their goals. For others,
traditional teaching methods used at school may have been difficult to follow due to
specific learning needs being undetected, such as dyslexia.

Learning styles inventory and assessment sheet

Type one learner: Reflector/Imaginative

Integrates experience with the 'self'

Seeks meaning, clarity and integrity

Needs to be personally involved

Seeks commitment

Learns by listening and sharing ideas

Values insight, thinking, works for harmony

Absorbs reality

Perceives information concretely and processes it reflectively

Interested in people and culture

Divergent thinkers who believe in their own experience and excel in viewing concrete situations from many perspectives

Model themselves on those they respect

Strengths: Innovations and imagination. They are ideas people. They function through social integration and values clarification

Goals: Self-involvement in important issues, bringing unity to diversity

Favourite question: Why?

Type two learner: Theorist/Logical.

Forms theories and concepts

Seeks facts and continuity

Needs to know what the experts think

Seeks goals attainment and personal effectiveness

Learns by thinking through ideas

Values sequential thinking, needs details

Forms reality

Perceives information and collects data

Thorough and industrious, re-examines facts if situations are perplexing

Enjoys traditional classrooms

Schools are designed for these learners

Functions by thinking things through and adapting to experts

Strengths: Creating concepts and models

Goals: Self-satisfaction and intellectual recognition

Favourite question: What?

Type three learner: Pragmatist/Practical

Practises and personalises

Seeks usability, utility, solvency, results

Needs to know how things work

Learns by testing theories in ways that seem most sensible

Values strategic thinking, is skills-oriented

Edits reality

Perceives information abstractly and processes it actively

Uses factual data to build designed concepts, needs hands-on experiences, enjoys solving problems, resents being given answers

Restricts judgement to concrete things, has limited tolerance for 'fuzzy' ideas

Need to know how things they are asked to do will help in real life

Functions through inferences drawn from their bodies

They are decision makers

Strengths: Practical application of ideas

Goals: To bring their view of the present into line with future security

Favourite question: How does this work?

Type four learner: Activist/Enthusiastic.

Integrates experience and application

Seeks hidden possibilities, excitement

Needs to know what can be done with things

Learns by trial and error, self-discovery

Seeks influence and solidarity

Enriches reality

Perceives information concretely and processes it actively

Is adaptable to change and relishes it, likes variety and excels in situations calling for flexibility

Tends to take risks, at ease with people, sometimes seen as pushy

Often reaches conclusions in the absence of logical justification

Functions by acting and testing experience

Strengths: Action, carrying out plans

Goals: To make things happen, to bring action to concepts

Favourite question: What if?

Specific learning need

Many adults were hampered from achieving their potential in school due to a lack of understanding of how to recognise and support such specific learning needs. This experience may have been accompanied with comments about an individual's ability with derogatory terms ('you're stupid' 'you can't learn') being applied or absence from school being sanctioned by parents due to the difficulties they were experiencing with learning. More recent research has uncovered ways to enable individuals with dyslexia, for example, to be taught in a different way using a range of strategies to meet their specific needs. For example, to assist those with **Irlen syndrome** changing the background colour upon which words are written can often benefit the reader.

Formal versus informal learning

Formal learning, such as that undertaken in a classroom, training session or workshop and sometimes referred to as 'talk and chalk', may have been useful for some aspects of learning, such as academic subjects or where the aim is to impart information with a view to increasing knowledge. However learning by doing is also important and opportunities to experiment and try out ideas are important too. Discussion and group work, experiential learning experiences such as role play or simulation provide the opportunity for informal learning. It is usual that more is achieved through these learning experiences than the intended learning outcomes identified by a tutor. Life experience provides many informal learning opportunities in relation to self-awareness and personal development as well as life skills. As Race's model suggests however, these are not necessarily effective unless the individual takes time to reflect and receive feedback as well.

Time and learning style

Being able to access learning opportunities that fit well with the individual's preferred learning styles is an important influence on their attitude and motivation to engage with learning. In addition, some individuals require more time than others in which to learn effectively. Having insufficient time or feeling pressured by time limits can influence learning effectiveness. Some learning also need to take place over a period of time and would be incomplete if the individual is not given that time, for example learning the complete process of an activity or gaining a skill may take time. The quality of the time spent is also a factor. If there is no consideration given to the individual's learning needs and preferred learning style, the amount of time may not make learning effective. Sometimes substantial learning can take place in a short time if the quality of the input is present, for example if an individual is shown a task accompanied by explanation and then given the opportunity to do the task, ask questions and receive feedback.

Learning environment

The learning environment is an essential ingredient in facilitating effective learning. Physical comfort is important in terms of warmth, ventilation and seating, a feeling of safety and security is achieved through ensuring individuals know what learning is planned and the expectations (in workshops this could be achieved through a 'working together agreement' or ground rules).

See page 283 in Unit 8 for more information about Maslow's hierarchy of need as regards psychological perspectives on personal growth and development.

Depending on the content, the individual must feel safe in terms of their competence and not be asked to do something they feel uncomfortable doing, such as talking about personal experiences. Although whoever is leading the learning has a responsibility to create a safe learning environment, the individuals involved also have a responsibility to keep to agreements and respect and support one another as an element of vulnerability is created when learning is taking place. For learning to occur, individuals need to become conscious of what they do not know and this can create concern or even anxiety if they feel others have expectations of them or have made assumptions about their knowledge or skill levels. Clear guidelines for activities and learning outcomes as well as a relaxed atmosphere with an element of fun also help to create a positive learning environment, as individuals are more likely to learn when they are relaxed than when tense.

Access to resources

Access to resources that are appropriate both to the individual's specific learning needs and to the area of learning are important influences on learning. Poor access can mean individuals fall into the negative attitudes they may have been exposed to during childhood or past learning experiences and become demotivated. Learning resources can be from a wide range of sources and include access to books, journals, interactive learning resources, such as CD ROMs or e-learning via the internet, audio-visual, intranet as well as individuals who have specialist knowledge or experience. Making sure individuals can access relevant information or resources to help them achieve their learning are therefore crucial.

Attitude and self-discipline

Individuals who have found learning to be a positive and enjoyable experience in the past or who have a clear sense of direction or goal they wish to achieve are likely to have a positive attitude which will motivate them. Poor past learning experiences where the individual felt incompetent because the style of teaching did not fit their learning style, where the challenges were too great or where their specific learning needs were not recognised or met are likely to have a negative attitude towards learning. An individual's attitude will have a significant influence on their motivation.

Feeling positive about learning and having a clear sense of purpose is likely to encourage an individual be motivated and self-disciplined in their approach. Balancing the demands of learning and timescales for completing tasks with other commitments, such as work and personal life, requires the individual to manage their time effectively. Many adult learners are excellent at finding a host of new distraction activities (ironing and cleaning, anything!) that have to be completed rather then settle down to get on with a piece of work they have been given to complete.

Fig 6.3 Attitudes to learning

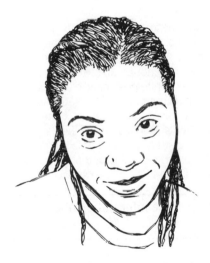

Aspirations and motivation

To achieve learning, the individual will need to apply some level of self-discipline and for some this will be difficult and may require support and strategies to keep them on track. An individual's priorities also play a part in both self-discipline and motivation. As Race suggests, the individual's desire to learn is often fuelled by having a clear sense of purpose for learning based on their ambition or aspiration. Knowing what you want to achieve, whether in terms of particular career choice and the entry requirements, work promotion, knowledge or skill (work-related or personal), is the best motivation possible. It will motivate them to engage in learning to begin with, as well as to keep going when the going gets tough so that they reach the end and enjoy the sense of satisfaction they will experience when they complete their learning and achieve their desired outcome.

Fig 6.4 Self-discipline is
a vital part of the learning
process

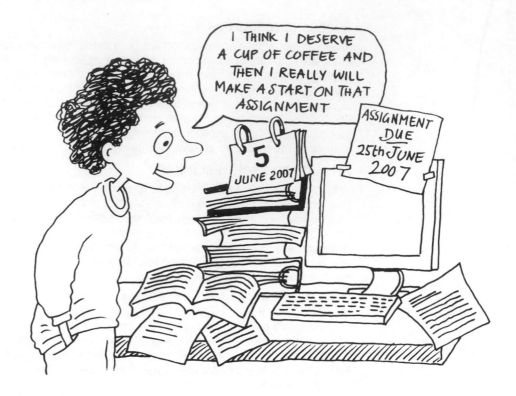

Priorities

However, an individual's other needs have to be satisfied before they are able to concentrate on meeting higher needs such as self-fulfilment and self-actualisation. If an individual's priorities are elsewhere, this will impact on their motivation as well and although they may have the desire to learn, they may not be able to engage with learning as meeting other needs take precedence. For example, personal circumstances such as caring for others, finding suitable accommodation, bereavement, relationship break-up or ill health will all impact on an individual's priorities and motivation. Other factors that may also impact on motivation are financial concerns, learning to live independently, stress, trying to balance and manage the demands of work, study, caring and family responsibilities. All of these will affect how the individual feels about their learning and at times some will become more of a priority than learning as they are required to be met to survive.

Link See page 278 in Unit 8 for more information about understanding psychological approaches to study.

activity
INDIVIDUAL WORK
6.1

P1

M1

1   Explain the main factors that may influence how adults learn.

2   Identify what has influenced your learning process and analyse the affect these factors have had on how you learn.

Skills for learning

So far we have discussed the different factors that may influence learning, but for an individual to be an effective learner they also need to develop study skills. Skills are generally considered to be physical in nature, for example being able to skip or use a keyboard. However, study skills are about the individual developing good study habits and routines, applying techniques and strategies to aid the process of their learning and understanding their learning process. Developing good study habits and routines helps maintain focus and avoid the many distractions that will be around or will be found!

Remember too that the amount of time spent on a task does not automatically equate to the quality of the time or to the outcome. For example, an individual may spend one hour 'studying', but on analysis they took fifteen minutes to get organised (make a drink, check the phone, tidy up, clear a space to work, decide what to do) ten minutes to find their assignment question and notes they have just decided to work on and five minutes arranging their pens on the desk, and so they actually only spent thirty minutes studying! Does this sound familiar to you?

Study skills

Planning time effectively and allocating specific tasks to time available will help an individual to use their study time wisely and achieve the goals they set themselves. Not all learning activities or study tasks take the same amount of time and sometimes a logical sequence of tasks needs to be followed to progress, for example planning research, research before assignment planning and writing. When planning time, consider all the parts of the activity. Fifteen minutes is a reasonable amount of time to spend on an activity, so consider all the 15-minute portions of time potentially available. Writing a weekly study plan will help to identify these. Allocate the available time appropriately rather than saying you don't have two hours so it is not worth starting anything (this is a common procrastination or excuse for not getting started!). When preparing material for assignments, it is useful to read information in smaller easily digestible chunks which can then be thought about rather than feeling overwhelmed by information overload. This also helps to raise questions and other ideas for research as well as helping you to process information and express ideas in your own words.

Literacy, numeracy, information and communication technology

Being able to use information effectively means being able to access it. This includes having appropriate literacy (reading, writing and comprehension ability) and **numeracy** (understanding numbers and how to work with numbers in everyday life) skills. Many individuals are concerned about these skills as poor past educational experiences or specific learning needs may have inhibited them from developing these to their potential. Further Education Colleges as well as larger employers will be able to offer courses and a range of flexible and open learning supports for individuals to enable them to develop these skills. Many individuals who embark on health and social care courses are concerned about their lack of experience in writing assignments and researching information. However, there are numerous opportunities to access practical advice regarding all aspects of study from research through to assignment writing and including study skills websites as well as books.

 Suupport 4 Learning www.support4learning.org.uk
This website lists a range of study skills

Understanding how to access and use information and communication technology are also important skills for learners at this level and for further studies. Using computers for writing assignments provides the learner with more opportunity to edit their writing as they go and to review and edit before completion. Some learners will, however, find this difficult as it does not suit their style of working. They may find they still use handwritten notes for planning and need to print out and read before they can edit their writing. Information technology enables learners to access information more quickly and easily than ever before, as well as being to find out where specific resources can be located without having to take precious study time travelling to a library only to find what they want is not there.

Fig 6.5 Study skills mindmap

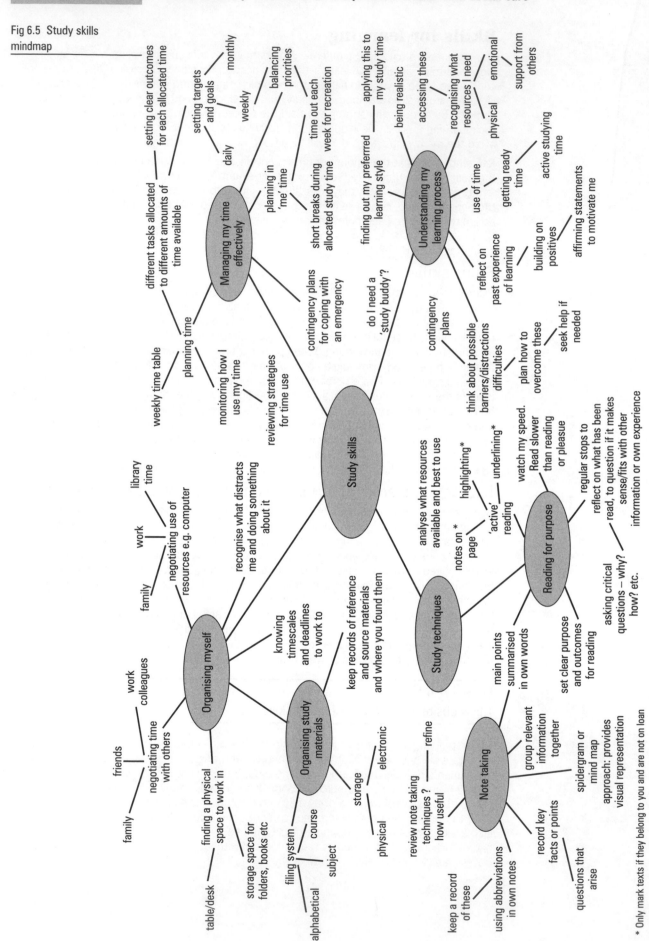

Research skills

Research skills are essential if the learner is to be efficient and effective in locating the information they require for a task or assignment without wasting time. Being able to recognise what information is required for the task set is the first step. This requires close examination and reflection on the task or assignment brief.

Research may involve observation or questioning in order to gather data for analysis. Observation would be used when researching a particular occurrence to understand more about it. For example, this may be observing how often something happens, how it is done or different techniques used for the same activity, such as taking a physical measurement or using a communicating aid.

The individual may also be able to ask questions and these should always be considered beforehand in terms of what information is required and how the information will be used and presented once it is gathered. Sometimes closed questions may be appropriate (those with yes/no/don't know answers), sometimes open questions are more appropriate (asking someone their views on a particular subject) and sometimes probing questions may be used to encourage the person to expand their answer or explanation. Being clear about what information is being sought is essential, otherwise the individual can find themselves with a lot of information of little use as it is irrelevant or unfocused.

The internet is a more immediate source of information and provides access to a seemingly never-ending amount of information from a wide range of sources. When using the internet it is important to remember that it is substantially unregulated except for obscene and illegal content and so it is imperative that when researching the individual checks the source of the information and establishes its validity, authenticity, currency, reliability and credibility. The internet provides a wide range of information of value to individuals studying and working within health and social care and which would otherwise be difficult, not to say time-consuming, to locate and access. Government websites, such as those referenced through this book, provide a wealth of information regarding legislation, policies, practice guidance, statistics, official reports and research findings. Many health and social care organisations also publish information on the internet, for example the Joseph Rowntree Trust, the Kings Fund, as well as universities and independent learning and research organisations. Another advantage to using the internet is that information is more up-to-date than that found in books and could have been posted the day you undertake your search. Using a search engine (a computer programme on the internet that searches for key words and produces a list to work from) such as Google will help you locate information when you are unclear where to start looking. However, individuals must be aware that typing some words into a search engine may lead them to places they had not intended going to, such as pornographic websites. This is particularly important to remember if they are using a computer in a public facility, such as a library or at work, where internet access is likely to be monitored and even unintentional access may contravene organisational rules or guidelines for use, or at home if parental controls are not in place to safeguard others who may be potentially vulnerable.

Feedback and reflection

Learning as discussed in the theories and models of learning involves using feedback from others. Feedback is a good source of information to stimulate reflection on what worked, how the individual felt, what they learned and how they may integrate that into what they do. As described in the study skills mindmap (figure 6.5), it is essential to monitor and review progress and evaluate if the strategies and techniques are working and enabling the individual to achieve their desired and planned outcomes. The individual can be helped in this process by others, especially those whose views the individual trusts and respects, and who are able to be honest with the individual. Individuals are motivated and maintain motivation if they can see some progress towards their goal. It is essential to review what is happening in reality against what was planned, reflect on this and then evaluate the effectiveness of techniques and strategies, in order that adjustments can be made if needed before motivation and confidence is lost.

Support for learning

As identified in the study skills mindmap (fig 6.5), support from others is an important part of being an adult learner. Different types of support are needed from different individuals and sources.

Tutors, peers, supervisors and mentors

Tutors are a primary source of support to help the individual understand the subject content as well as techniques for working with and studying the subject. They also provide invaluable support in understanding the criteria for assessment and the assignment tasks that are given. Before embarking on an assignment, the individual must check they are clear about what is being asked and what the expectations are in terms of quality and quantity of outcome (assignment brief, grading criteria and submission date and time). If an individual is struggling with any aspect of their course, it is imperative they seek advice and guidance from their tutor, supervisor or mentor (whichever is appropriate) as these people are unable to provide support if they do not know an individual needs it.

Finding a 'study buddy' for peer support may also suit many individuals. Peer support can be useful for joint projects, for discussing ideas or for sharing resources and coping with some of the practical issues that arise when studying, for example sharing transport to college or taking notes and sharing them with someone who is absent from a session. Discussions with peers can also help to open up a subject area especially if someone is finding it hard to get started or to understand a specific aspect of a subject. The bonus for someone involved in such as discussion is that explaining something to someone else is often a good way of checking your own understanding and reinforcing your own learning.

Supervisors may be allocated if an individual is studying within a college. This type of supervisor can offer generic support and act as a personal point of contact if the individual needs to discuss progress, practical aspects, issues or problems which may affect their learning. Supervisors may also be located within the subject specific area and able to offer advice on this too. Some learners will be employed and studying part-time for a job-related qualification which is either supported by their employer or by themselves. If their learning is supported by their employer then their workplace supervisor may also be able to provide support specifically related to how learning relates to practice.

Learners on work placements will also be allocated a work supervisor or a mentor who will be an invaluable source of support about workplace policies, procedures, guidelines and how all these relate to theory and practice. They will also provide advice and guidance and allocate tasks, if appropriate, as well as feedback on performance and progress.

Professional Practice

- Supervision is used in health and social care to support individuals to work effectively in meeting the needs of those they support as well as their own needs and to ensure the boundary between the two does not become blurred. Supervision should be available regularly and when requested, such as following a traumatic event or incident.

- Supervision either takes place as a group or individually (at least every six months)

- Supervision has three purposes:

    1 Allocating work tasks and responsibilities

    2 Discussion about work, progress and feedback on this

    3 Discussion regarding the individual's personal learning and development needs.

A mentor is someone who has considerable experience and is in a position to use their knowledge and experience to support the individual's learning. A mentor may set the individual specific tasks to undertake within the workplace setting to facilitate their practical application of learning and which supports their development.

Meetings

Meetings with tutors, peers, supervisors and mentors can all be useful for discussing issues, areas of uncertainty, dilemmas as well as sources of further information, advice, guidance, feedback and progress reports. Some meetings will be in groups where items that are relevant to all those attending are discussed. Individual meetings should be a two-way conversation and an opportunity for feedback and discussion on specific issues relevant to the individual. It is therefore, important that the individual prepares for the meeting beforehand, even sending the tutor, supervisor or mentor items for discussion, so that they get the most out of a meeting and it meets their learning and development needs.

Increased self-awareness

Receiving feedback from others increases self-awareness, as the way an individual sees themselves is not how others see them. As a health and social care worker involved in supporting others, it is imperative that an individual has self-awareness in order to recognise and understand how their behaviour impacts on those they come into contact with. A lack of self-awareness can lead to the individual becoming part of the problem and not part of the solution. For example, if an individual is unaware that their tone of voice is abrupt and their language negative and dismissive of others, they will find it difficult to understand why people they support appear withdrawn or reluctant to engage with them.

Accessing information and support on knowledge and best practice

Tutors, supervisors and mentors are all good sources of how and where to access information and support on knowledge and best practice. In addition, librarians can support an individual with research and accessing relevant documents or resources. The professional bodies for health and social care work, such as the Nursing and Midwifery Council (NMC) or the General Social Care Council (GSCC) for social work, government departments, standard setting organisations, such as the Commission for Social Care Inspection (CSCI) or the National Institute for Clinical Excellence (NICE), are all sources of information regarding best practice guidelines. A substantial amount of information is readily available on the internet so that saves time and cost of ordering publications without really knowing if the contents are appropriate to the need. Research into health and social care issues is undertaken in many universities in the UK and most publish information on the university website. In addition, organisations such as the Kings Fund and the Joseph Rowntree Trust also undertake research that then informs practice.

case study 6.1 — Johari window

While researching human personality at the University of California in the 1950s, psychologists Joe Luft and Harry Ingham devised the Johari window as a simple technique which can be used to think about how self-awareness can be increased. Below is an example of a Johari window.

Self-reflection and how others see us

Public self This part of our self is how we present ourselves to other people. It is the part of our identity that is **known to us** and **known to others**	*Constructive feedback from others can help us to know more about this part of ourselves*	**How others see us** This is the part of us that is **known by others** and **unknown by us**. It is about how others see us and the impact we have on them.
We can expand our public self by telling others more about our private self. To do this we must trust the other person. It is our choice as to whether we reveal more about our self or not.		*Observations and constructive feedback from others may help us to explore this part of our selves*
Private self This is the part of ourselves that we keep private. It contains our hopes, fears, desires, ambitions, etc. it is **known to us** and **unknown to others** unless we choose otherwise	*We can discover more about our deeper self through counselling if we choose to do so*	**Our deeper hidden self (subconscious)** This is the part of our self that is **unknown to us** and **unknown to others** – our subconscious. We only explore this if we choose to through active means such as psychotherapy

activity
INDIVIDUAL WORK

Reflect on this model and answer the following:

1 How different are your public and private selves?

2 How do you think wearing a uniform may change an individual's public persona?

3 How does this model help you to think about yourself?

Most health and social care organisations can be located via a website which will also contain information on alternative means of contacting them or local offices that can be accessed for information. Information sourced from the internet must be acknowledged and referenced like any other within assignments. Librarians can often access specific information as well which may be more difficult to source, for example articles from professional journals.

Within work placements or the work setting there will also be information relating to best practice within policies and procedures and specific professional journals.

Bath University Mental Health Research & Development
www.bath.ac.uk/mhrdu/intro.htm
Bristol University health and social care-related research centres
www.bristol.ac.uk/sps/research/hsc/default.shtml

Kings Fund	www.kingsfund.org.uk
Joseph Rowntree Charitable Trust	www.jrct.org.uk
Nursing and Midwifery Council	www.nmc-org.uk
General Social Care Council	www.gscc.org.uk
Commission for Social Care Inspection	www.csci.org.uk
National Institute for Clinical Excellence	www.nice.org.uk
Department of Health	www.dh.gov.uk

Learning opportunities

Adults are able to learn from a wide range of opportunities and are less dependent on more formal instruction such as that experienced during their school years. As the different learning styles indicate, adults are able to benefit from some opportunities more than others and the 'rounded' adult learner who does not have a strong preference for any one style is able to maximise their learning by engaging with a wider range of opportunities that may be available to them. Learning opportunities may be formal or informal. Formal learning opportunities are intentional from the learner's perspective whereas informal learning is more often unintentional and results from everyday life and activities such as watching, listening and copying, whether through work, family, friends or leisure pursuits. Sometimes the informal learning results from events that turn the individual's life upside down such as losing a job, relationship breakdown or the death of a loved one. When this happens, the individual is likely to re-evaluate their life and future which may lead them to undertake formal learning, such as a college course to gain a qualification.

Fig 6.6 Formal and informal learning

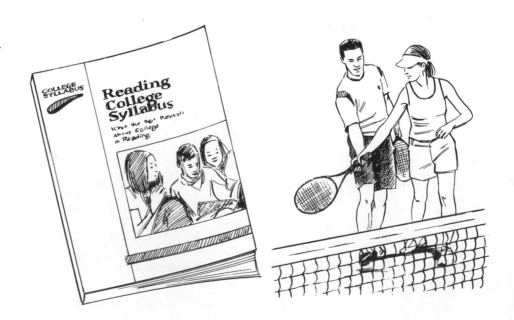

Formal learning opportunities:

- are organised, for example held at a college or training venue
- have a planned and prescribed learning framework, for example a syllabus or a BTEC specification
- are led by a teacher, tutor or trainer
- have identified learning outcomes, such as grading criteria or competences
- have an element of assessment which leads to accreditation for an externally recognised qualification, such as a BTEC National Diploma or National Vocational Qualification (NVQ)
- usually have a set timeframe, such as a day course or a number of terms or years.

Examples of formal learning opportunities are:

- Lectures
- Seminars
- Courses
- Workshops
- Vocational training programme e.g. NVQ
- Formal coaching or mentoring

Informal opportunities:

- are generally unstructured with no clearly defined learning outcomes, time or support
- are likely to result through life experiences and consequently can occur anywhere
- what is learned by the individual is generally under their control. However, it could be argued that informal learning through socialisation is subconscious and is not under individual control
- have no external criteria to guide or prescribe what is to be learned, to work towards or be assessed against
- is often given lower status as the outcome is widely variable and less controllable
- is almost incidental to other activities and can arise out of coping with incidents that are unplanned and subsequently reflected upon by the individual sometime with the support of others, such as debriefing after an incident at work.

Examples of informal learning are the many things that are learned as part of life experiences:

- setting up and using new appliances
- relationships with others
- reading and watching TV or films, listening to the radio
- doing quizzes or puzzles
- taking on a new project at work
- taking up a leisure activity such as arts or crafts.

Each of these opportunities provides the individual with a chance to learn new skills, increase their knowledge, their self-awareness and self confidence. Informal learning is therefore an important aspect of learning.

Classroom activities

Knowledge can be gained from a wide range of activities both formal and informal and sometimes the boundaries are blurred as to which type of learning is taking place. Knowledge gained through classroom activities such as teacher input is an example of more formal learning as there will be clear learning outcomes for each part of the session and each activity within it. The knowledge is likely to be subject-specific, contain facts, theories, concepts and ideas as well as explanations of how these are applied in reality if appropriate, for example, sociological perspectives and how these can be applied to understand social phenomena and develop social policy. Some subjects may be predominantly factual, for example history, although classroom activities and independent studies would be concerned with learners developing skills in research, critical analysis and writing. However, even within formal opportunities informal learning still occurs. For example, a tutor may ask individuals to form a group to discuss a topic. What is learned through that discussion is not just more about the topic content and different views about it but also information about group dynamics and the individual's strengths within group interaction. Individuals are generally unaware of this learning, but will carry it into future group work activities.

Placement experiences

Knowledge gained through placement experiences are likely to enable the individual to understand and experience how their theoretical classroom learning is applied in practice and the impact this has on health and social care service provision and the individual's being supported. For example, health and safety legislation taught in class will become 'real' when an individual sees how it applies within a work setting as well as the potential implications if it is not adhered to. As a result the legislation (which may have appeared as a rather dull litany of rules and regulations in class) changes from being theoretical into something more tangible for the individual as their knowledge and understanding has been grounded into practical application.

Independent studies

Independent study enables the individual to learn at their own pace, to set their own criteria and learning outcomes and to explore areas of particular interest, broaden and deepen their understanding of a subject area and open up new areas too.

remember

> Independent studies are often motivated by individual desire to learn.

The process of identifying, searching for and finding information often means the knowledge gained is retained longer. In addition, informal learning also takes place as research skills develop and incidental knowledge is gathered as well. Individual learning styles will also be a feature in how important this form of learning is to an person. This may not suit some people's learning style or they may struggle with self-discipline and find independent studies difficult as a result.

Life experience

Knowledge gained from life experience is, as discussed previously when considering informal learning, a really important part of learning and is taken into everyday activities as well as applied into work, such as working with others, self-discipline and a work ethic. Many adults find they cope with learning better than they expect to. Often this is because they have a wealth of knowledge and understanding from their life experiences that they can apply to courses of study. For example, adults often find studying sociology and psychology easier as they can apply what they have learned from life and other roles, such as being a parent, an employee or a volunteer, to the theoretical concepts which makes them easier to understand as well as helping them to make sense of their life experiences too.

Employment

Knowledge gained from employment includes the specific knowledge required to competently undertake the job tasks. In addition, the individual gains knowledge about how the organisation they work for functions, the systems and structures in place to manage the work and the workforce, as well as customers (if appropriate, although most employment will have an end user however remote they may be). The individual may gain knowledge about time management, using their initiative, following guidelines, what to do in the event of emergencies or unexpected occurrences, such as dealing with a complaint, working as part of a team, being supervised, supervising others and both effective and less effective management styles, and so on. An individual may also be given the opportunity to gain relevant qualifications through employment and this will add to their knowledge base.

Voluntary activities

Knowledge gained through voluntary activities may be in many ways similar to that gained through employment and life experience. However, significant informal learning will also take place and the individual is likely to learn not just more about the areas they are volunteering in but new skills and, importantly, more about themselves, their strengths and capabilities. Volunteers are often placed in situations that challenge and stimulate them to achieve things they would not have otherwise thought possible as well as gaining knowledge and insight into humanity. Undertaking voluntary work enables the individual to gain considerable personal growth experience in terms of knowledge, understanding and personal fulfilment.

Link

See page 238 in Unit 8 for more information about understanding psychological approaches to study.

case study 6.2

The Ghana volunteer experience: 10 fascinating facts

When you volunteer with VSO (Voluntary Service Overseas), as well as sharing your skills, you get an insider understanding of the country you work in, an experience you would never have as a tourist.

1   It is rude to arrive at work in the morning or leave in the evening without greeting every single person present

2   The national motto is: 'No hurry in life, this be Ghana'

3   If you take a taxi in Ghana, you share it with four other people.

4   If you go past people working and say 'ikoo', they will say 'yaa yea'.

5   You will be given a nickname in Ghana according to the day of the week on which you were born, for example the Kofi in the name of UN secretary general Kofi Anan means he was born on a Friday. If you want to check out which one yours will be they are:

   ■ Monday: Kojo (for a man), Adjoa (for a woman)
   ■ Tuesday: Kwabena, Abenaa
   ■ Wednesday: Kwaku, Ekuwa
   ■ Thursday: Ekow, Yaaba
   ■ Friday: Kofi, Efua
   ■ Saturday: Kwame, Aba
   ■ Sunday: Kwesi, Esi

6   Coffins in Ghana are crafted and painted to reflect the life of the dead person, so a seaman will be buried in a boat-shaped coffin and a seamstress will be buried in a sewing machine-shaped one.

7   Ghanaians wear white at a funeral and celebrate the life of the dead person with a party.

8   The national dish is groundnut soup (spicy peanut chicken or fish soup) with fufu (plantain and cassava pounded into a paste).

9   Christianity is very popular in Ghana and it is not uncommon for your local shop to be called 'Only God Knows Provisions and Cosmetics' or 'Thy Will be Done Snacks'.

10 Ghana was one of the only countries that sent troops to stop the Rwandan genocide.

activity
GROUP WORK

Discuss in a group what different learning experiences a tourist in Ghana would have compared with a volunteer worker in the country.

activity
INDIVIDUAL WORK 6.2

D1

Discuss within your group how personal learning and development may benefit others. Write up your own individual conclusions.

Planning for, monitoring and reflecting on, own development

An increasing feature of work, including health and social care work, is the recognition that individuals undertaking this work need to be able to plan, monitor and reflect on their personal and professional development in order to maintain the quality of their interaction with others and meet work standards and the expectations of those they support and work with.

Review at start of programme

An important first step when an individual begins a programme of study such as the BTEC National Certificate and Diploma in Health and Social Care is for them to review their current knowledge and skills, practice, values, beliefs, career aspirations and level of self-awareness. Learning is a journey of self-discovery and, as with any journey, the individual should be aware of the point at which they are setting out on that journey so that they able to measure how far their journey has taken them.

This review may be in the form of a skills audit document which asks the learner to indicate their knowledge, skills and practical ability in relation to the subject areas (or specifications) that make up the learning programme. This helps to identify specific areas for development. It will also enable the individual to identify those areas where they already have some knowledge, skills or practical ability. For a learner who lacks confidence in their ability to succeed, this is likely to be a considerably motivating and encouraging factor which gives them a positive approach to the programme.

Individual reflective activities, practice dilemmas and scenarios and group discussion may all be used to encourage the individual to recognise their values and beliefs. These activities should start them thinking about how these values and beliefs could impact on their practice and personal development, and how to reconcile them so that they do not hinder the individual's learning or their work with others. It is useful for the individual to review their career aspirations at the beginning of the programme as this may impact on their optional unit choices and enable them to target these so they can, for example, fulfil entry requirements. Wanting to learn is an important motivator. An activity such as Johari window may be used to encourage reflection and identify an individual's level of self-awareness, so they can consider how they may increase this through being open and actively seeking constructive feedback from others through their course and work placement. Reviewing may also be done through a one-to-one discussion with a personal tutor developing a personal learning plan and agreed with goals, monitoring processes and review dates.

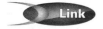 Refer back to page 203 to remind yourself about Johari window.

Fig 6.7 The learner's journey

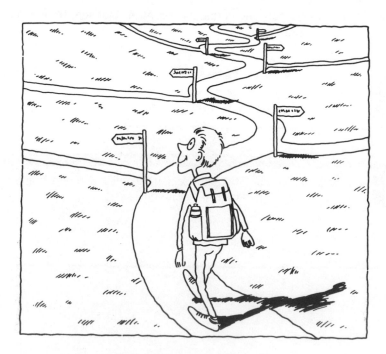

Knowledge

Relevant formal and informal learning to date

When reviewing knowledge, the individual may be given an activity which will ask questions about the ways they have gained knowledge as well as the different types of knowledge they may have. This may also have been included on a course application form. They may be asked to indicate the types of formal learning they have undertaken to date, such as school or college attendance, subjects studied and qualifications attained. They may be asked to write or talk about the knowledge they have gained through informal learning, such as life experience, employment, interests and voluntary work. Knowledge can be gained from a wide variety of learning opportunities and will to some extent depend on the individual's ability to engage with them which will be dependent on their individual learning style.

Current contemporary issues

When planning how to gain knowledge, an individual needs to consider both formal and informal opportunities. Knowledge can be gained from reading and exploration of current contemporary issues, for example about identity cards, immigration, welfare-to-work initiatives, health care rationing, equality and diversity issues, global warming and the effects of this and pollution on health and adult **abuse**, to name a few. These areas are consistently reported in the media (newspapers, journals and TV, especially current affairs discussions and programmes). Learners can consider how much access they have to this information and how they can achieve a balance in the information they absorb so that they have a sense of the differing viewpoints. This can be achieved by watching, listening and reading a variety of sources, comparing them and then considering why the same issue may be treated differently in terms of priority and perspective. This will encourage critical thinking and help the individual to monitor and reflect on their learning as well as how their values, beliefs and attitudes may be changing as their knowledge base widens and deepens. When planning development, it is important to find out where current contemporary issues relevant to health and social care are reported, discussed and debated, such as health and social care sections in daily newspapers, professional journals, TV and radio programmes.

Understanding of theories, principles and concepts

Within the BTEC programme, each unit will require individuals to develop their knowledge and understanding of theories, principles and concepts relevant to the subject area. For example, in Unit 8 there are a number of different theories regarding learning and motivation, while in Unit 2 there are principles and concepts regarding equality, diversity and anti-discriminatory practice. When planning study for each unit, the individual needs to consider the information they gathered through the reviewing process and focus their time and energy on the identified development areas. Applying study skills advice will also help in not only achieving the goal of gaining knowledge but also monitoring progress. Following study, it is equally important to reflect on what has been learned and a good way to do this is to consider how the theories, principles and concepts can be applied in practice and how the individual can apply them or how their learning will change what they do (depending on their circumstances and experience).

Understanding of potential careers

Part of the BTEC programme includes an opportunity to plan to develop knowledge and understanding of potential careers. Individuals embarking on this course will have indicated an intention to pursue a career within health and social care and, although some may have clear career aspirations, others may be undecided as to a specific career. Identifying careers of interest is important as the individual can then plan how they can investigate different careers as part of their course programme. This may be ideas for independent studies, voluntary work, visits and talks by different professionals or negotiating work experience placements. Adding this to their development plan helps with the monitoring process as well as helping to maintain focus. Following each encounter, the individual needs to reflect and analyse what they have learned as this will help them to make career decisions later.

Skills

A skill is the ability to do something well and is generally gained through experience or training, either informal (judging distances while driving a car) or formal (touch typing). Planning how skills will be attained as well as monitoring progress towards proficiency is dependent on the skill to be acquired.

Communicating

Communication skills such as verbal and non-verbal language are an example where a great deal of the learning is informal, as it takes place as part of human development and socialisation. However, adults continue to develop these skills the more they know about and develop their understanding of human interaction. In addition, an individual may have identified the need to develop their verbal skills in terms of oral presentations, interviewing and use of appropriate language. Active listening skills can be developed and this is an essential skill when supporting and working with people. Being able to interpret non-verbal language is also a skill that can be developed with practice. If an individual identifies this as an area for development, they need to think about the different opportunities they may have for development. This could include being an active participant in group and class discussions, presenting information, observing personal interactions and reflecting on the messages being conveyed, practising within the learning environment, for example in role play activities, and putting learning into practice when on work placements. Working with peers, whether in the classroom or while on work placement is another opportunity for developing cooperating, negotiation and group-working skills. Individuals will also benefit from actively seeking constructive feedback from those whose opinions they respect and trust. They can then use their comments as a basis for checking progress towards development goals and identifying new goals and then reflecting on how their learning is impacting on their interactions and practice.

See page 3 in Unit 1, page 289 Unit 8 and page 349 Unit 11 for more information about communication skills.

Working with others

Work placements, voluntary activities and employment which involves working with others such as service users and professionals provide good opportunities for developing a range of team-working and interpersonal skills. To get the most out of the experience in terms of learning, the individual needs to take time to identify what their development needs are in relation to working with others and to then consider these in terms of their desired outcomes. For example, the individual may want to develop their skills in communicating with service users who have communication differences or develop their practical skills in planning activities with service users.

It is useful to identify outcomes clearly as this makes the process of monitoring and reviewing to determine progress easier. Outcomes need to be SMART, that is:

- Specific: what exactly does the individual want to achieve?
- Measurable: how will they identify the difference (measure it)?
- Actionable: is it possible to achieve (within the opportunity and their capabilities)?
- Realistic: is achievement practical and reasonable?
- Timely: what is the right time to do this and what are the time limits?

Once outcomes have been decided, the individual can begin to plan how these can be achieved by identifying appropriate opportunities and how these can be accessed. Monitoring is easier because the individual has a clear guide to what they were expecting to achieve. Following the identified opportunities, the individual also needs to take time to reflect on what happened, what was learned and how this will change what they do. New goals may be identified through this process.

See page 16 in Unit 1 for more information about models of reflection.

Technical skills

Learners increasingly require technical skills in terms of using information technology (IT). These skills are invaluable for the purposes of learning, when researching and presenting work for assessment. However, they are also vital within health and social care work, where the use of computers, email and the internet are commonplace practices and increasingly a necessity as more organisations move towards paperless systems for record-keeping. If the individual has identified IT skill as a development need, they need to plan how to meet this need. This could be through accessing a course at a local college or through their employer. On-line courses are also available, for example, through Learn Direct.

Learn Direct	www.learndirect.co.uk

Planning how to develop skills in relation to use of equipment will depend on the type of equipment. To develop these skills with equipment used within health and social care settings, such as hoists, communication aids and equipment used to undertake physiological measurements the individual needs to specifically identify these as learning outcomes within their development plan for their work placements. Working with more experienced staff, the workplace supervisor or mentor will also assist in developing these skills which are usually taught through demonstration and practice with supervision until competence is demonstrated.

Becoming familiar, confident and competent in using creative and craft skills generally develops through demonstration and practice with constructive feedback to monitor progress and adapt techniques if required to achieve the desired outcome. These may be useful skills to develop as they are used within areas of health and social care work, such as therapeutic activities with older people and adults with learning disabilities or mental health issues. If the individual identifies these are development needs, they should find out where they can learn specific skills, for example at college or within a work placement.

> **remember**
>
> According to Phil Race, feedback is essential to effective learning.

Research skills

Research skills are essential for anyone undertaking study at this and at a higher level as assignments will require individuals to research and draw from a range of sources in order to present their knowledge and understanding for assessment. Research skills are also an important part of reflective practice and problem solving within the health and social care worker role. Research skills include being able to undertake primary research (undertake research themselves), source, interpret and use secondary data (information researched by others, such as census statistics) as well as handle data.

Undertaking primary research requires skills in constructing a research brief and devising questions (multiple choice, open, and so on) to include in a questionnaire or for structured or unstructured interview. Once either primary or secondary data is collected data-handing skills (organising, analysis and evaluation) are required to interpret and apply the findings to the original brief. Organising skills are essential to research as considerable amounts of time can be wasted trying to locate a research source. Undertaking small projects to begin with are a good way of developing these skills. The individual needs to monitor how effective they are in applying their skills as they progress through a project and at the end take time to reflect on what was learned so that their skills can develop and their process become honed (improved through making adjustments) to increase their effectiveness and time management. The study skills websites suggested earlier in this unit will also have information regarding research skills.

Personal skills

Studying requires individuals to develop a range of personal skills in order to be effective in their study and application of learning. As discussed in the section about study skills, having good organisational skills is really important if a learner is to use the time available to them effectively. Getting organised and staying organised requires self-discipline but it will prove to be beneficial in both studying and work. Organisational skills are a fundamental part of the health and social care worker's job role. They will need to be able to plan and carry out activities independently and efficiently while actively demonstrating that they value and respect those they work with. This is true of routine tasks as well as management tasks. For example, organisational skills are essential when supporting a service user with their personal care. The worker needs to think through the activity and ensure they are organised in collecting everything required before starting so the service user is valued, respected and their dignity preserved. If the worker is not organised then they will find themselves leaving the service user unsupported (or undressed) while they collect things they have forgotten, which falls below the expectations of good care practice. If this is an area for development then the individual may find it useful to set themselves SMART outcomes as a starting point with regular monitoring, feedback from others and reflection in one-to-one tutorials.

Another aspect of personal skills is personal presentation. This can be in relation to dress as well as manner, attitude and behaviour; in other words, how an individual presents themselves to others. Health and social care workers need to present themselves to service users, **carers** and other professionals in a manner which instils confidence in their knowledge, skills and abilities. Understanding the health and social care worker role and responsibilities as well as the boundaries within worker-service user relationships and between different professionals are important aspects of this. Again, identifying what needs to be achieved when on work placements and through other learning opportunities will help the individual to plan this development as it comes with learning and experience. Receiving constructive feedback from someone the individual respects and trusts is an essential part of this development area as is personal refection and reflective discussions with a tutor, supervisor or mentor.

Practice

At the beginning of the BTEC programme, the individual will have reviewed their development needs in relation to health and social care practice. Before undertaking study and work placements, they should have written a development plan which identified SMART outcomes to meet those development needs. As they go through their programme of study and work placements, they will have regular opportunities to consider their health and social care practice and the outcomes they have set for themselves. This could be through individual reflection as well as reflective discussions and feedback during their one-to-one discussions with their tutor, supervisor or mentor. These will all help them to monitor and reflect on their progress and identify where they may need to make appropriate adjustments to their original development plan.

When planning, monitoring and reflecting on practice the individual needs to consider:

- how they will and do demonstrate their respect for the **care value base**
- how they will become effective and can demonstrate their effectiveness in professional interactions with others
- how they will become effective and can demonstrate their effectiveness in co-operative working with others
- how they can become effective and can demonstrate their effectiveness in team work
- the influence personal values and beliefs have on their practice
- how they can demonstrate their awareness of the need to develop their personal value base in order to support and promote good practice
- how they can develop and demonstrate their awareness of the impact of legislation, codes of practice and policies on their own practice
- how to develop and demonstrate their understanding of the responsibilities and limitations of their role in practice.

As suggested previously, there are a number of opportunities the individual can use in order to achieve these. Identifying current practice and planning how development needs will be met by setting SMART outcomes is an important starting point. Assignments and work placement objectives may provide guidelines and opportunities on how these are to be achieved within the individual's programme of study. Monitoring development progress through discussions with others, individual reflection and actively seeking and responding to feedback from peers, tutors, workplace supervisors or mentors will all aid this process so that appropriate adjustments can be made to the original plan.

Values and beliefs

When receiving feedback from others and undertaking individual reflective activities, another aspect to consider is the individual's personal values and beliefs and how these relate to the care value base.

See pages 48 in Unit 2 and page 349 Unit 11 for more about the relationship between personal values and beliefs and the value base of care.

Personal values and beliefs are not always aligned with the value base of care and this can have a considerable impact on practice. If a health and social care worker is to be effective, they need to take time to consider how their own socialisation process and factors that have influenced their development and their perspective on life impact upon their attitude towards a range of different issues they may encounter in their work. They need to consider, for example, the influence of their culture, ethnicity, gender, race, age, sexuality, nationality, education, life experience, employment experience, religious or spiritual beliefs, the media and friends and family on their personal values and beliefs and how this translates into their attitudes towards and interactions with others. Personal values and beliefs may not always align with those of others or the individual's employer and there may be aspects of the value base of care which require reconciliation if the individual is to be effective in their role as a health and social care worker.

Career aspirations

Career aspirations will have been reviewed at the start of the programme and the individual should have identified potential career options. They may well have identified their preferred choice as well, although many individuals may still be uncertain of this at the start of the programme. Writing a plan to identify how each option is to be explored, for example through research, visits, careers events, work placements or voluntary work, is important. First-hand experience is more likely to assist the individual to make informed choices about which career they wish to pursue than remote information, so whenever possible plan early in the programme to find opportunities to explore career options as being able to identify a preferred choice is a really positive motivator for study.

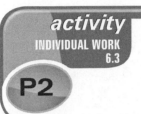

activity
INDIVIDUAL WORK 6.3

P2

Complete the table on pages 214–5 to describe your knowledge, skills, practice, values, beliefs and career aspirations at the start of the BTEC Health and Social Care programme.

Plan for own development

Once the individual has compared their current knowledge, skills, practice, values, beliefs, career aspirations and self-awareness and matched this to the programme content they will be in a position to plan their development.

When planning development, the individual needs to consider their targets or goals both in the short term and long term. Thinking about targets or goals as something to aim for is an effective factor in learner motivation. Short-term targets or goals are usually considered to be those to be achieved within a six-month period, while long term targets are those to be achieved over a minimum of an 18-month period. Short-term targets may relate to the acquisition of knowledge or a practical skill, such as learning about sociological perspectives or learning how to measure a pulse rate. Long-term goals may relate to attitudinal changes, such as applying and demonstrating the value base of care. They may relate to the application of knowledge and understanding into practice, such as active listening or understanding human behaviour. The acquisition of more complex practice skills or the ability to transfer knowledge and skills into a range of different contexts or situations will certainly be long-term goals, the achievement of which can only be determined over time and the opportunity to demonstrate this consistently before competence can be confirmed.

For targets and goals to be effective in terms of the individual being able to demonstrate their achievement they need to be SMART (specific, measurable, actionable, relevant and timely).

Link

Refer back to page 210 to remind yourself about defining SMART outcomes.

Consider personal goals

Planning your development requires you to consider your personal goals in terms of knowledge, skills, practice, values, beliefs and career aspirations. Use the format in activity 6.4 as a template for recording your development goals and devising your action plan to monitor your progress towards achieving those goals. Remember to make your goals SMART. When writing your goals, you may find it helpful to think about how you will monitor and evaluate the plan, as if it is difficult to identify this it is likely that the goal is not a SMART one.

Monitor and evaluate plan in terms of own development

When completing the development or action plan, identify at least three goals for each area as well as how you plan to monitor and evaluate progress against target or goal set.

Career aspirations

Area reviewed	Description
Knowledge	
Skills	
Practice	

Career aspirations

Area reviewed	Description
Values	
Beliefs	
Career aspirations	

case study 6.3

SMART Goals

John has been on the BTEC programme for a month and has been asked to set himself some development targets. He wrote the following:

- Meet my tutor within the next two weeks to discuss arranging work experience placements to explore my career options in nursing older people and adults with physical disabilities
- Research local health and social care provision for older people and adults with physical disabilities before meeting with tutor
- Identify other career options that I want to explore

activity
INDIVIDUAL WORK

1 Which of the three targets is SMART? Explain the reasons for your decisions.
2 How could you rewrite the target or targets that are not SMART?

You will need to consider what methods you will use to monitor and evaluate your progress against the targets or goals set. The methods used will depend on the nature of the targets. For example, with knowledge, it may be through completing assignments, answering questions or a self-assessment progress check such as are found at the end of each unit in this book. If the target relates to values and beliefs, this may be monitored and evaluated through reflection or a reflective discussion with a peer, tutor, supervisor or mentor.

Changes

Regular progress checks undertaken as part of a monitoring and evaluation process enable the individual to identify early if changes need to be made to plans. These changes may be in response to ongoing development needs, goals and reflection. Changes may be in relation to asking for additional support with an area the individual is finding difficult, or they may be trying different approaches to evaluate which one is better suited to their learning style or development needs. If an individual does not identify difficulties early enough, they risk falling behind in their studies, becoming demotivated and, as a result, may decide to give up the course rather than pursue their aspirations. Identifying when support is needed and being able to ask for that support is a sign of maturity and a self-directed learner, not of weakness, as everyone needs help with something at some time in their life. Asking for help from someone can give another perspective or reassurance that you are making progress, and that may be all that is needed to get the individual back on target.

Contexts

There are a number of different contexts in which development will be taking place and these all need to be considered as each context offers different opportunities and challenges.

Work experience placements

These provide an excellent opportunity for learners to experience the reality of working within health or social care and are invaluable in assisting them to make decisions about their career choices. Work experience placements provide the opportunity for the individual to plan how to develop, monitor and reflect on their care practice and practical skills. It also provides the opportunity for the individual to receive feedback and reflect upon how their values and attitudes impact on their behaviour within the context of health and social care work.

activity
INDIVIDUAL WORK 6.4

Complete the action plan on pages 218–9 for self-development and the achievement of your personal goals which demonstrates how you will monitor your progress.

P3

Action plan for personal goals

Area for development	Target or goal		How will you monitor and evaluate progress?
Knowledge	1		
	2		
	3		
Skills	1		
	2		
	3		
Practice	1		
	2		
	3		

Action plan for personal goals

Area for development	Target or goal		How will you monitor and evaluate progress?
Knowledge	1		
	2		
	3		
Skills	1		
	2		
	3		
Practice	1		
	2		
	3		

case study 6.4

Monitoring and evaluation

Grace applied for the BTEC National Diploma in Health and Social Care programme as she had always wanted to work with adults with learning disabilities. Her first work placement experience was in a supported living home for adults with mental health needs which she was a little disappointed about as she had hoped to work in her preferred area. She was also uncertain about whether she would cope with working with adults with mental health needs and was apprehensive when she began her placement. However, she was surprised how quickly she gained confidence and how much she enjoyed the work and felt she was able to make a difference, albeit in a small way, while on placement. By the end of the placement, Grace was no longer convinced she had made the right career choice. Grace decided to discuss how she felt with her workplace supervisor and also ask them for feedback in relation to her aptitude for this area of work. She also discussed it with her tutor when she returned to college. They both suggested she reflect on her experience and then look again at her goals in relation to her career aspirations. Grace did this by reflecting on the reasons for her initial choice, the factors that led her to question that choice and how she felt while on placement that had made her uncertain about her initial choice. Following this Grace met with her tutor and discussed her new development plan.

activity
GROUP WORK

1   How was monitoring and evaluation valuable to Grace?
2   What changes might she make to her development plan as a result of her reflection and discussions?

Although time will have been spent during the programme on values, beliefs, attitudes and the care value base, putting it all into practice may well raise unforeseen issues, dilemmas and conflicts. For some, the rhetoric and the reality may not be congruent (matching) and so discovering this while on a work experience placement provides the opportunity to re-evaluate career options sooner rather than later.

The individual's development of practice through work experience placements will be monitored through discussion with their supervisor, tutor or mentor. They may also be asked to keep a diary or learning log which they will use to reflect on their learning. Following each placement, the individual should review their development targets and set new ones for the next placement. Targets may relate to specific knowledge gained related to the specialist area as well as care practice.

There may be a variety of work experience placements available locally for learners to access and being able to spend time in a number of different health and social care settings is important, as it ensures future career decisions are informed ones. It enables the learner to see first hand how different care provider services, professionals and organisations relate to one another and work together in the best interests of the people they seek to support.

Visits

Visits are another opportunity for learners to gain some insight into the range of different employment opportunities that may be available and of interest to them. Again, it also helps to place different organisations and services into context with one another and will provide a good overview of how health and social care services are organised in the UK. If an individual is uncertain which career to choose, or which work experience placement may be relevant to their chosen career, it is important for them to plan visits to a variety of services as this will help them to make some decisions which can then be explored further. As part of the initial review and setting of development targets related to career aspirations, the individual should have identified specific visits they wished to undertake in order to research career options and work experience placements. Following each visit, the individual needs to spend time reflecting on what they have gained and monitoring their original plan and adjusting as required.

Study environment

Learning, as discussed previously, can take place in a number of environments. This could be in a college, the workplace, or both, as well as the range of places in which informal learning takes place. The individual needs to be open to learning occurring in any of these and to grasp the opportunity when it arises.

Refer back to page 199 to remind yourself about study skills.

The study environment is important to individuals and it needs to suit their needs. If the individual is to find an environment they feel comfortable in and one which is conducive to their learning they may need to plan carefully and negotiate conditions with others, such as physical and emotional space, time, quiet and resources such as computer time. They will also need to consider what they want to learn within a study environment such as a college class. Knowledge is a predominant feature of more formal learning. However, experiential learning opportunities within formal learning, such as role play, group work and discussions will also enable the individual to learn new skills, for example team working, communication, resolving conflict or diffusing situations of conflict. The study environment enables the individual to not only observe a number of different approaches, but also the opportunity to test ideas out, receive feedback and reflect on their personal effectiveness before having to apply the approaches in practice.

Life events

Life events, including employment, provide a range of informal learning opportunities and so the individual needs to be open to these occurring and to recognise events as learning. Some things may just happen and so cannot be planned. There may be prior notice of other events, such as a new work project or change at work, and these may provide the individual with the opportunity to plan for their development, for example developing planning, organisational and co-ordinating skills, all of which may be part of their wider development plan. When such learning opportunities arise, the individual should discuss their plans with their supervisor and tutor as both may be able to make suggestions about how the individual can maximise their learning from an opportunity.

Professional development portfolio

Each individual working in health and social care is now required to maintain a record of their ongoing professional development, as learning is a lifelong process. For an increasing number of professions, evidence of continuous professional development is required to secure registration to practice and so keeping a record is viewed as an essential part of professional health and social care practice.

The professional development portfolio or professional practice logbook can take any form, for example a ring binder folder or a folder stored on computer. Key contents should include an overall record of every learning opportunity undertaken by the individual containing as a minimum the following information:

- Start date of activity
- Type of activity (attendance at event, reflective diary, reading, assignment, etc)
- Length of time taken to complete activity (in hours, days or)
- Purpose of activity (planned learning outcome)
- Relevance of activity to personal development plan
- Summary of the activity (what the individual did)
- Summary of what was learned through undertaking the activity
- Changes the individual plans to make as a result of their learning

Keeping the logbook up to date is important. It should be completed as soon after completing the activity as possible, when the activity is easy to remember and the detail of what was done is still recent in the individual's thinking.

The professional development portfolio also needs to be structured appropriately for assessment of each unit and the nature of the evidence. One suggestion would be to divide the portfolio into sections according to the type of evidence, for example, separate sections for reflections, reading notes, research, work experience placement reports, courses, assignments, and so on. Each section needs to be clearly indexed so that it is easy to locate information and cross-reference this with the professional practice logbook. It may be more appropriate to divide the portfolio according to the units being studied. The key thing is clarity and ease of locating information in a logical manner.

Supporting evidence should also be included in the portfolio. This may include authenticated records to demonstrate personal progression in developing knowledge, skills, practice and career aspirations over time within a variety of context for learning and development. The individual can ask for records to be authenticated by their tutor, supervisor or mentor. The individual needs to take their portfolio to each meeting with their tutor, supervisor or mentor so they can review their progress against their development goals and targets and discuss and agree any adjustments and changes that may be required to stay on track. The portfolio provides a good evidence of the individual's personal development over a period of time and this is useful in developing self-confidence as both a learner and a health and social care worker. It will also act as a positive motivation for further learning.

Relevant evidence

Evidence to support personal and professional development may come from a range of sources. Any type of evidence must be clearly identified against the development goal, target or programme criteria it relates to as this confirms its relevance. Evidence can be formal or informal.

The individual must ensure that all evidence is:

- authentic: generated by the individual or belonging to the individual or about the individual
- current: up-to-date and within the timescales required
- valid: appropriate evidence to the criteria or goal that it is claimed to be evidence for
- sufficient: enough in terms of quantity and quality

Fig 6.8 Formal and informal evidence

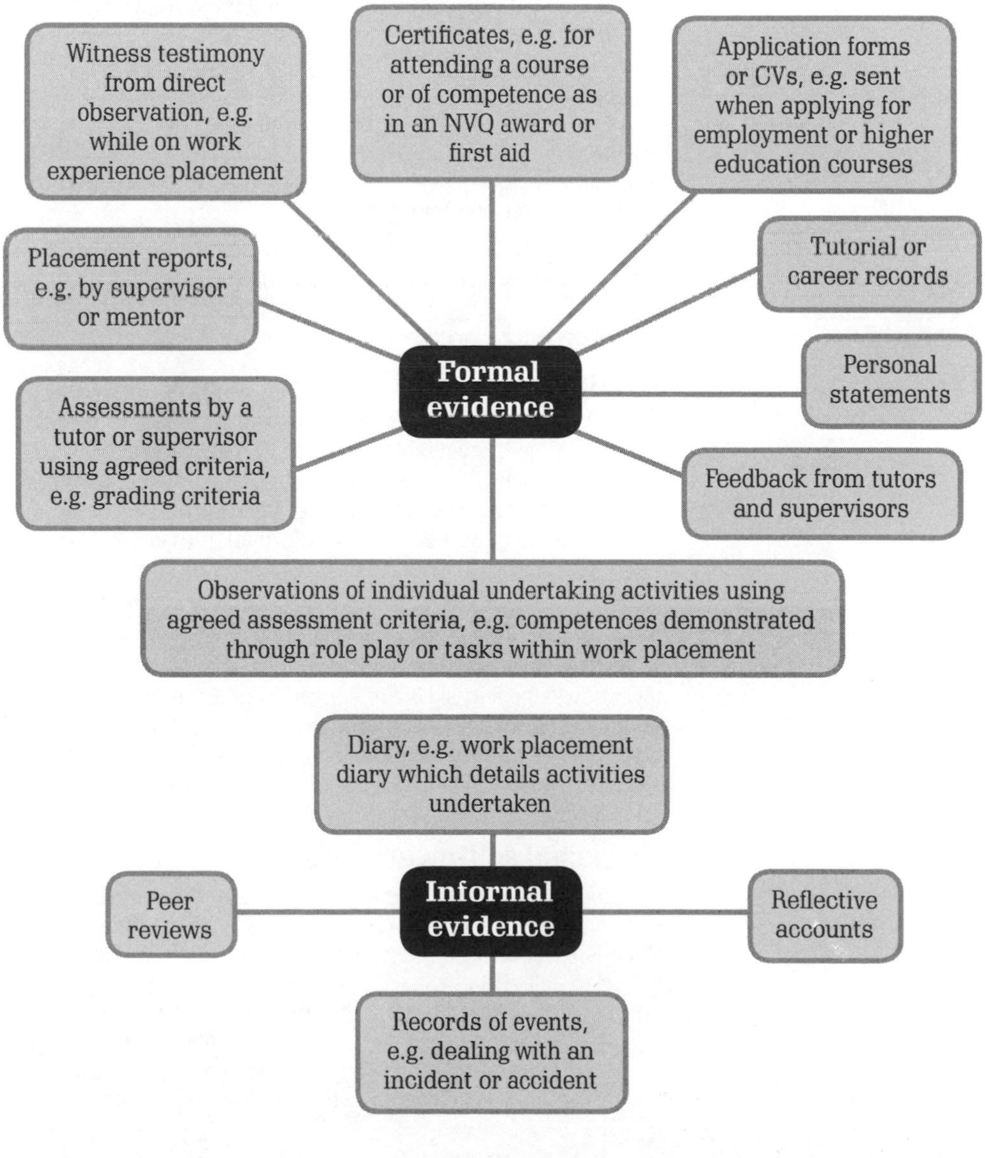

Witness testimony from direct observation, e.g. while on work experience placement

Certificates, e.g. for attending a course or of competence as in an NVQ award or first aid

Application forms or CVs, e.g. sent when applying for employment or higher education courses

Placement reports, e.g. by supervisor or mentor

Tutorial or career records

Formal evidence

Personal statements

Assessments by a tutor or supervisor using agreed criteria, e.g. grading criteria

Feedback from tutors and supervisors

Observations of individual undertaking activities using agreed assessment criteria, e.g. competences demonstrated through role play or tasks within work placement

Diary, e.g. work placement diary which details activities undertaken

Peer reviews

Informal evidence

Reflective accounts

Records of events, e.g. dealing with an incident or accident

Any of these sources of relevant evidence are valuable as they demonstrate how the individual is developing and can be used as a measure to quantify the individual's development when monitoring and reviewing progress against their original personal development plan. Before presenting any of these sources as evidence, it is important to check it against the criteria detailed above to ensure credibility and integrity is maintained.

Support for development

Tutors, peers, supervisors and mentors

The individual can access support from a range of different people to assist them in achieving their development goals or targets. Their personal tutor is a key source of support as tutors can provide both academic and pastoral support in terms of helping the individual to adjust to the level of study required and managing learning within their life. Tutors are also a valuable resource as well as someone to talk through options and dilemmas that may occur through the programme. They are however, unable to help if they are unaware that the individual requires support, so it is important to talk to them sooner rather than later if problems occur as negotiations with others may be required to maintain progress. For example, if the individual has personal issues that are creating stress in meeting deadlines. Tutors are a good source for constructive feedback and encouragement which will all motivate the individual and guide them in the right direction.

Peers are another valuable source of support as they are experiencing the same things as the individual in terms of making adjustments to their lives and managing study commitments. Having peers to share resources and information with is helpful as this can assist with time management as well as learning. Peers are also a valuable source of support at those times in the course of the programme when energy, enthusiasm and confidence are low and when the individual needs encouragement and reassurance that their goal is worth the hard work and commitment and that they can achieve it. Peers may also be able to offer other practical support, such as help with transport to college as well as sharing notes if sessions are missed. Being able to discuss coursework is useful as this often a good way to embed learning as well as opening out debate and widening an individual's perspective, as discussion often involves challenging assumptions and seeking to understand another's interpretation. Some projects may also require working with others and so to complete these successfully individuals will need to support one another.

Supervisors and mentors are also good sources of support as they can provide both opportunities for discussion and learning through this, as well as providing constructive feedback on the individual's practical application of knowledge and problem solving within work experience placements.

Meetings

The individual is likely to have one-to-one meetings with their supervisor or mentor. This individual time is invaluable for discussion about specific issues and areas of development that may be difficult to discuss in a group setting. Meetings with tutors, supervisors or mentors enable the individual to receive feedback, discuss issues and concerns and check out their learning as well as learn information that is of specific use to their individual needs. Meetings provide an opportunity to monitor progress, review goals or targets and discuss options and adjustments that may be required to maintain progress.

Other types of meeting can also support development, such as team meetings when on work experience placements. Team meetings often contain an opportunity for discussion of how knowledge and skills are applied in practice in terms of problem solving, for example managing behaviour or supporting an individual who is moving to another service or who is dying. These discussions provide an opportunity to listen to a range of ideas, perspectives and possible solutions which the individual can learn from and this will further support their development.

Increased self-awareness

Discussion and feedback from supervisors and mentors will often include information regarding personal effectiveness and this is an essential part of increasing self-awareness which is required if an individual is to be effective within a health or social care role. This increased self-awareness will support development in a number of ways. For example, individuals may feel more able to try new things or to take on more responsibility as the feedback they have received from others confirms their feeling that they are capable of more than they are currently involved in. An increased self-awareness may give the individual more confidence in their abilities as well as being able to recognise and accept their limitations.

Increased self-awareness supports development as it increases insight and this increases personal effectiveness so that the individual knows what they need to do to maximise their strengths and minimise their weaknesses, for example they know when to ask for help rather than muddle through and make mistakes.

How and where to access information and support on knowledge and best practice

A successful learner is one who knows what questions to ask rather than one who knows all the answers. Research skills are more valuable in supporting development than just having the information, as they provide the individual with a greater potential for accessing more answers. Keeping records of where and how to locate information is an important aspect of managing learning to ensure easy access and effective time management.

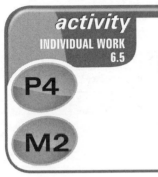

activity
INDIVIDUAL WORK
6.5

P4

M2

1   Give an account of your progress against your action plan over the duration of the BTEC programme.

2   Explain how your action plan has helped to support your own development throughout the BTEC programme.

Reflect on own development

Reflection is an important part of the learning process. For health and social care workers, reflecting on their own development is a crucial aspect of professional practice as the need to integrate their learning into their practice is essential in maintaining effective and up-to-date practice.

 Link

Refer back to page 192 to remind yourself about learning styles.

Donald Schön considered that reflection took place when individuals encountered unique situations they were unable to apply previous learning to. He identified two types of reflection:

■ 'Reflection-in-action' takes place during the event while in the process of responding and is sometimes referred to as 'thinking on your feet'. Reflection in this situation is limited as there is neither the space nor time to answer all the questions raised by the situation.

■ 'Reflection-on-action' takes place after the event and provides an opportunity to consider the reasons for actions and the impact of those actions on the individuals and the situation.

To be effective, health and social care workers need to be able to utilise both types of reflection so that they can continue to develop their knowledge, skills and practice. The result of reflection should be learning and change within the person and their perspective of the situation which will inform their actions if the same or a similar situation should occur again.

Different models of reflection can be used for linking theory to practice and practice to theory. Reflecting involves the individual in consciously taking notice of what is happening in a situation, asking questions and then making sense of the experience and determining what it means to them. Many individuals find it difficult to know where to start when considering reflection, so having a framework or a set of trigger questions to structure reflection is useful. One framework for reflection is Gibbs' reflective cycle.

Gibb's model can be used for reflection either verbally, within a meeting with a tutor, supervisor, mentor or peer, or in written form, within a reflective account or diary. This model enables the individual to link theory to practice during the analysis stage of the process, as it requires the individual to draw upon their previous learning in order to make sense of what happened and to explain their feelings and responses in the situation. Linking practice to theory also happens at this stage as well as the action plan stage when different approaches may be considered in light of learning.

Fig 6.9 Gibbs' reflective cycle

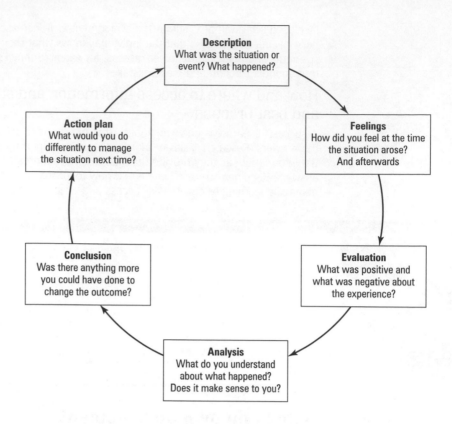

Undertaking reflection either in meetings, through maintaining a learning log or reflective diary all contribute to the individual's personal development as each achievement of personal goals in terms of knowledge, skills, practice, values, beliefs and career aspirations will be considered and documented. As each achievement is entered and acknowledged, there will be reflection on how the individual knows this has been achieved, for example what evidence they have to support it as well as what other informal and possibly unplanned learning was also achieved.

As part of the reflection process, the individual needs to ask themselves questions about what they were trying to achieve in terms of knowledge, skills, practice, values, beliefs and career aspirations as these are key motivations for change. When considering the evaluation and conclusion parts of the reflective cycle, the individual will be questioning the influence of their personal values and beliefs on the situation and the impact of their behaviour on others involved and the outcomes of the situation. If the individual is to increase their self-awareness, these are crucial questions they must seek to answer. Seeking, receiving and responding to feedback from others is an important aspect of this part of reflection as this can enable individuals to gain insight into how others perceive them. For this to be an effective process, the individual needs to recognise the impact of others on evolving development of self.

activity

INDIVIDUAL WORK 6.6

D2

Reflect on your development during the BTEC programme and consider the value and importance of your development in helping you achieve your goals and aspirations.

Feedback from others is not the only way others can impact on development. A significant factor in the processes of learning and development is imitation and individuals have the capacity to choose which characteristics they have observed in others to imitate and integrate into their own character, attitude and behaviour. As an emerging health and social care worker, the individual will see both positive and negative practice and attitudes and the impact these have within different health and social care settings. For example, a positive role model can provide a framework by which to measure the individual's development and attitude, for example in terms of managing others. Experience of poor practice or negative attitudes and the destructive influence of these on others may either lead the individual to see this as an easy way to progress and therefore lead them to imitate poor practice, or they may develop a stronger sense of their own beliefs and attitudes and be determined not to undertake this type of behaviour.

 Link

See page 278 in Unit 8 for more information about social learning and the effects of other individuals, groups, culture and society on the behaviour of individuals.

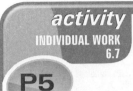
activity
INDIVIDUAL WORK 6.7
P5

Produce a personal and professional development portfolio and write a reflective account of the value of this record to your development.

activity
INDIVIDUAL WORK 6.8
M3

Reflect on three experiences you have had as a part of your work in health and social care which demonstrate how theory has been linked to practice.

Service provision in the health or social care sectors

As part of the BTEC Health and Social programme, individuals will be investigating a range of occupational areas to help them decide on future career options. A part of this is gaining an understanding how health and social care services are arranged both on a national and local level.

Provision of services

Health and social care services are provided through a national framework relevant to each country within the UK. These more local arrangements are overseen by central or devolved government departments. Most services are provided locally and are either primary, such as GPs, community-based services, pharmacists, opticians, or secondary services, such as acute hospitals. Some services are referred to as tertiary services as they are provided on a regional or sub-regional basis. Tertiary services are specialist services dealing, for example, with a disease or condition that is rare within the population and for which specialist skills or equipment are required to diagnose, treat and support patients. Tertiary services include those for patients with rare cancers, burns, plastic surgery, rare diseases or genetically inherited conditions.

 Link

See page 241 in Unit 7 for more information about how health services are arranged within England and Wales in terms of primary and secondary care services within the statutory sector.

England and Wales

In England and Wales, health care provision is overseen by the Department of Health.

Fig 6.10 Department of
Health services

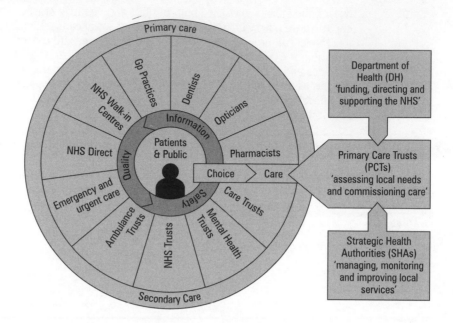

In England and Wales, joint health and social care Partnership Trusts have been established to provide specialist services, such as services for people with learning disabilities, mental health needs (children and adults), secure and forensic services and substance misuse. Partnership Boards have also been set up to support people with learning disabilities through bringing together statutory, voluntary, independent agencies and the wider community to implement the vision for learning disability services in the 21st century set out in 'Valuing People'. This document was published by the Department of Health in 2001 following wide consultation. It sets out the strategy and actions to be undertaken to improve the lives of children and adults who have a learning disability to ensure they access the same opportunities to participate and live full and independent lives as part of their local community.

| Valuing People Support Team | www.valuingpeople.gov.uk |

Social services in the UK are generally provided through the local authority, although there may be joint health and social care services in some areas of the country. Policy and guidance is provided through government directives, objectives and targets. NHS services are free at the point of delivery apart from some services such as prescription charges, eye tests and dental check-ups. Social services provision differs from those of the NHS as they are means-tested (based on financial status) and subject to Fair Access to Care Services eligibility criteria. This guidance published in January 2003 provided local authority social services departments and councils with a framework for setting their eligibility criteria for funding adult social care through the consideration of an individual's needs and risks. It was implemented in April 2003. The aim was to ensure that fairer and more consistent eligibility decisions regarding adult social care funding across the whole of England and Wales. Fair Access to Care Services identifies risks and needs and categorise these into those that are critical, substantial, moderate and low. In most areas, the local authority social services department will provide funding to support those people whose needs are determined to be critical or substantial. If the individual's needs are moderate but likely to deteriorate to become either substantial or critical within a six-month period if support is not provided then services may be provided. The individual will be required to complete a financial assessment to determine their ability to contribute to the cost of their support.

Scotland

In Scotland, it is the Scottish Executive that oversees the work of the fourteen Health Boards in Scotland which cover different regional areas. The Scottish Executive, like the Department of Health, determines the national objectives for health services and offers guarantees on behalf of patients. It also provides the statutory and financial framework for NHS Scotland and is accountable for its performance. The Health Boards manage acute and community-based hospital provision (provided by independent Trusts as in England and Wales) as well as mental health and physical disabilities services. Community Health Partnerships (CHP) or in some places joint Health and Care Partnerships (CHCP), are responsible for community-based services which include social services in CHCP. CHPs and CHCPs may oversee a number of different provisions, including:

- healthy living centres: to provide a one-stop shop for advice and support to maintain health and well-being
- podiatry services
- smoking cessation services
- community learning disability team
- intensive community treatment team: to provide short-term rehabilitative services to prevent hospital admission or assist early hospital discharge.

Northern Ireland

In Northern Ireland, health and social care services are overseen by the Department of Health, Social Services and Public Safety. Responsibility for services is devolved to a local level with four Area Boards. The Area Boards are responsible within their area for assessing needs of individuals who may require their support and services as well as commissioning services to meet those needs. Each Area Board is responsible for setting key objectives, developing policies and priorities to enable them to meet these key objectives and in doing so meet the health and social needs of their population.

In Northern Ireland there are also a number of health agencies which support the diverse range of health and social care needs within the population. They include services such as the ambulance service, cancer services, such as screening and treatment, and children's services, such as Guardian Ad Litem. As in all parts of the UK, there are also health councils that act as independent consumer organisations through which public views and interests are represented. They are responsible for reviewing health and social care services and are able to make recommendations for improvements in service delivery as required. Generally health councils are within the same geographical area as the corresponding Health or Area Board.

Services are also provided by a range of voluntary and independent organisations and these may be part-funded through health or social services.

Regulators

Health and social care services are regulated through inspection authorities who are required to provide regular inspections of services in terms of quality and meeting service standards. There are a number of regulators responsible for ensuring expected standards are met by all health and social care services. As well as those organisations that regulate health and social care organisations there are also regulators specific to occupations such as the professional bodies.

Department of Health	www.dh.gov.uk
Commission for Social Care Inspection	www.csci.org.uk
Commission for Health care Audit and Inspection	www.healthcarecommission.org.uk
Scottish Executive	www.scotland.gov.uk
NHS Scotland	www.show.scot.nhs.uk
Health Improvement in Scotland	www.healthscotland.com
Social Work in Scotland	www.socialworkscotland.org.uk
Scottish Social Services Council	www.sssc.uk.com
Social Work Inspection Agency (Scotland)	www.swia.gov.uk
Scottish Commission for the Regulation of Care	www.carecommission.com
Health & Personal Social Services in Northern Ireland	www.healthandcareni.co.uk
Department of Health, Social Services and Public Safety in Northern Ireland	www.dhsspsni.gov.uk

Regulators of health and social care services

Regulator	Function
Commission for Health care Audit and Inspection	The health watchdog for England which is responsible for checking that health care services meet the standards that have been set in a range of areas, e.g. health and safety, cleanliness and waiting times. They have a statutory duty to assess the performance of health care organisations (through the annual health check process which considers the quality of service and the use of resources), award a rating based on the results (excellent, good, fair or weak) and coordinate reviews of health care by other organisations. Concerned with provision of health care as described in section 45(2) of the Health and Social Care (Community Health and Standards) Act (2003) and the provision of independent health care services within the meaning of section 5A (A) of the Care Standards Act (2000).
Health care Inspectorate Wales	Responsible for review and investigation into the provision of health care by and for Welsh NHS bodies as defined under the Health and Social Care (Community Health and Standards) Act (2003).
Commission for Social Care Inspection	Responsible for the registrations and inspection of social care services as defined under the Care Standards Act (2000) (e.g. residential care homes, domiciliary care services, etc) and the performance assessment of English local authority social services as defined in section 148 of the Health and Social Care (Community Health and Standards) Act (2003). CSCI produces reports which are accessible by the public.
Care Standards Inspectorate Wales	Responsible for the provision of services as described under section 8 of the Care Standards Act (2000) and the Children Act (1989).
Social Services Inspectorate for Wales	As for English CSCI.
Scottish Commission for the Regulation of Care	Responsible for the provision of services as described in the Regulation of Care (Scotland) Act (2001), e.g. adult placements, residential care homes, day centres, supported housing services, domiciliary care services.
Regulation and Quality Improvement Authority	Responsible for regulation of standards of both statutory and independent health and social care services in Northern Ireland.
Commissioner for Children and Young people	There is a commissioner for each of the four UK countries, and they are responsible for matters relating to the rights and best interests of children and young people.
Social Care Councils	There is a social care council for each of the four UK countries. These are responsible for the registration of social care workers as described under the Care Standards Act (2000).

See page 372 in Unit 11 for more information about regulation of health and social care workers.

Local health or social care service providers

Health and social care workers need to have a good understanding of local provision if they are to adequately support and advocate for the individuals they work with. To do this, they need to know what type of provision is available locally (supported living, tenancies, residential care, domiciliary or day services), what type of funding is need to support attendance or access (through means-tested social services funding, charitable funds) and how individuals can access both the provision and any funding to support their use of the provision. It is important to also know what potential barriers to access there may be, such as a waiting list, limited transport available, lack of funding or eligibility criteria.

The health and social care worker also needs to have an understanding of the organisational policies and procedures of each organisation as this may impact on choice and compatibility with the individual's values, beliefs, interests and priorities. It is also important to understand how the different services fit within the national frameworks and how they relate to other organisations and are regulated. These are all safeguards when choosing appropriate health and social care provision to meet the individual's needs and circumstances.

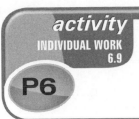

1   Describe the services provided by a local health or social care service provider.
2   Explain how this provider fits into the national framework of health or social care provision.

Health and social care workers

There is a diverse range of occupations within the health and social care services, including health and social care professionals such as nurses and social workers, professions allied to medicine, technical support professionals such as medical and non-medical laboratory staff and other support professionals such as managers and administrators.

Health and social care professionals

Nursing staff

Nurses work in a variety of settings and with anyone with health care needs whether they are a child or an adult. They may work in acute hospital settings or within the community, including in schools. To practise they require a nursing qualification which they gain through a university where theory and practical experience are combined within the course. Nurses provide a range of support to individuals including practical nursing care, health screening, undertaking routine measurements and observations and assisting doctors and others in providing health care. Some nurses undertake additional training and qualifications to become specialists, such as midwives, nurse prescribers (who have the authority to prescribe some medications) or clinical nurse specialists. Once qualified and registered with the Nursing and Midwifery Council (NMC), nurses and midwives are required to maintain their registration through re-registration and evidence to demonstrate continuing professional development and practice.

Social workers

Social workers undertake a 3-year social work degree either before embarking on their role or while they are undertaking their social work job. Social work courses include work placements to enable the individual to apply theory to practice and practice to theory. Social workers work in variety of settings from fieldwork to residential care.

Field social workers work with individuals living in the community and provide advice, guidance, support and protection. This may be through assessment of their needs, direct provision of support (emotional and social) to children and families or assisting young adults to live independently. Field social workers commission services from others to provide support to individuals living in the community once eligibility for services has been identified and agreed.

Residential social workers work within care homes, children's homes, hostels and youth centres. They too assess needs and circumstances and provide emotional and social support to individuals. They may also manage residential care provision and ensure individual's rights and choices are upheld and they are treated with respect for their individuality and dignity.

Fig 6.11 A nurse

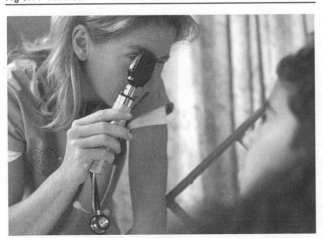

Fig 6.12 A social worker

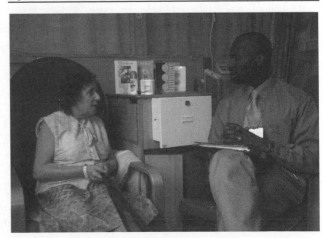

Professions allied to medicine

There numerous allied professions including arts, drama and music therapists, psychologists and psychotherapists.

About the range of careers within the NHS	www.nhscareers.nhs.uk
About careers in the care services	www.skillsforcare.org.uk
About other careers in health services	www.skillsforhealth.org.uk

More details about a number of allied professions are included in the table below:

Professions allied to medicine

Profession		Function	Workplaces	Training
[HDI 6-5]	Physiotherapist	Assesses and treat physical problems that affect movement and function which they regard as central to health and well-being. They identify and maximise movement potential through the use of appropriate therapies including exercise	Works with anyone who has physical problems resulting from illness, accident or ageing; works in a variety of settings	3- or 4-year degree course
[HDI 6-6]	Speech and language therapist	Assesses and treat speech, language and communication problems in people of all ages to enable them to communicate to the best of their ability. Also supports people with swallowing and eating problems	Works in schools, hospitals and community settings	4-year degree course
[HDI 6-7]	Occupational therapist	Assesses and treats physical and psychiatric conditions using specific purposeful activity to prevent disability and promote independent function in daily activities	Works with all ages and in a wide range of settings	3-year degree course
[HDI 6-8]	Dietician	Interprets and communicates the science of nutrition to enable individuals to make informed choices about their diet and lifestyle	Works within hospital, community, in education and the food industry	4-year degree + 2-year post-graduate course
[HDI 6-9]	Chiropodist, podiatrist	Diagnoses and treats abnormalities of the lower limb. Give advice on foot care and how to prevent foot problems	Works within both hospital and community settings	3-year degree course
[HDI 6-10]	Radiographer	Two types of radiographer: diagnostic radiographer undertakes radiology and imaging (e.g. X-rays, ultrasound). Works mainly in hospitals or clinics with people of all ages. Therapeutic radiographer generally involved in providing radiotherapy treatments for people with cancers. They work closely with oncology (cancer treatment) teams	Works with people of all ages within a hospital or specialist centre	3- to 4-year degree course
[HDI 6-11]	Operating department practitioner	Provides care to patients undergoing operations during the administration of the anaesthetic, during and after surgery and in the recovery phase	Works as part of a team within the operating department of a hospital and will work with people of all ages: assesses patient needs and provides appropriate care and intervention	2-year diploma course
[HDI 6-12]	Prosthetist and orthotist	Provide care and support for individuals who require an artificial limb (prosthesis) or a devise to support or control part of the body (orthosis). They provide advice and support related to rehabilitation. They work as part of a team with individuals who have either lost a limb through birth defect, accident or amputation (e.g. due to a disease such as diabetes)	Works with individuals of all ages; works within specialised companies or within large NHS hospitals	4-year degree course at either the University of Salford or the University of Strathclyde

Technical support professionals

Technicians, both medical and non-medical, provide vital support to professionals and allied professionals within health care. Medical staff require clinical investigations that they undertake in the course of diagnosis to be processed and sometimes interpreted, in order to prescribe the appropriate treatment or intervention. Medical and non-medical laboratory staff are essential to the diagnosis and treatment of patients. They may take blood samples for a range of tests (phlebotomy), process the samples to detect the presence of disease and report the outcomes of tests (haematology). They may also be involved in the microscopic study of body tissues to aid diagnosis of disease (histology), study of the immune system to identify allergies, disease resistance and acceptance or rejection of tissues following bone marrow or organ transplant (immunology), examining cells such as cervical cells following a cervical smear as part of health screening (cytology). Medical and non-medical laboratory staff play an important role in health care and disease prevention and treatment. These areas of work are particularly of interest to individuals who are interested in science and health care rather than direct care of individuals. Training for medical and non-medical laboratory staff is mostly work-based, for example NVQs. Individuals can progress to become a trainee biomedical scientist and then on to further study.

Other support professionals

Other support professionals include managers and administrators. Some health care practitioners, such as nurses and allied health professionals progress their career from clinical work into management and may undertake management courses to assist them in their career progression, such as leadership and management courses, management degrees or MBAs. Other NHS managers enter through the NHS Graduate Scheme following successful completion of a first degree at university or as an experienced manager from another area of work, such as personnel management. In social care, most managers progress from social care practice into management positions and, like their counterparts in health care, are likely to undertake management qualifications while employed as a manager as part of their continuing professional development. Managers working in residential care services are required to have attained recognised care and management qualifications at level 4 or above and many hold the NVQ Level 4 Registered Manager Award (RMA) (for adults or residential childcare) in order to comply with the CSCI registration requirements. Managers are involved in every aspect of health and social care work and are likely to be involved in managing both services and people who work within those services. They will be responsible for budgetary management, maintaining the quality of service provision, recruiting and developing staff, managing staff performance, work activities and information. They may also be involved in developing new services.

Administrators are also essential to the effective running of health and social care services as they are often responsible for managing the information flow required to document health and social care activities, producing reports for other organisations for funding purposes and managing the administrative activity involved in supporting individuals to access and use health and social care services, for example arranging out-patient appointments and sending individual's assessment records and care plans. Administrators are also be involved in managing the administrative processes involved with employing staff, such as recruitment and paying salaries. Administrators will often have qualifications, for example related to IT skills, or receive work-based learning opportunities, such as Office Administration or Customer Services NVQs.

Role of professional bodies

Professions are supported by professional bodies which regulate the profession through qualification requirements, registration, codes of conduct and continuing professional development requirements, and provide advice and professional practice guidance. They produce this guidance in line with changes in legislation which have a direct impact on policy, practical procedures, roles and responsibilities and accountability, for example, adult protection guidance. Professional bodies also provide professional codes of conduct which detail the role, responsibilities, attitudes and accountability of individuals within the profession. In their role as regulators, professional bodies also have professional conduct and complaints committees which hear evidence regarding complaints or cases of professional misconduct, and make decisions regarding an individual's fitness to practice and be maintained on the professional register. Professional bodies hold details of all individuals who have been removed or suspended from the professional register. At present only specific groups within health care, such as registered nurses, midwives, and other allied health professionals, for example physiotherapists and speech and language therapists have to be registered with professional bodies in order to do their jobs. Within social care, social workers and student social workers are the only groups who have to be registered with the General Social Care Council. In those professions where there is a registration requirement, this means that individual would be unable to work within that profession if for some reason they were removed from the register.

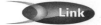

See page 372 in Unit 11 for more information about professional bodies and codes of conduct.

Career pathways

There is recognition within health and social care that career pathways are essential if individuals are to remain working in the sector.

Training and qualifications

For those individuals who enter health and social care through an academic route, such as a nursing or social work degree, the career pathway is clearly defined. For example, a social worker once qualified can continue their professional development by undertaking a Post-Qualifying Award in Specialist Social Work, Higher Specialist Social Work or Advanced Social Work. They could specialise in one of five areas: mental health, adult social care, children, young people, their families and carers, practice education or leadership and management.

Individuals entering social care via a vocational route can access training from their initial induction through to health and social care NVQs, the level of which will depend on their job role and responsibilities. For a care worker undertaking routine tasks that are generally supervised, NVQ Level 2 would be appropriate. For a senior care worker or support worker who undertakes fewer routine tasks, works with less supervision and may supervise others, NVQ Level 3 is likely to be appropriate. For an individual working as an assistant manager or in a post that requires they undertake management tasks, such as managing staff, services or budgets, an NVQ Level 4 is likely to appropriate. The registered manager or a social care service will undertake the NVQ Level 4 Registered Manager Award (RMA) for adults or residential childcare depending on their work setting. A Foundation Degree in Health and Social Care is also available in many universities and colleges and individuals may be able to access this with some credit towards a shortened course if they have an RMA.

In health care, it was recognised that to achieve the NHS plan to modernise the NHS and improve the patient's experience of receiving health care, staff needed to have relevant opportunities to learn and develop their knowledge and skills. As a result, the Skills Escalator was developed to enable individuals to plan their development so they can develop their skills and knowledge in readiness for promotion. The Skills Escalator shows how qualifications (National Qualifications Framework) and job responsibility (Career Framework) are linked or overlap and gives an impression of how learning links to progression in the NHS. Having a career pathway is a significant motivator for many people and the Skills Escalator provides a clear progression route linked to qualifications and job roles and responsibilities.

Fig 6.13 Skills Escalator

Career framework

National Qualifications Framework	Career Framework
9	More senior posts
8 — Doctoral level	Consultant practitioner
7, 6 — Post-graduate level	Advanced practitioner
	Senior or specialist practitioner
5, 4 — Degree/Diploma level	Qualified practitioner
	Assistant practitioner
3, 2 — NVQ 1–3, GCSE and A-Level	Senior assistant
1	Assistant
Entry	Supporting roles

National qualifications and the careers framework

NQF level	Level description	Sample qualifications	CF level	CF level name	CF level description
Entry	Entry level qualifications recognise basic knowledge and skills and the ability to apply learning in everyday situations under direct guidance or supervision. Learning at this level involves building basic knowledge and skills and is not geared towards specific occupations.	Entry level	1	Initial entry level jobs	Jobs such as 'domestics' or 'cadets' requiring very little formal education or previous knowledge, skills or experience in delivering, or supporting the delivery of healthcare.
Level 1	Level 1 qualifications recognise basic knowledge and skills and the ability to apply learning with guidance or supervision. Learning at this level is about activities which mostly relate to everyday situations and may be linked to job competence.	NVQ 1; GCSEs Grades D-G	2	Support workers	Frequently with the job title of 'health care assistant' or 'health care technician' – probably studying for or has attained NVQ Level 2.
Level 2	Level 2 qualifications recognise the ability to gain a good knowledge and understanding of a subject area of work or study, and to perform varied tasks with some guidance or supervision. Learning at this level involves building knowledge and/or skills in relation to an area of work or a subject area and is appropriate for many job roles.	NVQ 2; GCSEs Grades A*-C	3	Senior healthcare assistants/ technicians	This is a higher level of responsibility than support worker, probably studying for or have attained NVQ Level 3, or Assessment of Prior Experiential Learning (APEL).
Level 3	Level 3 qualifications recognise the ability to gain, and where relevant apply a range of knowledge, skills and understanding. Learning at this level involves obtaining detailed knowledge and skills. It is appropriate for people wishing to go to university, people working independently, or in some areas supervising and training others in their field of work.	NVQ 3; A levels	4	Assistant/ associate practitioners	Probably studying for Foundation degree, BTEC higher or HND. Some of their remit will involve them in delivering protocol-based clinical care that had previously been in the remit of registered professionals, under the direction and supervision of a state registered practitioner.
Level 4	Level 4 qualifications recognise specialist learning and involve detailed analysis of a high level of information and knowledge in an area of work or study. Learning at this level is appropriate for people working in technical and professional jobs, and/or managing and developing others.	NVQ 4; Certificate of Higher Education	5	Practitioners	Most frequently registered practitioners in their first and second post-registration or professional qualification jobs.
Level 5	Level 5 qualifications recognise the ability to increase the depth of knowledge and understanding of an area of work or study to enable the formulation of solutions and responses to complex problems and situations. Learning at this level involves the demonstration of high levels of knowledge, a high level of work expertise in job roles and competence in managing and training others. Qualifications at this level are appropriate for people working as higher grade technicians, professionals or managers.	Diplomas of Higher Education and Further Education; Foundation Degrees; Higher National Diplomas; BTEC	6	Senior/ specialist practitioners	Staff who would have a higher degree of autonomy and responsibility than 'Practitioners' in the clinical environment; or who would be managing one or more service areas in the non-clinical environment.

►

NQF level	Level description	Sample qualifications	CF level	CF level name	CF level description
Level 6	Level 6 qualifications recognise a specialist high level knowledge of an area of work or study to enable the use of an individual's own ideas and research in response to complex problems and situations. Learning at this level involves the achievement of a high level of professional knowledge and is appropriate for people working as knowledge-based professionals or in professional management positions.	Bachelor's Degrees; Graduate Certificates and Diplomas	7	Advanced practitioners	Experienced clinical professionals who have developed their skills and theoretical knowledge to a very high standard. They are empowered to make high-level clinical decisions and will often have their own caseload. Non-clinical staff at Level 7 will typically be managing a number of service areas.
Level 7	Level 7 qualifications recognise highly developed and complex levels of knowledge which enable the development of in-depth and original responses to complicated and unpredictable problems and situations. Learning at this level involves the demonstration of high level specialist professional knowledge and is appropriate for senior professionals and managers.	Masters Degrees; Postgraduate Certificates and Diplomas	8	Consultant practitioners	Staff working at a very high level of clinical expertise or have responsibility for the planning of services.
Level 8	Level 8 qualifications recognise leading experts or practitioners in a particular field. Learning at this level involves the development of new and creative approaches that extend or redefine existing knowledge or professional practice.	Specialist awards; Doctorates	9	More senior staff	Staff with the ultimate responsibility for clinical caseload decision-making and have full on-call accountability.

Source: www.lnrhwd.nhs.uk/wdc/skills_escalator/priorities.php

Training and qualification frameworks are developed by the Sector Skills Councils, such as Skills for Care and Skills for Health, following development and agreement regarding National Occupational Standards (NOS). The NOS describe health and social care tasks and include the skills, knowledge, understanding, attitudes, values and beliefs required to competently carry out those tasks. The NOS are reflected in the NVQ standards as well as within individual's roles and responsibilities as described in their job description. In fact, many job descriptions are now written to reflect the appropriate NOS. Organisational polices and procedures also provide the health and social care worker with information about their role and responsibilities in relation to specific tasks or events, such as when providing personal care support or in the event of an emergency.

Workforce development

Every health or social care organisation has a responsibility to plan the development of their workforce to endure individuals remain interested and motivated by their work as well as up-to-date in their knowledge and skills in order to deliver the best quality care possible. As discussed earlier, organisations are also required by nature of their registration or funding to demonstrate how they ensure workforce development occurs. It is important also for organisations to ensure they are planning for the future so that if individuals leave the organisation others are able to be promoted into those positions to ensure continuity and maintained quality of service provision. Continuing professional development is a feature of health and social care work in the 21st century and organisations are more active in workforce development activities as they rise to the challenge of meeting increased public expectations of health and social care services and provision. Within social care, Skills for Care have actively promoted workforce development thought the qualifications framework and providing funding to enable individuals to access appropriate qualifications. The NHS Agenda for Change scheme has actively encouraged workers to develop their practice through linking professional development to pay scales so that there are tangible incentives to engaging in learning and development activities.

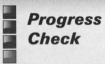 Link

Refer back to page 232 to remind yourself about the Skills Escalator.

Multi-disciplinary teams

Multi-disciplinary teams bring practitioners from different disciplines (areas), such as social work, nursing, physiotherapy, speech and language therapy, psychology and occupational therapy, together to enable them to work more effectively with individuals whose needs and circumstances are complex and which require coordinated assessment and care planning to support those needs from a number of different health and social care practitioners in order to improve or maintain their well-being. This is particularly true for individuals with short term intensive needs, such as those who require rehabilitation either in hospital or in the community, or who require **palliative** care, or individuals with longer-term complex needs such as individuals with long-term chronic health conditions, for example chronic respiratory or heart disease; individuals with learning difficulties or mental health needs. In recognition of this, multi-disciplinary teams have developed to ensure the individual is supported in a coordinated and effective manner so that their well-being is maintained and is not subject to fluctuations and crises as a result of delays in various practitioners getting involved in their support.

The composition of a multi-disciplinary team will depend on the area of work or the particular needs of the individual they support. For example, a community mental health team for older people is likely to be made up of a psychogeriatrican (specialist psychiatrist for people over 65 years old), a social worker, a community psychiatric nurse (CPN), an occupational therapist, a psychologist and community support workers who provide home support. Multi-disciplinary teams are invaluable to the individual who then receives a seamless service which is coordinated with all those practitioners involved in supporting them aware of the interventions being undertaken by others and a clear sense of the goals and outcomes being worked towards.

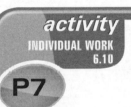

activity
INDIVIDUAL WORK
6.10

P7

Describe the roles, responsibilities and career pathways of:

- occupational therapist
- registered nurse
- social worker.

Progress
Check

1 What is the experiential learning cycle as described by David Kolb?
2 How might individuals' aspirations and motivations influence their learning?
3 How can supervisors and mentors support learning?
4 Give three examples of informal learning.
5 How can self-awareness be used to review values and beliefs?
6 How would you monitor and evaluate your development plan?
7 How would you ensure that evidence to support development is relevant and valid?
8 Use an example to explain how you would link theory to practice.
9 What are tertiary health care services? Give examples.
10 What is meant by workforce development?

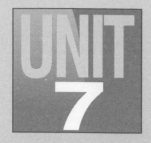

Sociological perspectives for health and social care

This unit covers:

- Sociological approaches to study
- Applying sociological approaches to health and social care

To be effective in their role, health and social care workers need to have an understanding of sociology, that is how society works and the factors within society that impact on individual's lives. Understanding sociology and how sociological perspectives are applied in practice will enable health and social care workers to develop that understanding. In particular, health and social care workers need to understand how the biological, social and cultural concepts of health and illness, are constructed in society and how this social construction influences people's attitudes towards them. This unit will also explore the health inequalities that exist between different groups and the range of explanations sociologists have for these.

grading criteria

To achieve a **Pass** grade the evidence must show that the learner is able to:	To achieve a **Merit** grade the evidence must show that, in addition to the pass criteria, the learner is able to:	To achieve a **Distinction** grade the evidence must show that, in addition to the pass and merit criteria, the learner is able to:
P1 use sociological terminology to describe the principal sociological perspectives Pg 251		
P2 describe different concepts of health Pg 253	**M1** use two sociological perspectives to explain different concepts of health Pg 253	
P3 describe the biomedical and socio-medical models of health Pg 225	**M2** explain the biomedical and socio-medical models of health Pg 255	**D1** evaluate the biomedical and socio-medical models of health Pg 255
P4 describe different concepts of ill health Pg 259		

To achieve a **Pass** grade the evidence must show that the learner is able to:	To achieve a **Merit** grade the evidence must show that, in addition to the pass criteria, the learner is able to:	To achieve a **Distinction** grade the evidence must show that, in addition to the pass and merit criteria, the learner is able to:
P5	**M3**	**D2**
compare patterns and trends of health and illness in three different social groups Pg 272	use sociological explanations for health inequalities to explain the patterns and trends of health and illness in three different social groups Pg 275	evaluate the four sociological explanations for health inequalities in terms of explaining the patterns and trends of health and illness in three different social groups Pg 275

Sociological approaches to study

Sociology is one of the social sciences. Social sciences are concerned with understanding human behaviour and include psychology (which often overlaps with sociology), economics, politics, history and anthropology. Both sociology and psychology explore how we learn, how we make sense of the world around us and how social conditions affect behaviour and life experiences. Sociology is particularly interested in the social dimensions of health and illness; health inequalities and the impact of these in society, for example in terms of how the structure of health and social care services impact on individuals. To gain an understanding of sociology, it is important to understand social structures, diversity and the process of socialisation.

See page 278 in Unit 8 for more information on psychology.

Terminology

Social structures

The family

A family is generally considered to be a group of individuals who are closely related to one another either through birth, marriage or adoption. Family relationships are complex and they are probably the place where individuals experience their greatest joys as well as their greatest pain. For many of us, family is a place of acceptance and where we feel we can be truly ourselves. However, that shared heritage can also create conflict, not least because assumptions are made about individuals getting along with one another purely because they are members of the same family. Even though individuals may experience **abuse** at the hands of their family, they often remain loyal which suggests that blood ties are strong. For sociologists the family is both influenced by society as well as an influence on society.

Fig 7.1 Families

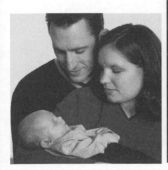
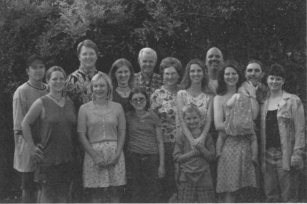
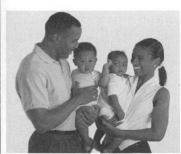

The most common family system is known as the 'nuclear family' with a father, mother and a child or children (biological or adopted) all living in and sharing the same household. An 'extended family' includes the nuclear family's other relatives, such as parents or older children and their families. During the 20th century, the idea of the nuclear family as the norm was challenged by the emergence of a variety of different types of family due to changes in social attitudes and circumstances. Although marriage and the idea of the nuclear family created as a result remains popular, changes in legislation and religious attitudes have meant that access to and acceptance of divorce (the UK divorce rate in 2005 was 13 percent) has led to the existence of other types of family which in some communities represent more the norm than the traditional nuclear family.

National Statistics Office   www.statistics.gov.uk

One variation is the 'reconstituted family', which results when divorced individuals form couples to create a new nuclear family made up of the couple and their children from their previous relationships, so that there is at least one step-parent relationship within the household. Another type of family that often arises due to divorce and changes in social attitudes, for example in relation to unmarried mothers, is the 'single (or lone) parent family', with a child or children living with only one of their parents. Lone parent families are not a homogenous group as they are made up of individuals who are widowed, separated, divorced or single. Also more recently people who are single have been able to both foster or adopt a child. Information from the Office of National Statistics (ONS) shows that, in 1998, the trend indicated a decline in the number of lone parent families resulting from divorce and the death of a spouse and an increase in single parents as a result of separation from a partner (both for males and females). The average number of lone parent families in the UK in 2005 was 25% with nine out of ten lone parents being lone mothers. Some would argue that a single parent family is an incomplete nuclear family as opposed to a distinct family type. Women are no longer economically dependent on their husbands or male family members and this, as well as support through the welfare system, has contributed to changes in family composition. The welfare system is considered by many to have replaced some of contributions made by the nature of **kinship** to family life and which united the nuclear family, for example when older people are supported by health or social care services rather than by relatives.

Changes in ideas about how best to care for and support children whose birth parents are unable to look after them has also meant more children being fostered in the short or long term, in order to enable them to live within a family environment which is still considered to be the best in terms of a balanced and nurturing upbringing. The dominant idea of the nuclear family as being a heterosexual couple with a child or children has also been challenged by couples in same-sex relationships. Some same-sex couples will have a child or children from a heterosexual relationship before 'coming out' (openly expressing their sexuality), while others will choose to have children through assisted means, such as in-vitro fertilisation (IVF), by donor or by adoption. The advent of IVF has also enabled many single women to actively choose motherhood as their desire to have a child is greater than their need to be in a relationship with the child's father. Within the UK, marriage is still **monogamous** although in other cultures, religions such as the Mormons or parts of the world, **polygamy** (having more than one spouse) is still accepted. The way that some individuals form relationships, marry and divorce several times during their lives is sometimes referred to as serial monogamy, that is being in one relationship at a time but numerous relationships over time. As a result of changes in social attitudes and behaviour, some families are even more complex as they include children with the same mother but with different fathers.

This complexity of family make-up may create moral dilemmas regarding relationships between 'siblings' where there is a non-blood relationship. Such moral dilemmas also occur when young unmarried mothers give a child up for adoption with no further contact and then later in life the mother and son or siblings meet and form relationships, unaware of their blood relationship. There remain both biological (genetic inheritance issues) and moral concerns and objections to these types of relationship.

Other cultures have different ideas regarding family where for example the responsibility for children is viewed as a collective one, as in the kibbutzim in Israel and state-run nursery provision in China. The benefit of these systems is that they also release women from child care duties to work and contribute to economic productivity.

Link

See page 248 for information about Marxists and feminist perspectives on the family.

Education system

The education system has an important role to play within any society and is a significant influence on individuals' framework for living and making sense of the world. Today, it is compulsory for young people to spend a minimum of eleven years in the educational system, and those who progress to further or higher education could be in the education system for nineteen years.

Fig 7.2 Educational establishments

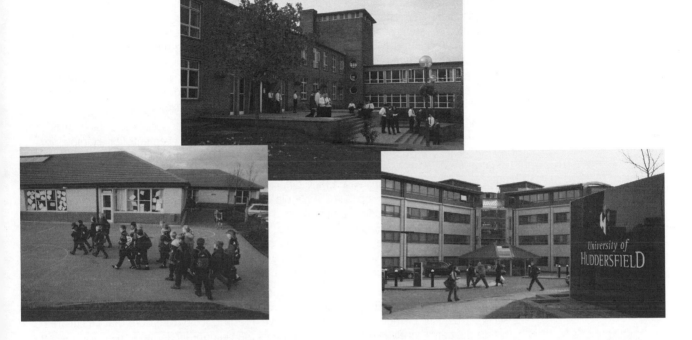

In the UK, there are state schools which receive funding from the Local Education Authority (LEA) and independent fee-paying schools. In England and Wales, all children aged 4 to 16 are entitled to a free place (3 to 16 years in Scotland) and nine out of ten children attend a state school.

Types of school and educational establishment

Type	Information
Community schools	■ Managed by the local authority and responsible for employing all staff ■ School premises owned by the local authority
Foundation or trust Schools	■ Managed by a governing body which is responsible for employing staff and setting the admissions criteria ■ Land and buildings usually owned by the governing body or charitable trust
Voluntary-aided schools	■ Usually faith-based schools managed by a governing body which is responsible for employing staff and setting the admissions criteria ■ Land and buildings usually owned by the governing body or charitable trust
Voluntary-controlled schools	■ Similar to voluntary-aided but run by the local authority ■ Land and buildings usually owned by a religious organisation or a charity

Admission to schools depends generally on geographic location although some schools will have other admissions criteria, such as religious observance. Fee-paying schools set criteria based on not only ability to pay but often on academic ability, such as through entrance examinations. Some fee-paying schools offer bursaries or scholarships for children whose parents are unable to pay tuition fees but who have either the academic ability or special ability in a subject such as music or sport. In primary education, children are taught in mixed ability age groups. When children reach secondary education, they are generally taught in ability groups for different subjects.

Further education colleges provide both academic and vocational post-16 education and qualifications. Higher education colleges and universities provide under- and post-graduate degrees as well as doctorates.

There is a national curriculum for each of the four countries of the UK. Each country has similar but also specific requirements. Within English schools, the National Curriculum is the framework for education used by all maintained and state schools. It is designed to provide consistency and a balanced education throughout a child's school life. The National Curriculum sets out the subjects to be taught including the knowledge, skills and understanding required at each stage for each subject. It also sets targets for achievement and regularly measures these through standardised tests. Schools can decide how subjects are taught so that children's learning needs are met. In Scotland, the Scottish Curriculum is flexible and open to interpretation by individual areas and not fixed by law.

One major issue in the education system is equality and whether social class, race, ability, disability and gender create inequalities of opportunity and achievement. For example, for many decades, children with disabilities were excluded from education or, when they were able to access it, the expectations and therefore standards of education and achievement were low which in effect increased their difference from others in society and reinforced negative ideas about the capability of people with disabilities. Since the 1944 Education Act, many laws have tried to address the question of equality and all have resulted in changes to the education system structure. For example, changes to selective entry system to secondary education which used the eleven-plus examination to determine children's suitability to enter grammar schools, the advent of comprehensive schools for all and the increase in university places to encourage wider access and participation in higher education.

Parents are responsible for their child's education although in most cases this is deferred to the local authority. Although education is compulsory between the ages of 3 or 4 and 16, school attendance is not. Local authorities have a responsibility to ensure that all children within their area receive education that prepares the child for life in modern civilised society and which enables them to achieve their full potential. An increasing number of parents are opting for home schooling as they do not feel the education system achieves these aims for their child. Legislation such as the Special Educational Needs Act (2000) (which relates to the Disability Discrimination Act) re-emphasises the rights of children and adults to be educated within mainstream education at all levels with appropriate provisions being made to enable this to occur. However, does this automatically mean equality is achieved for those with a disability? Although many children with disabilities do attend mainstream schools, schools are not always able to meet their needs adequately and many children achieve more through attendance at a school that understands and provides for their particular needs and circumstances.

University students were traditionally predominantly drawn from grammar and public (fee-paying) schools even up until the 1980s. During the 1990s, the government legislated to widen opportunity and access to higher education and set the prestigious universities, such as Oxford and Cambridge, targets to widen participation in terms of socio-economic groups and intake from state education. This agenda was intrinsically linked to the economic imperative for the UK to have a skilled and educated workforce able to compete effectively in an increasingly competitive and globalised marketplace. To achieve this, Britain needed to respond to the changes in the world of work. Britain was becoming less a manufacturing country as more of its wealth was being generated by the financial and service sector industries as well as knowledge and high-tech industries. These required higher levels of education and the skills and the ability to innovate and achieve lifelong learning. These changes have placed a greater emphasis on vocational learning and achievement (partly as a means to measure workforce capability), but the status of an academic university degree remains dominant over the equally demanding vocational qualifications now being achieved.

Education has an important role to play in socialising individuals into the accepted ways of society. This is important if the status quo is to be maintained. In addition, since the 1990s, education has also become closely aligned with employment as it has become focused on preparing young people for their role as economically productive individuals. This has also meant an emphasis on lifelong learning to equip them for the demands of work as well as the reality that many people will undertake several changes in their occupation during their lifetime.

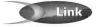

See page 239 for more information about different sociological perspectives relating to education.

Health care services

Fig 7.3 The health care system

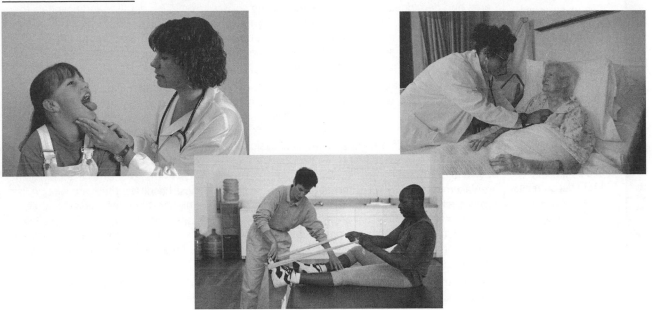

Since the advent of the welfare state in 1948, health care services have gone through a number of changes in organisation. The National Health Service (NHS) has increased in size (it is the largest organisation in Europe) and provides numerous services which add it its complexity. As a publicly funded organisation, the policies, strategies, national standards, working practices, funding, monitoring and regulation of the NHS are determined by the Department of Health within the government. Local policy implementation and performance management is the responsibility of the Strategic Health Authorities.

The National Health Service consists of primary and secondary care services.

Primary care services are those that individuals encounter within their community and include the following:

Fig 7.4 Primary care services

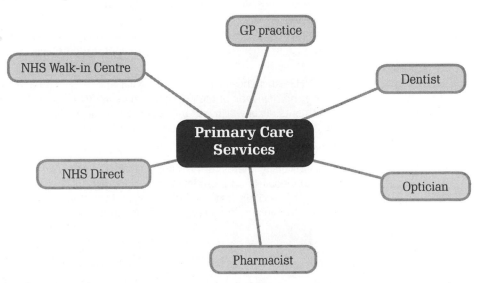

Primary care services are responsible for the identification and treatment of routine injuries and illnesses as well as providing services designed to maintain general good health and prevent illness and disease, for example stop smoking services and regular dental check-ups. Some primary care services also provide specialist services. For example, dental practices may include dental hygienists and GP practices may carry out simple surgical procedures. Individuals have some choice regarding accessing these services although many GP practices will only accept patients from within a designated geographical area. Individuals can access most of these services free at the point of delivery although there may be charges for some services, such as eye tests, prescription charges or holiday vaccinations. GPs and dentists can also be accessed through private means when a fee would be charged for their services.

The Primary Care Trust (PCT) is responsible for determining the levels of health need in their area and developing plans and commissioning services from GPs, dentists and hospitals to meet those needs. PCTs are responsible for improving the general health of the population they serve and ensuring access to services in order to achieve the health improvement targets set by the government. They are responsible for monitoring service quality and listening to patients' views and concerns.

Secondary care refers to acute care provision, either elective or emergency care, which usually takes place within an NHS hospital. Emergency and urgent care can be access either through a primary care out-of-hours service, such as a doctors on call service or an NHS Walk-in Centre, the ambulance service or a hospital. NHS Trusts provide emergency and planned hospital treatment and are commissioned by PCTs to provide care and intervention. This includes any in-patient care or day surgery undertaken at treatment centres, either run by NHS or private companies which provide speedier access to treatment (for example, joint replacement or cataract surgery) or diagnostic tests. In most hospitals, there are waiting lists to access consultations and treatments as the demand is higher than the available supply, either in terms of financial or physical resources, such as operating theatre staff or availability. Secondary care includes the provision of A&E departments for acute medical emergencies (accidents or trauma requiring immediate treatment) and this area of specialist health care remains solely within NHS provision.

Secondary care services also include specialist services for people with mental health problems, learning disabilities and for older people. A wide range of staff as well as doctors and nurses are employed within secondary care NHS services including allied health professionals such as physiotherapists and speech and language therapists, and ancillary staff including administration, catering, domestic, security and maintenance services.

Ambulance Trusts respond to the emergency calls prioritising them into immediately life-threatening, urgent or non-urgent. They also provide transport to and from hospital and first aid out of GP practice working times. Paramedics are now able to provide on-the-spot medical interventions, for example, administering blood clot-dissolve medication which increases survival rates for people who have heart attacks. Private ambulances exist, but they are used only for transport, not for paramedic treatment.

Although the NHS is the main health care provider in the UK it is not the only one. Many services are available through private organisations. Many of these private organisations are commissioned by PCTs to provide routine health interventions, such as joint replacements or diagnostic tests, in order to expand access to care and provision. Many services are accessed by individuals independently and they pay each for consultation and treatments. However, since the 1980s there has been an increase in the number of people who pay health insurance in order to access private treatment when they require it rather than waiting to be seen within the NHS.

The NHS experiences change on a regular and on-going basis as it seeks to meet the increasing demands of the public for preventative medicine as well as new innovative treatments, all of which was unpredicted at its inception in 1948. Heath and attitudes to health and care have dominated the debate around the NHS since that time.

Social diversity

Social diversity relates to the differences that exist between individuals within society and can lead to inequality and discrimination. A just and fair society attempts to take into account the impact of social diversity on individuals and to attempt to configure social structures in such a way as to minimise the inequalities that can result.

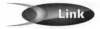 See page 48 in Unit 2 for more information about the benefits of social and cultural diversity.

Social class

Social class refers to different groups (classes) people can be divided into according to their social or economic status. Ideas about social class resulted from the development of capitalism as an economic model within industrialised societies. Social class is an economic division as an individual's occupation determines their income, economic wealth and capacity to consume goods and services. However, although two individuals may earn similar amounts of money, this does not mean they belong to the same social class. For example, a doctor has a higher status in society than a manual worker. Social class is therefore dependent on other factors, including social status or the importance given to particular occupations within society and the relative power that results from this. As individuals from the same social class tend to mix with one another, it is likely they will share similar values, beliefs and behaviours in terms of lifestyle and consumption and all of these reinforce their sense of belonging to that particular group. Since 2001 the National Statistics socio-economic classification (NS-SEC) has been used to reflect the changing occupational structure within the UK.

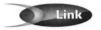 See page 49 in Unit 2 for more information on National Statistics Socio-economic Classification.

Gender

Gender relates to those characteristics, qualities, behaviours and social roles that have been attributed by society as belonging particularly to men or to women. Within society, women and men are perceived as being different in terms of their roles and functions within society. These differences however are not just biological but are subject to social construction. For example, in many societies men are the breadwinner or 'hunters' and women are the homemakers or 'gatherers'. However, in some societies, it is the women who hunt and the men who remain at home and those societies function equally well. 'Gender' is not something you are born with. It results from the process of **socialisation** (the process of growing up to think and behave according to the expectations of family and society). Gender differences impact on an individual's life experience, their expectations and the opportunities available to them. As a consequence, this influences their perception of their world. For example, we know that if occupational roles are only attributed to one gender this has a strong influence in terms of attitudes and expectations so that roles become gendered leading to stereotypes, for example only men can become plumbers, engineers and doctors while women are teachers, nurses and secretaries. Social constructions of gender differences, such as characteristics attributed to being masculine (assertive, tough, competitive, logical, and rational) and to being feminine (intuitive, compassionate, emotional and irrational), have created divisions as masculine attributes may be viewed as having greater importance than feminine attributes. This has created a situation where male ideas, values, interests and priorities have been able to dominate society, consequently reinforcing those ideas and embedding them so that they appear to be natural (biological and so irreversible) differences, as opposed to socially constructed differences.

 See page 62 in Unit 2 for more information on the impact of gender stereotyping.

Culture

The idea of culture is a contested one with different views as to its meaning. Cultures are systems of shared meanings, representations and practices that make up social life. It is the perspective an individual has and through which they view and make sense of the world as well as live within it. Cultures therefore relate to where individuals come from (nationality, ethnicity, home) what they believe (religious, political or other beliefs) and what they do (dress, behaviour, identity). People's cultural backgrounds provide a framework by which they live their lives. Different cultures have different customs and traditions, for example, relating to celebrations, dress or hospitality, that have been handed down through generations or which members of that group respect and adhere to. There is a tendency to think that culture relates only to people who are from different ethnic or religious groups. However, people from different areas of the UK have different cultures in that there are behaviours, customs and traditions that are not universal across the UK.

Ethnicity

Ethnicity relates to an individual's cultural or nationality and the distinctive characteristics attributed to that group. Ethnicity is bound up in all the factors that contribute to national identity for example, language, customs, religion, history and shared meanings, all of which are passed from generation to generation. Ethnicity is more widely used today as opposed to 'race' in recognition that the differences related to nationality, origins and influences are more than physical characteristics and differences of for example stature or skin tone.

The 2001 Population Census categorised ethnic groups in the UK as the following:

Ethnic groups in the UK

Ethnic group	People within this group
White	British, Irish and other White
Mixed	White and Black Caribbean, White and Black African, White and Asian, other mixed backgrounds
Asian or Asian British	Indian, Pakistani, Bangladeshi, other Asian background
Black or Black British	Caribbean, African, other Black background
Chinese or other ethnic group	Chinese or other ethnic group

Within the UK, about 7 per cent of the population belong to ethnic minority groups according to the 2001 census. The largest ethnic minority group are Indian.

Age

Society is made up of people from all age groups and this provides balance in terms of constantly regenerating the human species. Having a balance is important if society is to keep functioning so that there are enough people to support those who are unable to support themselves (children, older people and people with disabilities). At different times in history, the balance of age groups has shifted and this has an impact on society. For example, following the 2nd World War there were fewer young men to work to rebuild the country and Britain actively recruited people from the Commonwealth to boost the labour force.

Life expectancy has increased considerably since the 1950s and although, on average, women still live longer than men, the gap between them is decreasing. The advent of better health care has meant that fewer babies die in the first years of life and people are living longer. Britain, like most of the Western world, is seeing the overall population aging faster than it is reproducing so the balance is changing. This means there are fewer people actively involved in economic productivity than the number who require support. On the 2001 census the number of people over 60 years of age was 12.4 million which is 21 per cent of the total population. This has implications not just for the economy but for health and social care policy and services in terms of planning for the future.

Locality

The locality or the areas where people live in the UK are diverse. The UK is made up of cities, towns, villages and hamlets. Some areas are highly populated, such as London and the south-east of England, while others are sparsely populated, such as the highlands and islands of Scotland. The population spread is determined partly by geography (for example, due to accessibility), partly by choice (for example, for different lifestyle or retirement) and partly by employment opportunities and facilities.

The demographic profile of a locality, that is the size and characteristics of the population, ethnicity, age, growth, and on, has an impact on the individuals who live there. Different localities have different cultures, customs as well as opportunities for education, employment and lifestyle. Employment opportunities vary across the UK, sometimes as a result of natural resources, such as the coal, fishing or farming industries, sometimes as a result of economic incentives and population density, for example there are fewer (in number and type) employment opportunities in rural communities than in cities, and sometimes as a result of historical construction, such as the creation of the City in London which is the centre of the financial services markets in the UK. Areas of high employment or opportunities for high salaries will increase opportunities for employment due to higher consumption of goods and services and this attracts a wider range of facilities and services. In areas of high unemployment or lower wages, there will be less money for consumption and the quantity and type of services and facilities will be affected.

The population profile varies across the UK. For example, people coming into the UK from other countries are more likely to settle near family or friends or people from their own culture or nationality or where their particular skills are in demand. This creates even more diversity across the country.

Socialisation

Socialisation is the process whereby an individual's behaviour is shaped through experience within different social situations. It is the process by which individuals learn the socially accepted values, attitudes and behaviours and what is expected of them by their family and within society so they can contribute and participate fully. Socialisation takes place initially within the relationships individuals have with their parents, family, primary care givers, peer group and other close knit social groups, such as neighbours or community network. Through these relationships and the teaching that accompanies them, the individual learns through personal experience about values such as love, trust, loyalty, honesty, justice, fairness and sharing. This aspect of socialisation which occurs in the early part of an individual's life is considered to be fundamental in laying the foundations of a person's character and providing a framework to live their life by.

Secondary socialisation is more informal and occurs as part of an individual's everyday experience. It takes place in larger, more impersonal and formal organised groups, such as school and college. It describes how individuals learn how to behave in different social settings and with people of different social status and authority. Professional bodies, for example, may have a code of conduct which formalises the expectation of membership and so influences the individual's behaviour. Another strong influence on socialisation is the media in all its forms.

Norms

Through socialisation, individuals learn about their society's norms, that is the guidelines for what is considered to be acceptable behaviour. Some of these norms are formal and are in the form of written rules or codes of practice, while other are informal and unwritten. Examples of informal norms are what to wear in different social and everyday situations, such as warm clothes when the weather is cold. Norms will vary between cultures and within a culture especially within generations. For example, many older people in the UK would still wear dark or black clothing and a hat when attending a funeral as a sign of respect. Younger generations may disregard the strict observance of this custom while still showing respect.

Values

Values are the fundamental standards that are generally accepted within a society and which inform the behaviour of those within that society. Values such as love, trust, loyalty, honesty, respect for others, justice, fairness and sharing are taught and reinforced from an early age. Other values such as hard work, achievement, enterprise or individualism may also be features of early influences through the dominant ideas within society and the process of secondary socialisation. Values also differ between and within cultures. Values are an important part of an individual's framework for living. Organisations may also have a set of values they expect employees to hold and adhere to and this may be what attract both the employee and the customer to that organisation, for example ethical investment or environmentally friendly polices.

See page 54 in Unit 2 for more information about values in relation to health and social care.

Beliefs

Beliefs are those things that an individual accepts in their mind to be true. Beliefs are most often associated with religious and spiritual principles or related cultural understandings passed through generations. Beliefs underpin the way an individual perceives the world and consequently affect how they interact with those within it. Beliefs can be based on personal experience, for example, a belief that people will let you down and so cannot be trusted if your life experience is one of this happening repeatedly. Beliefs can be hard to understand and hard to change as they are often irrefutable (difficult to prove or disprove). Beliefs have a considerable impact on an individual's behaviour towards themselves, others and society.

Roles and Status

Status refers to an individual's position in society relative to others. A person with higher status generally has more responsibilities than a person with lower status and may be in charge of people with lower status. For example, members of a family have different statuses such as parent or child, and within a school a teacher and a student have different statuses. The behaviour or duties expected of each of these individuals within a particular status or social position is known as their role. For example, a teacher's role is to facilitating learning while a student is expected to learn. Roles are governed by certain expectations or norms, so, for example we know how parents or teachers are expected to behave. However no two parents or teachers will behave in exactly the same way as their behaviour will be subject to the socialisation processes and this will impact on how they interpret their role. 'Role models' are those individuals who provide unambiguous examples of how to behave that are also consistent with an individual's values and beliefs and whose behaviour other emulate. Uniforms are a clear way of denoting role and, by inference, status.

Principle sociological perspectives

In an attempt to try and understand society, the founders of sociology developed a number of different perspectives and these have been added to as society has changed.

Functionalism

This perspective was proposed by one of the main founders of sociology, Emile Durkheim (1858–1917). The main tenets of this perspective are that society is made up of a number of social institutions organised to fulfil certain functions, for example the nuclear family. The number and complexity of institutions increases (differentiation), as society develops. Institutions are grouped into four sub-systems.

Functionalists believe that society functions like a biological **organism**, that is, that the individual parts function in conjunction with one another for the benefit of the whole of society and as a result is more than just the sum of the individual parts. For example, according to the functionalist perspective, schools and employment have an interdependent relationship as schools provide education which prepares young people for employment and if the function to be achieved there must be a structure to both those social institutions.

Equally, the individual is seen to be a product of society. Society influences individuals through their lives and experiences of the various social institutions they connect with, such as family, school, work, and so on. Therefore, individuals are viewed as being unable to control their lives or change society.

Fig 7.5 Sub-systems of society

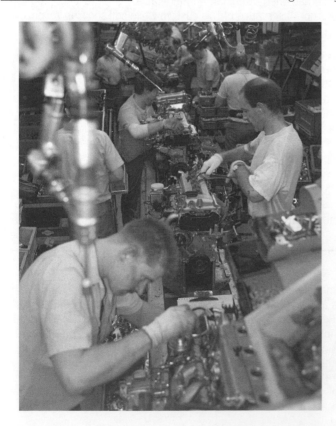
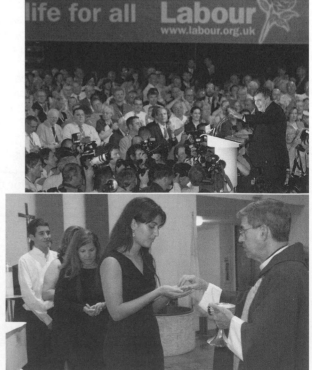

Society is normally controlled and balanced and if that balance is disrupted, for example through civil unrest, this is like a sickness in a living organism. Social equilibrium is achieved through moral consensus with the majority of people sharing the same values and moral codes of behaviour. Functionalists also argue that for society to function effectively and without chaos there must be leaders and so a level of inequality in terms of power and influence is an accepted inevitability of society.

According to Functionalists, social change is an evolutionary process that occurs as necessary through adaptation or integration. An example of this is the need since 1980s for workers to have greater levels of skills and knowledge in order for the UK to compete in a globalised economy. This led to significant changes in the education system and the merging of the UK Government Departments of Education and Employment in the 1990s.

For Functionalists the purpose of sociology is to analyse and explain how society functions both normally and abnormally through the exploration of the relationships between the different institutions in society.

case study 7.1

The family

George Murdock is a British sociologist who studied 250 small societies across the world and came to the conclusion that the basic human grouping across the world is the nuclear family, that is a father, mother and their child or children. Like other functionalists, Murdock considers the family to be universal and 'the body' of society responsible for four basic functions; sexual, reproductive, socialising and economic. With regards to the sexual and reproductive functions, marriage and the nuclear family were viewed as providing the best way to control the expression of sex drive socially. In addition, marriage and family also provided the stability required to successfully nurture and bring up a child which was considered to require support from more than one person.

American anthropologist Margaret Mead (1901–1978), another functionalist, contended that the nuclear family is not inevitable or biologically determined but instead a social and cultural construction. She believed that greater understanding of your own life could be achieved through understanding the lives of others especially in helping to understand the variations is family groupings that are a feature of 20th century. She believed that careers and motherhood should go together and that building support networks outside the nuclear family would achieve a greater sense of well-being.

Although individuals now experience greater sexual freedom before finding a life partner or marriage, there is still a strong belief that the relationship should then become monogamous. This arrangement also attempts to ensure the men do not father more children than they can support which also helps the continuation of the human species. The advent of more effective contraception however, has altered this situation.

The family's economic function is to provide food and shelter to its members and, unlike the self-sufficient times of pre-industrial Britain, it also plays a major role in both the production (through paid employment) and consumption of goods and services. The family is also instrumental in socialisation both in terms of passing on values and beliefs to its own members as well as participation in society and community life, for example in terms of adherence to laws and community activities. Teaching and learning also take place within the family both in terms of education and life skills. Functionalists have been criticised for presenting a model that assumes the existence of harmonious relationships whereas in fact families can be full of conflict and tension.

activity
INDIVIDUAL WORK

1   How well does this sociological perspective and explanation of the family fit with your experience?

2   What questions does this perspective not answer in relation to families?

Marxism

Karl Marx (1818–1883) was another of the founders of sociology. He was born in Germany and studied law and gained a PhD in philosophy. He was a revolutionary thinker and his ideas formed the basis for communism. The basis of Marxism is social class in terms of the different levels of power each class has, the relationship of each class to the means of production, the conflicts this creates and the impact these conflicts have on society. In Marxism, there are two major social classes within a capitalist society of private enterprise economy. These are the powerful ruling class (bourgeoisie) who have the means of production. These are the owners of property, land and factories, who, as a consequence of their position, are able to subordinate the working class (proletariat). The working class have to 'sell' their labour to the ruling class in order to earn wages to live. As a result of this situation of business ruling labour, Marxism considers that, while there may be times of equilibrium from which the powerful and wealthy benefit most, the norm in society is disequilibrium due to class conflict.

Class conflict causes society to change as each class is motivated to pursue their own interests which will bring them into conflict with the other. For example, business owners and shareholders are interested in maximising their profits and this may be by keeping wages low to reduce the cost of production. On the other hand, workers are interested in a fair wage and acceptable working conditions which may potentially drive the price of the goods up resulting in reduced profits for owners or shareholders. Hence conflict occurs.

Marx did not believe that class differences were natural, inevitable or necessary and considered socialism as the means by which a more equal sharing or power, wealth and property and as a result society, could be achieved. Some Marxists consider that the individual is powerless to effect change as class conflict is inevitable whatever happens. Others, however, hold a view that the individual does have a significant role to play in society albeit as a result of belonging to a class. Marxists see sociology as analysing and explaining class conflict.

Feminism

This is a movement which is committed to ensuring women have and retain rights and opportunities equal to those enjoyed by men. Feminists believe that women experience discrimination because of their sex and they also have specific needs that remain unmet as to meet them would require radical change in the social, economic and political order in society. Within the feminist movement, there are varying perspectives of what is of prime importance. Some feminists hold Marxist views and consider that capitalist society is patriarchal (dominated by men). They believe that these two factors are constantly reinforcing the other so cementing and embedding their position as the natural order of society, thus perpetuating female **oppression** both ideologically and economically. Liberal feminists seek equal opportunities for women while radical feminists consider patriarchy as the central issue for women. For radical feminists, men oppress women using the biological inequality and the nuclear family and through controlling the female roles of reproduction and childrearing as these make women dependent on men for the means to live. Some feminists argue that women also become willing collaborators in their oppression.

During most of the first part of the 20th century, many women remained predominately occupied in the private world of the home maintaining those roles deemed natural and so there were fewer women in the public world of work, although there were also many women in the workforce as a result of the industrial revolution working in factories and mills. During World War 2, there were too few working men left in Britain to meet production demands and women were then deemed suitable and able to undertake jobs previously only considered suitable for men. After the war ended, women were expected to return to the confined world of home and give up their new-found freedom to rebuild the country through reproduction and home-making. As a result, many women questioned and challenged this definition of their 'natural' role.

For feminists, the power of patriarchy lies in the way the world is defined in masculine terms, for example through language, with society's systems and structures at every level dominated by male concerns and interests to the extent that it is presented as natural and so difficult to challenge as any challenge is viewed with suspicion and presented as deviant. Feminism has, like anti-racism, had an impact on society from the 1960s with changes in legislation and greater awareness of equality issues. However, inequalities and male **hegemony** (dominating influence) remains a feature of capitalist societies.

See page 52 in Unit 2 for more information about sexism.

Interactionism

This perspective has its roots in the work of American philosopher and social psychologist George Mead (1880–1949). He developed ideas about the development of self through the play and the game stages. Before this a child's interaction with others is based on imitation without being fully aware of the meaning underlying actions. The play stage involves the child trying out familiar roles, such as parent, teacher, doctor or nurse, within imaginative play. The child plays only roles within their experience either direct or indirect through the media. They are generally unaware of how these roles interact with one another. In the game stage the child is able to see wider roles as well as situations from different perspectives, resulting in the development of social awareness. This process enables children to learn the rules of the game and of society in general.

Mead considered that human beings were distinctive because they have the ability to reflect on their own thoughts and actions. Interactionism looks at society on a small scale, refusing to generalise and apply its ideas to the whole of society. It focuses on individuals and how they interact with others.

Interactionism emphasises the way individuals gain shared understandings of the meanings attached to objects and phenomena. These meanings only exist as a result of social interaction and interpretation and are then shared through language, labels, symbols and signs. For example, uniforms convey different meanings so while a police uniform conveys authority, power and strength, a nurse's uniform conveys caring, sensitivity, femininity and vocation. These meanings are reinforced through images and experience, such as pictures and characters in television and films.

Interactionists are interested in how individuals create the social world through their behaviour rather than how society creates the individual. As opposed to thinking of society as a living organism, Interactionists consider society to be a fiction created to maintain life in an orderly and predictable way. They believe that society is unable to force individuals to do anything as it is only real for as long as the individual's pretence of its reality lasts. This pretence is assisted by the fact that individuals involve themselves in social relationships and roles with rules and routines. The focus of Interactionism is the consideration of individuals and their part in wider social groups.

Interactionism has particularly been applied to the study of changes in identity in different social circumstances. In particular, Goffman's work on **stigma** reveals how identity forms as a result of interaction with others, their perceptions of the individual and how these are reflected back to the individual through language and behaviour. Difference from others if perceived negatively by them creates a stigma will impact negatively on the individual's sense of identity.

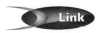

See page 66 in Unit 2 and page 361 in Unit 11 for more information about the impact of discrimination and abuse on identity.

Collectivism

This perspective considers that society and its members have a general responsibility to meet the needs of individuals and should be responsible not just for social activities within society but also for ownership and control of the means of production and that the benefits of this should be shared by all in society. Pure collectivism is generally considered to be impossible to achieve. However, degrees of collectivism do exist. For example, members of society transfer responsibility to the state or government for some social and economic activities and collectively contribute to pay for these through taxation. The principle of collectivism underpins the welfare state in that individuals pay tax to the government who then provide education, health and social care services which individuals then access on the basis of rights as opposed to the ability to pay.

This approach also aims to address the inequalities in society that result from different levels of wealth and social status. Through collective provision of education and welfare, the state can in some way compensate those on lower incomes to enable them to access education and welfare services in order to maintain health and improve their circumstances.

Postmodernism

Modernism was a movement which believed in linear progress and essential truths such as power of reason over ignorance, order over disorder, and science over superstition. Postmodernists reject this perspective and also sociological perspectives such as Marxism that seek to understand society by using a unifying **ideology** or a universal truth. They consider that such universal truths fail to explain society. Postmodernists consider that in a post-industrial world, progress is fragmented and it is **pluralism** with its variety of groups and subcultures that help us to understand society. Within a postmodern society, those groups that helped create a sense of belonging, solidarity and identity, such as the nuclear family, become fragmented and this creates uncertainty about not only who the individual is but also their place within society. Postmodernism considers it necessary to embrace a range of ideas in order to understand contemporary society as diverse perspectives are seen as a positive contribution.

New Right

This is a political movement with a considerable cultural influence with its emphasis on individualism and distrust of the state as controlling and interfering in what is essentially the private world of the individual. It came to prominence internationally during the 1980s. Some believe that individuals should have the maximum amount of freedom and to that end society does not exist. Former Prime Minister Margaret Thatcher famously commented that 'there is no such thing as society', something which had a fundamental impact on ideas and behaviour during the time of successive Conservative governments in the 1980s and early 1990s. The New Right ideology particularly relates to economics and a free market approach. Individual enterprise and the rewards of the free market are of paramount importance and any state intervention seen as curbing this natural order. In the 1980s, this led to privatisation of nationalised industries such as the railways and utilities and an increase in share ownership, previously the preserve of the wealthy upper and upper middle class.

The New Right view capitalism, the free market and competition to achieve the best returns both socially and economically as the only economic system that allows individual freedom. New Right ideas were introduced into the NHS with the creation of internal markets and individual choice regarding treatment. During this time, attempts were made to reduce the state control of education and health and the New Right ideology of individualism encouraged ordinary working people to think they could create their own welfare state through insurance and savings policies to pay for education and health care rather than be at the mercy of state controlled decision-making and funding. The reality remained that this was still out of reach of most.

activity
INDIVIDUAL WORK 7.1
P1

Describe the main ideas (using sociological terms) of each of the following sociological perspectives:

- Functionalism
- Marxism
- Feminism
- Interactionism
- Collectivism
- Postmodernism
- New Right

Applying sociological approaches to health and social care

Application of sociological perspectives to health and social care

Link See Unit 24, in BTEC National Health and Social Care Book 2, for more information about sociological perspectives to health and social care.

Applying principle sociological perspectives will help the health and social care worker to understand the different concepts of health and illness held by individuals, organisations and society and how these impact on attitudes and behaviour. Sociological perspectives can also be applied to assist the health and social care worker to understand the patterns and trends in health and illness among different groups. This is essential for identifying needs and planning care.

Understanding different concepts of health and ill health

An important starting point when trying to understand what is meant by health is to consider the different definitions and ideas associated with health. Ideas about what is meant by health have been found to differ according to, for example, a person's age, their state of health, culture, beliefs and their social circumstances. Health was considered to be a divine gift before the Greek philosopher Hippocrates, known as the 'father of medicine', changed people's perceptions and advocated that doctors should use observation as the basis for acquiring knowledge about health. He also advanced understanding of how external factors would impact on health and well-being, for example sanitation, diet and personal hygiene. He believed that to achieve health four fluids within the body, blood, yellow bile, black bile and phlegm, needed to be in balance and if they were not ill health would result. The idea of internal balance remains a strong one even today, particularly in alternative and Eastern traditional medicine, such as acupuncture. The idea of health being a divine gift however persists with many religions, for example Muslims and Christians believe that health is aligned with spiritual well-being and granted by a divine power and that healing also results from divine intervention. This concept will impact on how individuals understand their well-being and respond to ill health as well as their part in achieving and maintaining health.

Concepts of health

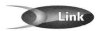

See Unit 20, in BTEC National Health and Social Care Book 2, for more information about concepts of health.

Negative concepts of health

Many people do not really consider their state of health or think of themselves as being 'healthy' in their daily lives. They find the concept of health difficult to quantify or describe as it is so much as part of their normal experience. Many people therefore have a negative concept of health, thinking of it as the absence of ill health. For these people, being healthy means not having anything wrong with you, no illnesses, diseases or injuries. Concepts of health appear to change with age with many older people describing being healthy in these negative terms whereas younger people talk about health in terms of eating the right things and taking exercise. The individual's state of health at any one time will also impact on their concept of health. If they are experiencing symptoms of disease or illness or are injured, they are more likely to apply a negative definition than a positive one. However, research by Blaxter (1990) found that even if people had a disease they could still consider themselves to be healthy as they framed this in relation to how they coped with or managed their disease within their lives. Sometimes health is seen in relation to how well people recover from illness. For example, people may say 'I got better quicker because I'm healthy'. Gender also appears to have a bearing on concepts of health with women conceptualising health as being in control of their physical bodies through taking positive action, such as taking care of themselves by eating sensibly and taking exercise, while men in particular tend to consider health as the norm and so do not think they have to play an active part in achieving this state of well-being.

Positive concepts of health

More positive concepts of health are often described in relation to being able to do things, being resilient to stress, disease and being able to cope with life rather than an absence of ill health. Those who have positive concepts of health might describe the feeling of being healthy as having energy to be active and being physically fit. Health may also be viewed in terms of the body's condition or appearance, for example, having clear skin and feeling slim (especially as this is a socially constructed and reinforced as the preferred body type in Western society).

However, as well as physical well-being emotional well-being should be considered. Living a healthy lifestyle including balancing all the factors in our lives which potentially cause stress with those that can help us to relax is a dominant idea in the late 20th and early 21st centuries. The promotion of health encourages positive concepts as it focuses on the benefits to health of lifestyle choices and behaviours. Expressions regarding energy levels also relate to emotional well-being and how enthusiastic people feel about life, what they are doing or going to be doing. Being physically fit as well as emotionally fit is viewed as equally important by many.

Women are more likely to use the word healthy relating to their social relationships with others and being able to cope with these, such as looking after the family or managing children's behaviour positively. Many people also consider that being healthy means being able to work, play an active role within their family, community or society, being useful and helping others.

There has been a tendency in the past to focus on physical well-being when thinking about health. However a greater awareness of mental health issues has produced positive concepts of health that focus on what a person is able to do rather than what they are not. Tudor (1996) describes mental health as having six dimensions: affective, behavioural, cognitive, socio-political, spiritual and psychological. While in 1997 the Health Education Authority (now the Health Development Agency) defined mental health as 'the emotional and spiritual resilience which enables us to survive pain, disappointment and sadness. It is a positive sense of well-being and an underlying belief in our own and others' dignity and worth'.

The Mental Health Foundation defines a mentally healthy person as someone who can:

Fig 7.6 Definition of mental health

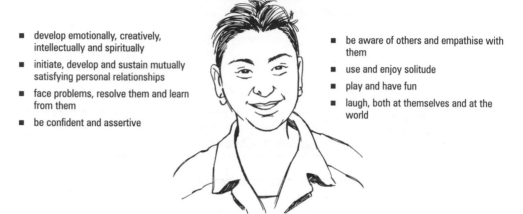

- develop emotionally, creatively, intellectually and spiritually
- initiate, develop and sustain mutually satisfying personal relationships
- face problems, resolve them and learn from them
- be confident and assertive

- be aware of others and empathise with them
- use and enjoy solitude
- play and have fun
- laugh, both at themselves and at the world

Another positive view of health is that it is a commodity that can be supplied, for example by providing health screening services, and bought, for example buying healthy foods or products to reduce stress.

Holistic concepts of health

Increasingly, concepts of health take a holistic view. To be healthy means considering the whole person, their physical, psychological, emotional and spiritual well-being as well as how they function within their environment and social relationships. Holistic concepts consider the need to balance the different facets of an individual in order to achieve a state of health. Ideas relating to holistic concepts have arisen out of critical analysis of the impact of western medicine on disease and illness. For example, in Ivan Illich's book *Limits to Medicine* (1976), one of the recurring themes is the concept of holistic health and the need to consider the spiritual and personal dimensions of an individual's life in order for them to cope with illness and disease. Holistic concepts of health underpin much of current practice as there is a recognition that to enable an individual to improve their health, manage their disease or recuperate from illness, practitioners need to understand the whole person, their values, beliefs, priorities, social relationships and environment as well as their physical and mental well-being. Person-centred approaches to health and social care are based on holistic views of health and the interdependent relationship of the different facets of an individual's life.

World Health Organisation definition

In 1946, the World Health Organisation (WHO) defined health as 'a state of complete physical, mental and social well-being and not merely the absence of disease and infirmity'.

The first international conference on health promotion was held in 1986 in Ottawa, Canada. The conference clarified the definitions regarding health and health promotion as well as what was required for health to exist in society. Participants pledged a commitment to health promotion and international action. The Ottawa Charter for Health Promotion came up with a holistic view of health which took into consideration the active and changing nature of health and the impact of social and environmental factors. It said, 'To reach a state of complete physical, mental and social well-being, an individual or group must be able to identify and to realise aspirations, to satisfy needs and to change or cope with the environment. Health is, therefore, seen as a resource for everyday life, not the objective of living. Health is a positive concept emphasising social and personal resources, as well as physical capacities.' The Ottawa Charter and identified as prerequisites for health:

- peace
- shelter
- education
- food
- income
- a stable ecosystem
- sustainable resources
- social justice and equity.

[Permission 7.5]

WHO define mental health in this way: 'Mental health is a state of well-being in which the individual realises his or her own abilities, can cope with the normal stresses of life, can work productively and fruitfully and is able to make a contribution to his or her community.'

[Permission 7.6]

---

activity
GROUP WORK
7.2

P2

M1

1   Describe what is meant by each of these different concepts of health:
   - Negative concept
   - Positive concept
   - Holistic concept
2   Explain these three different concepts of health from:
   - a Functionalist perspective
   - a Marxist perspective

World Health Organisation	www.who.int

Models of health

Link   See Unit 20, in BTEC National Health and Social Care Book 2, for more information about models of health.

The dominant model of health in western medicine and health care is the biomedical model which applies the principles of sciences, such as biology, to medicine and medical diagnostics. This medical model is however a negative one as it is concerned with ill health rather than health. As a consequence, an alternative model, the social (or socio-medical) model, emerged which places ill health into the context of occurring as a result of complex interactions of individual and external environment factors. These models help in the analysis of health problems and solutions.

Biomedical model
The biomedical model emerged at the end of the 19th century and presents health as the absence of disease. The emphasis is on the facts that result from the theoretical testing associated with science and considers biomedicine as the only appropriate response to ill health. Biomedical models assume that the complexity of individuals can be reduced so that by accumulating facts about the parts that make up their body a decision about how to 'fix' that part will result in health.

The biomedical model of health is one where:
- the state of health is a biological fact and the norm
- the body is a machine and ill health results from dysfunction of that machine
- ill health is a deviation from the norm
- ill health is caused by biological factors, such as viruses, bacteria, genetic characteristics or trauma

- the cause of ill health is identified through the process of diagnosis, considering the signs and symptoms
- medical knowledge is based on facts which legitimises and privileges it as superior to all other types of knowledge. It is the exclusive domain of the expert medical practitioner (this has ensured the high status of doctors in society)
- alternative approaches are invalid and inferior
- biomedical treatment as the only valid and appropriate response to ill health
- individuals play little or no part in the interventions to restore the body to health
- there is no consideration of the individual's interpretation of health and ill health or of social factors that may contribute to ill health
- finding a cure is a greater concern than preventing ill health.

Socio-medical model

The socio-medical model challenges the assumptions made through the medical model and although not suggesting a total rejection of it emphasises the need for wider considerations. The socio-medical model suggests that the facts presented in the biomedical model are interpretations and that they deny a number of key factors. Ill health results from the interaction of the complex, ever-changing social environment. It is a holistic model which is concerned with the context in which people live their lives identifying the impact of lifestyle choices, social factors such as deprivation, poverty, education, employment, housing and social relationships on health and illness.

The socio-medical model of health is one where:

- the state of health is socially constructed resulting from historical, social and cultural influences that have shaped perceptions of health and ill health
- the root causes for disease and ill health are to be found in social factors, such as the way society is organised and structured
- root causes are identified through beliefs and interpretation, for example, from a feminist perspective, root causes relate to patriarchy and oppression
- knowledge is not exclusive but has a historical, social and cultural context as it is shaped by those involved.

The socio-medical model recognises the power that has been vested in the medical profession through social construction of health and illness. The socio-medical model recognises the opportunity for health prevention and community-based approaches as it identifies the importance of individuals in maintaining their own health.

---

activity
INDIVIDUAL WORK
7.3

P3

M2

1 Describe the biomedical and socio-medical models of health.

2 Explain the difference between the biomedical and socio-medical models of health.

---

activity
INDIVIDUAL WORK
7.4

D1

Evaluate benefits and drawbacks to the biomedical and socio-medical models of health, making a judgement of the value of each to health and social care provision.

Ill health

As we have seen through considering the different concepts of health, ill health can be viewed in different ways.

Illness

This is an individual and therefore subjective feeling associated with the experience of changes within the individual and expressed as feelings of pain, discomfort or unease. If the individual has a medical examination, these symptoms are named and this forms the basis of medical diagnosis. For example, an individual is feeling unwell and this feeling is based on their feelings of a headache, pain in their ear and pain when swallowing. A medical examination might confirm this illness by identifying the symptom of the headache is due to a raised body temperature, the pain in the ear and when swallowing due to inflamed and enlarged tonsils. The diagnosis is made based on these symptoms and using a biomedical model the cause determined as being due to an infection of their tonsils by either bacteria or a virus (tonsillitis). Treatment would be based on reducing the discomfort of the symptoms (due to the action of the body's natural defence mechanisms) and destroying the infecting agent if possible (if it is thought to be a bacterial infection then antibiotics would be suggested).

However, sometimes individuals express feeling unwell or ill when there is an absence of disease. Illness is not just about physical symptoms and can have a social or psychological aspect. Sometimes this is associated with imbalance with the individual 'feeling out of sorts' as they compare their current state to their norm. Individuals may hold different views about the causes of illness. For example, some may take a biomedical view that tonsillitis was caused by bacterial infection while a socio-medical model view may be that it was caused by working too hard, stress and not taking care of their health. Individual attitudes to illness will be based on the cause; the length of time they may have to experience the symptoms; the limitations placed on their life as a result and the potential for a cure and its effectiveness.

Disability

Definitions of disability differ depending on the perspective or model being applied. It is widely accepted that disabled people generally have fewer opportunities and a lower quality of life than non-disabled people. Any actions taken to deal with or remove the disadvantage experienced by disabled people depend on what is believed to be the cause of the disadvantage.

There are two different ways of explaining what causes the disadvantage:

- an individual (or medical) model of disability, which encourages explanations in terms of the features of an individual's body
- a social model of disability, which encourages explanations in terms of characteristics of social organisation.

Under the medical model of disability, disabled people's inability to join in society is seen as a direct result of having an impairment and not as the result of features of our society which can be changed. Disability is seen as an inability to function physically or mentally within the range of accepted standards of normal functioning within daily life, since the norm is to be able-bodied. When people such as policy makers and managers think about disability in this way, they tend to concentrate their efforts on compensating people with impairments for what is 'wrong' with their bodies by, for example, targeting special benefits at them and providing segregated 'special' services for them.

The medical model of disability also affects the way disabled people think about themselves. Many disabled people internalise the negative message that all disabled people's problems stem from not having 'normal' bodies. Disabled people too can be led to believe that their impairments automatically prevent them from participating in social activities. This attitude can make disabled people less likely to challenge their exclusion from mainstream society.

The social model of disability makes the important distinction between 'impairment' and 'disability'. The social model has been worked out by disabled people who feel that the individual model does not provide an adequate explanation for their exclusion from mainstream society because their experiences have shown them that in reality most of their problems are not caused by their impairments, but by the way society is organised.

In a social model of disability, 'impairment' is defined as an injury, illness or congenital condition that causes or is likely to cause a long-term effect on physical appearance or limitation of function within the individual that differs from the commonplace. By contrast, 'disability' is defined as the loss or limitation of opportunities to take part in society on an equal level with others due to social and environmental barriers. In this model, the individual model definitions of impairment and disability are combined as 'impairment'. This means that both the cause of functional limitation and the functional limitation within the individual itself are separated from external factors. Disability is shown as being caused by 'barriers' or elements of social organisation which take no or little account of people who have impairments. Society is shown to disable people who have impairments because the way it has been set up prevents disabled people from taking part in everyday life. It follows that if disabled people are to be able to join in mainstream society, the way society is organised must be changed. Removing the barriers which exclude (disable) people who have impairments can bring about this change.

Barriers can be:

- prejudice and stereotypes
- inflexible organisational procedures and practices
- inaccessible information
- inaccessible buildings
- inaccessible transport.

Also, disabling barriers experienced in the past can continue to have an adverse effect. For example, those disabled people who attended segregated schools may have gained lower academic qualifications than their non-disabled peers, simply because their 'special' school failed to provide a proper mainstream curriculum. These barriers have nothing to do with individual disabled people's bodies, they are created by people which means it is possible to remove them. Individuals can take a social approach to disability by identifying and getting rid of the disabling barriers which are within their control.

Disease

A disease is a medical condition which results from a specific disorder or change which has recognisable signs and symptoms and a recognisable cause. A medical practitioner can examine the signs and symptoms and compare these with the normal functioning ranges as well as the symptoms agreed as relating to particular conditions and diseases in order to form the basis for medical diagnosis and to identify the appropriate treatment. The medical diagnosis defines an illness as a disease although not all diseases make individuals feel ill. For example, individuals with long-term conditions such as asthma have a diagnosis but do not feel ill all the time. Also some diseases such as the sexually transmitted disease chlamydia can create no symptoms to alert the individual to its presence as a disease.

Diseases have certain recognisable characteristics that assist in identification and differentiation. They are seen as universal as they create the same or very similar symptoms in individuals regardless of their individual characteristics and circumstances. As a result, the WHO produces the International Statistical Classification of Diseases and Health-related Problems (ICD) which is used in most countries to classify and code mortality and morbidity (death and the presence of illness and disease).

WHO International Statistical Classification of Diseases and Health-related Problems

Chapter	Title
I	Certain infectious and parasitic diseases
II	Neoplasms
III	Diseases of the blood and blood-forming organs and certain disorders involving the immune mechanism
IV	Endocrine, nutritional and metabolic diseases
V	Mental and behavioural disorders
VI	Diseases of the nervous system
VII	Diseases of the eye and adnexa
VIII	Diseases of the ear and mastoid process
IX	Diseases of the circulatory system
X	Diseases of the respiratory system
XI	Diseases of the digestive system
XII	Diseases of the skin and subcutaneous tissue
XIII	Diseases of the musculo-skeletal system and connective tissue
XIV	Diseases of the genitourinary system
XV	Pregnancy, childbirth and the puerperium

Chapter	Title
XVI	Certain conditions originating in the perinatal period
XVII	Congenital malformations, deformations and chromosomal abnormalities
XVIII	Symptoms, signs and abnormal clinical and laboratory findings, not elsewhere classified
XIX	Injury, poisoning and certain other consequences of external causes
XX	External causes of morbidity and mortality
XXI	Factors influencing health status and contact with health services
XXII	Codes for special purposes

Although there is a strong tendency to view disease as a biological deviation from the norm, a socio-cultural interpretation of disease would also consider that what is viewed as normal and abnormal is subject to social and moral judgement as they are set by individuals and society. As a result, disease differs across cultures and circumstances. From a socio-cultural perspective, it is the significance of biological changes rather than just the biological changes that contribute to understanding disease.

Iatrogenesis

This is a term developed by Ivan Illich to describe where medical intervention results in ill health rather than effecting a cure, for example the effects of medication overuse or side effects. Illich felt that medicine and medical intervention created a dependency in individuals which stopped them from relying on their own resources. He expands his explanation further to include the wider implications of relying on medical solutions to 'cure' all ills including social and spiritual ones. He considers that iatrogenesis has resulted from **medicalisation** where the role, power and value of medicine within society has been expanded to include the use of technology in diagnosis and where doctors make decisions on a wider range of issues not previously considered as relating to illness, such as moral dilemmas.

Refer back to page 252 for more information about Ivan Illich.

Three types of iatrogenesis have been identified. These are:

- clinical, where medical practitioners and hospitals are the cause of illness, for example when interventions result in side effects that are worse than the original illness

- social, the way in which modern medicine is organised so that it labels the individual's experience of illness as deviant

- cultural, the emphasis is on technological solutions and relief from symptoms. The expectation that all symptoms should be relieved rather than enabling individuals to understand the significance of symptoms and enabling them cope with these and to decide when intervention is appropriate. In effect, this dominance of health by medicine has created a situation where individuals have lost confidence in their own ability to understand their body, manage sickness through the use of non-invasive or traditional solutions or remedies.

The sick role

Talcott Parsons (1902–1979) was a sociologist and the founder of modern functionalism. He developed the model of the 'sick role' in the 1950s and it was the first theoretical concept that explicitly concerned medical sociology. This model is in contrast to the biomedical model, which pictures illness as a mechanical malfunction or a microbiological invasion, Parsons described the sick role as a temporary, medically sanctioned form of deviant behaviour. Parsons' theory shows that illness is not just a natural event but one which can be motivated as well as reflecting the social definitions of sickness and wider cultural values. According to Parsons, people who are ill enter into a 'sick role' which provides the individual with certain rights and obligations. For example, within the sick role, an individual's right not to go to work and to receive help from others is legitimised. In addition, the individual has an obligation to do that which is suggested to recover quickly, for example stay in bed or at home, rest, seek help or take medicine as prescribed.

According to Parsons, the sick role legitimises and regulates illness so that it creates the minimum amount of disruption to others and normal life. Sickness is disruptive to normal functioning and so is social constructed as undesirable and ideally a temporary state. For example, in some organisations the culture is that those who are absent are 'letting their colleagues or service users down'. However, an individual can legitimately enter into the sick role when they are sick. Although the sick role views sickness as a social deviance rather than a diagnosed state it avoids blame or responsibility for being sick.

It is further legitimised through the visible roles undertaken of doctor and patient. The obligation to seek and conform to medical advice and help within the sick role does create a power imbalance between doctor and patient. If the obligations of the sick role are not met or it has not been granted (through diagnosis) or if the individual remains within the role longer than is legitimate they are likely to be viewed by society as weak, or a malinger or a difficult patient. There are also some medical diagnoses that are associated with assumptions of responsibility and blame and as a result are **stigmatised**, such as HIV/AIDS, and hepatitis C. These may result in the individual being discriminated against.

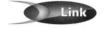

See page 64 in Unit 2 for more information about discrimination, stereotyping, labelling, prejudice and disadvantage.

However the medical profession is powerful and can act as a 'gate-keeper' controlling who enters the sick role and as a result the social relationships that result. For example, where illness is difficult to diagnose, for example in post-viral conditions such as ME (myalgic encephalomyelitis), individuals may have a legitimate reason for entering the sick role which is denied as it is not confirmed through medial diagnosis. This may have devastating implications for the individual, resulting in greater levels of ill health. Chronic and mental health issues create difficulties in applying the sick role as it lends itself more to short-term acute episodes of sickness rather than long-term conditions. Pregnancy too has created contradictions in the social role of women during this time where many view this as a natural state and not sickness, but there is nonetheless disruption to normal functioning which impacts on roles and responsibilities before, during and after birth of the baby.

Functionalists view the sick role as providing an example of behaviour which is encouraged or discouraged, punished or rewarded. Most individuals will be socialised in the sick role as they are growing up when responses to childhood illnesses will cement attitudes and behaviours. For example, if a child grows up where the sick role is discouraged through the emphasis on robust good health and little changing when they are ill, they view the sick role having little benefit and so only adopt it when necessary. If, however, adopting a sick role comes with more rights than obligations, such as being the centre of attention and cosseted by others, this may create a learned response that the sick role can be manipulated to meet emotional and psychological needs even when illness is not present.

The clinical iceberg
As with all icebergs, this describes a situation where what is seen is only a small part of the total picture. In relation to illness, this means that the numbers of people who present with ill health to their GP or hospital are only ever a small proportion of those in the population who are experiencing ill health. The reason for this is that in most cases individuals will choose to either ignore what is happening, consider it part of a normal range of well-being or dismiss it as being not important enough to take action. Individuals learn to accommodate and live with minor symptoms and it is only when these symptoms become so severe that they interfere with their day-to-day life, for example when pain intensifies or they collapse, that they will seek medical help. This does not mean they necessarily seek no advice or support. Many individuals will seek to alleviate symptoms through a variety of means, such as by self-medicating with non-prescription medicines or home remedies, for example using steam inhalations to relieve upper respiratory tract congestion, by seeking advice from a pharmacist, family, friends, literature, the internet, self-help websites and books. Other popular sources of support are alternative therapies such as reflexology, homeopathy, acupuncture or osteopathy.

The implications of the clinical or illness iceberg is that many people are experiencing symptoms that limit their capacity, functioning and potential when often they could be treated and return to a quality of life and function they have lost. It also suggests that individuals do not see the biomedical response as the only route to well-being and that they are capable of managing their own health. However, it is also a reality that should all those individuals within the population who are experiencing ill health choose to seek support from the NHS it would be overwhelmed.

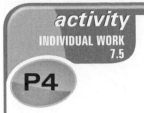

activity
INDIVIDUAL WORK
7.5

P4

Describe what is meant by the each of these different concepts of ill health:

- Illness
- Disability
- Disease
- Iatrogenesis
- The sick role
- The clinical iceberg

Understanding patterns and trends in health and illness among different social groupings

Any society will not have a homogeneous population. It will be made up of people of different ages, genders, abilities, ethnicities and social class. This diversity within society will be particularly noticeable when considering health and well-being.

Measurement of health

As the biomedical model of health dominates thinking in the West, health is generally measured in negative terms, such as the level of disease and the number of deaths within a population, rather than by analysis of positive indicators, such as the presence of health. Epidemiology is the study of disease origins or cause and how diseases are spread within the population. Epidemiological data provides valuable information about the number of people within a population that are affected by ill health, who die as a result of particular health problems and which groups of individuals are most at risk of developing and dying from particular types of illness or disease. This information is used to identify and plan appropriate health and social care services as well as health-promotion activities. The most commonly used indicators are morbidity (presence of illness or disease) and mortality (death).

Morbidity rates

Morbidity is more difficult to measure as the information is gathered from a range of different sources. Data is collected by the government as well as the NHS and local authority social services departments through direct surveys of the population such as specific health surveys, and as a result of administrative processes, for example, when an individual visits a GP or A&E department or has an assessment of needs. Some diseases are required to be reported, for example, cancers and communicable (infectious) diseases and so data is collected via this process. The problem with this information is that to some extent it reflects services that are available rather than the true picture of disease incidence. Also, as discussed in the clinical iceberg, individuals have to express their needs through actively seeking medical (or social care) services and this is again not a true picture of the actual incidence of disease in the population.

The General Household Survey (GHS) is a continuous government population survey and it does include questions about people's experience of illness both acute and chronic within the two weeks prior to the person completing the survey. The individual GHS 2002 interview includes questions regarding health and the use of health services.

National Statistics Online
www.statistics.gov.uk
General Household Survey

This provides information about the individual's view of their health and, as discussed previously when considering different models of health, the individual interpretation of what is meant by health makes this a subjective rather than objective measure.

The measurement of working days lost due to sickness can also provide a measure of morbidity for those who are in paid employment. As a measure, it is limited as it only relates to paid employment and this excludes many women who are at home caring for children or older people as well as those who are retired or unable to work through disability.

Mortality rates

The Office for National Statistics is responsible for collecting and analysing data collected from a range of sources including the ten-year national population census, the GHS and specific health information gathered through, for example, deaths and disease incidence reporting

Fig 7.7 Questions included in the General Household Survey (GHS)

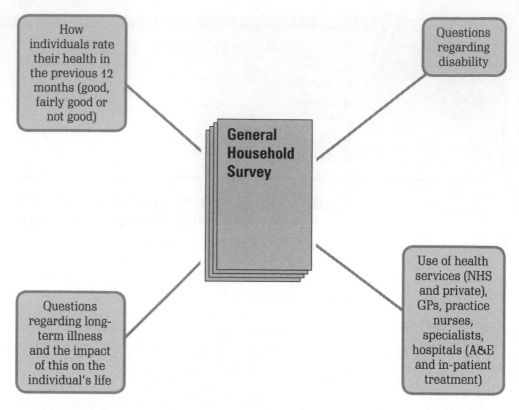

How individuals rate their health in the previous 12 months (good, fairly good or not good)

Questions regarding disability

General Household Survey

Questions regarding long-term illness and the impact of this on the individual's life

Use of health services (NHS and private), GPs, practice nurses, specialists, hospitals (A&E and in-patient treatment)

undertaken by GPs and strategic health authorities. Mortality rates can be compared internationally because most countries hold similar information. Mortality rate are expressed in several different ways. A basis measurement is to express mortality as the number of deaths per 1000 people per year. However this does not allow for the diversity of age within the population which varies over time and between geographical areas. For example, mortality rates in the south-east of England will appear high as there are a high percentage of older and very old people living there. The Standardised Mortality Ratio (SMR) is the method used to compare mortality levels across different years or for different sub-populations within the same year. It also takes into account the different age structure of the population. The ratio is of actual or observed to expected deaths, multiplied conventionally by 100. So if mortality levels are higher in the population being studied than would be expected, the SMR will be greater than 100. A standard set of age-specific mortality rates is chosen, and these are applied to the population for each year. This gives the expected number of deaths in each case, that is, the number of deaths there would have been if these rates had applied. The SMR is useful because it can be used to identify trends and for comparisons.

Infant mortality rate (IMR) are also used as a measurement of health as this provides information about the number of deaths that occur in the first year of life per 1000 live births per year. The IMR is strongly associated with adult mortality rates as it is sensitive to changes in preventive medicine and improvements in health services. Gender, age, social class and cause of death are variables that can be accessed through analysis of the mortality rates.

Infant mortality rates, 1976–2005

England and Wales				
	Neonatal		Post neonatal	
Year	Under 4 weeks Numbers	Rates*	4 weeks–1 year Numbers	Rates*
1976	5,663	9.7	2,671	4.6
1981	4,226	6.9	2,795	4.4
1986	3,489	5.3	2,824	4.3
1991	3,052	4.4	2,106	3.0
1993	2,796	4.2	1,446	2.2

England and Wales				
	Neonatal		**Post neonatal**	
1994	2,749	4.1	1,371	2.1
1995	2,698	4.2	1,284	2.0
1996	2,645	4.1	1,314	2.0
1997	2,517	3.9	1,282	2.0
1998	2,418	3.8	1,207	1.9
1999	2,435	3.9	1,186	1.9
2000	2,335	3.9	1,042	1.7
2001	2,137	3.6	1,103	1.9
2002	2,126	3.6	1,001	1.7
2003	2,264	3.6	1,042	1.7
2004	2,209	3.5	1,009	1.6
2005	2,220	3.4	1,028	1.6

* Per 1,000 live briths

Health events
As indicated previously, health services collect data as part of their administrative processes. This will include GP visits and other primary care interventions, such as consultation and treatment by a GP practice nurse, chronic respiratory disease nurse specialist, cardiac nurse specialist or community nursing services, visits to A&E departments, out-patient clinics or hospital admissions. In addition, work-related injuries and communicable diseases are reported by employers through the RIDDOR (Reporting of Injuries, Diseases and Dangerous Occurrences Regulations 1995) requirements and incidence of food poisoning, for example, are reported by Environmental Health officers. Each of these health events provides data which is reported and collated by the government and which all add to the picture of morbidity and mortality within the population.

Disease incidence
Within epidemiology, the term 'disease incidence' is the proportion of a group that is free of a condition but who develop it over a given period or time, such as a day, week, month, year or decade. In other words, it measures the number of new cases that occur in the population.

The four most common cancers, breast, lung, colorectal and prostate, accounted for just over half of the 233,600 new cases of malignant cancer (excluding non-melanoma skin cancer) registered in England in 2004. Around 117,800 of the total were in males and 115,800 in females. Breast cancer accounted for 32 per cent of cases among women and prostate cancer for 25 per cent among men. Cancer is predominantly a disease of the elderly. Only 0.5 per cent of cases registered in 2004 were in children (aged under 15) and 26 per cent were in people aged under 60. Between 1971 and 2004, the age-standardised incidence of cancer increased by around 21 per cent in males and 41 per cent in females.

incidence of HIV/AIDS   www.statistics.gov.uk

Disease prevalence
This approach is where a defined population is surveyed and its disease status determined at a particular point in time. Prevalence studies therefore provide a snapshot of how many people in the given population have the specific disease being measured at a given point in time. Disease incidence and prevalence are related but measure different aspects of disease within the population. The prevalence of a disease will depend not only on the incidence of new cases within the given group but also on the course of the disease in terms of how long it lasts, whether it can be treated and whether people die as a result of having it.

Health surveillance

Heath surveillance is generally related to occupational health screening methods used to identify occupational health hazards for workers. The description has been widened to include the range of routine health screening strategies and methods which begin before birth and throughout an individual's life. The Child Health Surveillance Programme has been replaced by the Child Heath Promotion Programme as part of the Children's National Service Framework. However it still includes such actions as child screening and immunisation programmes and the information from these can help to measure the prevalence and incidence of illnesses and diseases that are either genetically inherited or specific to babies and young children within the population.

Health surveillance is increasingly available, such as screening for specific cancers (breast, cervical, prostate), diabetes, high blood pressure (hypertension), raised blood cholesterol levels and bone density. All of these are aimed at early detection of treatable conditions and may be targeted at specific 'at risk' groups within the population. In the course of carrying out this surveillance, information about the incidence and prevalence will be gathered as many of these treatable conditions may be asymptomatic (without symptoms) and so not alert the individual to the presence of a problem.

Much occupational health surveillance is a legal requirement for employers to ensure the health and safety of their employees. This includes specific monitoring related to work activities, for example, work involving heavy lifting, working with computer screens, x-rays or blood tests for workers who may be exposed to potential irritants such as chemicals which could cause skin conditions or asthma. In addition, employers will carry out sickness absence monitoring as a means of identifying potential occupational health conditions. The information gathered through these processes will not only be the means ensure early intervention to treat and prevent further disease and ill health but will also provide another measure of health within the employed population.

The clinical iceberg and the number of people who have symptoms and do not act upon them by seeking medical advice is greater than those who do.

Fig 7.8 Cancer occurrence

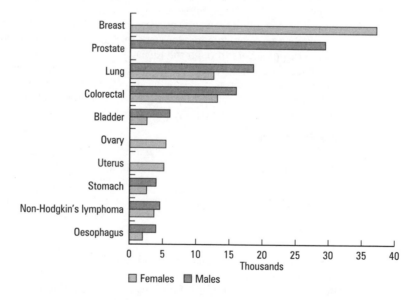

Difficulties in measuring health

The measures most frequently used currently to measure health have limitations as they rely on a negative model which measures ill health and disease and does not measure health or the quality of health experienced by the population. Also some of the measures used are subjective measures based on the individual's perception or reporting of their health status. However, there are a number of positive and objective methods which taken together can provide a measure of health within a population.

Health measures that are routinely undertaken at different points in an individual's life, such as height, weight and dental health status, are by proxy indicators of health. For example, the average height of the population can indicate their nutritional status and well-being. Also the percentage of low birth weight babies can indicate the healthiness of women. Another indicator is health behaviour, for example the number of people in the population who smoke, drink alcohol, are drug users, take regular exercise, and so on. These can be measured within particular populations and used in relative comparisons. This could also include the number

case study 7.2

Rheumatism

The prevalence of arthritis and rheumatism is higher in women than in men and also increases with age in both sexes. In 2003, the rates for men and women in the UK were less than 25 per 1,000 of population up to age 44. After that, there was a rapid increase in prevalence, with rates increasing sixfold to age 64. The rates for women then rose more sharply than for men. Among those aged 65 to 74, the prevalence rate for women was twice that for men (227 per 1,000 compared with 113).

Fig 7.9 Arthritis/ rheumatism prevalence by age and sex in UK, 2003

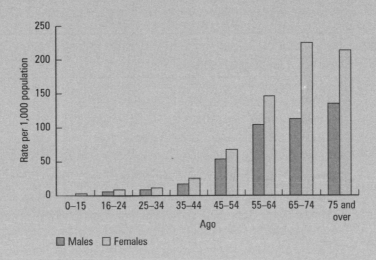

□ Males □ Females

activity
GROUP WORK

1   What might account for the differences in prevalence between men and women?

2   What factors might explain the sharp rise in prevalence over the age of 44years?

3   How might this information be used in relation to health and social care?

of people who access health screening opportunities, such as immunisations; breast cancer screening and been seen as an indicator of health within the population.

Environmental indicators, such as the measurements collected by environmental health departments of air and water quality, housing types and density, can also be used as indicators of health. Finally, socio-economic indicators, such as wealth, can also be viewed as an indicator of health as the more equitable the distribution of wealth the healthier the population is likely to be overall. The government uses these positive measurements to set targets from improving health, such as the National Service Frameworks, Public Service Agreements (PSA) and Health Inequalities targets.

The Scottish Health Survey used a number of different positive health indicators to form an understanding of the healthiness of people in Scotland. In Wales, the report 'Inequalities in Health – The Welsh Dimension 2002–2005' describes the outcomes and improvements of initiatives to readdress health inequalities as well as identifying targets for further improvements. In Northern Ireland, the research paper 'Measuring Poverty and Social Exclusion in Northern Ireland' considers the same areas of need and targets for addressing health inequalities.

The Scottish Government   www.scotland.gov.uk
Scottish Health Survey 2003
Welsh Assembly Government   new.wales.gov.uk
Inequalities in Health – The Welsh Dimension 2002–2005
Northern Ireland Assembly   www.niassembly.gov.uk
Measuring Poverty and Social Exclusion in Northern Ireland

Patterns and trends in health and illness

Being able to identify patterns and trends in data is an important part of the analytical process as they indicate regular occurrences which can be used as a basis for predicting future behaviour. Statistical information is presented in a number of different formats, for example, as bar charts, pie charts, tables or graphs, as well as a written commentary which provides some interpretation of the information presented. Bar charts and graphs provide the reader with a lot of information which is often less specific, that is, it is usually rounded numerical data, unless it has labels giving the exact numerical data. This can be used to make comparisons as well as making it easy for the reader to clearly identify in a visual format any patterns and trends. Tables are generally used to provide a lot of detailed specific data from different categories. Most presented data will provide several different types of information.

Refer back to the data on mortality rates page 260 to see how tables are used to provide a lot of detailed data.

When analysing data presented in visual formats:

■ read the labels on each axis

■ look at the scale, especially the starting point

■ look for any wide variations

■ read any supporting or explanatory notes

■ look at the data source.

Statistics can be misleading and so it is important to always read them with a critical eye, asking yourself questions about their validity, currency, authenticity and reliability.

Measures of health, whether in negative terms, such as mortality rates, or positive terms, such as health behaviours, can be analysed to provide a wealth of information about different groups or sub-populations which can then inform actions.

The Office for National Statistics (ONS) graphs reproduced in this unit provide information about gender, age and health-related behaviour statistics which relates to risk behaviour (smoking and alcohol consumption). The Office for National Statistics is a major source of statistical information that informs us about social patterns and trends in relation to all aspects of life in the UK, not just about health.

Social class and gender

A government-appointed research working group led by Sir Douglas Black looked at inequality and health in Britain in the 1970s, and published their findings in the Black Report (1980). The government of the day tried to minimize the impact of the report's findings (especially the causes of ill health identified through research) and recommendations. The Health Divide written by Margaret Whitehead was commissioned by the Health Education Council to update the evidence from the Black Report and to update the 37 recommendations made in the Report. The Health Divide was published in 1987 and confirmed the findings of the Black Report. Again the government of the day sought to 'bury' the 'controversial findings'.

It is clear from analysis of ONS information that the health inequalities first identified in the Black Report and The Health Divide, are still apparent in the UK today. Both the Black Report and The Health Divide identified the health inequalities that existed in relation to social class (based on the Registrar General's Social Class (RGSC)) with higher mortality rates being seen in the lower social classes (manual and unskilled workers).

Today, life expectancy at birth remains lower for those in the lower social classes (for men more so than for women) than in the professional and managerial classes. Although life expectancy at birth has increased for all social classes over the past thirty years, inequality has increased. In 2004, life expectancy at birth was 77 years for men and 81 years for women (ONS 21-02-06). In 1996, the difference in life expectancy at birth between social classes was significant for both men and women. For men, the difference in life expectancy at birth between those in the Registrar General's Social Class I (professional) and those in Class V (unskilled manual) was 9.5 years. For women, the difference was 6.4 years. Although life expectancy at birth has changed over the past 25 years, a differential remains and figures show that similar patterns are emerging for women as for men. However, it is important to remember that allocating social class to married women is problematic as the current system is based on the spouse's occupation which may be lower than indicated by the women's occupation. Death of people of working ages (35–64) from specific causes, such as ischemic heart disease, cancers or respiratory diseases, are indicating a widening divide between social classes (ONS 1999).

National Statistics Office　　www.statistics.gov.uk

'Trends in life expectancy by social class – an update' (Office of National Statistics, 1999)

Locality

In addition to gender and social class, locality is also significant factor in inequalities in health. In 1999–2001, a reported 10-year difference in life expectancy at birth for men living in Glasgow City (69 years) than those living in North Dorset (79 years). According to the findings reported in the 'Inequalities in Health – The Welsh Dimension 2002–2005', Wales has the highest rates of cancer registrations not just in the UK but in Western Europe. Although mortality rates for cancer are worse than for England and Northern Ireland, they are better than for Scotland. Within Wales, where you live has a bearing on mortality with death rates being 50 per cent higher in the South Wales valleys than in Ceredigion (West Wales).

Ethnicity

People from minority ethnic groups were found to self-report poor health more frequently and visit their GP more frequently (especially if from the Indian subcontinent). People from South Asia (in particular of Pakistani and Bangladeshi origin) have moderately higher incidence of coronary heart disease. There is also a higher prevalence of diagnosed non-insulin dependent diabetes among South Asians and people from the Caribbean, with mortality directly associated with diabetes amongst South Asian migrants around three and a half times that of the general population.

Another key indicator of health, the Infant Mortality rate (IMR) fell considerably over the 20th century as a result in part of improved living conditions and technological advances and improved healthcare. However, the father's socio-economic status (highest IMR occurring in lower social classes), parents' marital status and mother's country of origin as well as birth weight are factors that all increase the chances of infant death.

Risk behaviour

Patterns and trends in risk behaviours, such as alcohol consumption, smoking, illegal drug use, poor diet and lack of exercise, are areas of considerable concern to government and health and social care services. For many years, research has clearly shown the links between these particular behaviours and poor health and the evidence grows stronger each day. The impact these risk behaviours have on health is not just morbidity but increasingly mortality

remember

stillbirth
born dead after 28 weeks of pregnancy
early neonatal
within 1 week of birth
neonatal
the first 28 days after birth
post neonatal
from 28 days to 1 year old
infant
less than 1 year old

Fig 7.10 Age-standardised limiting long-term illness: by ethnic group and sex in England & Wales, 2001

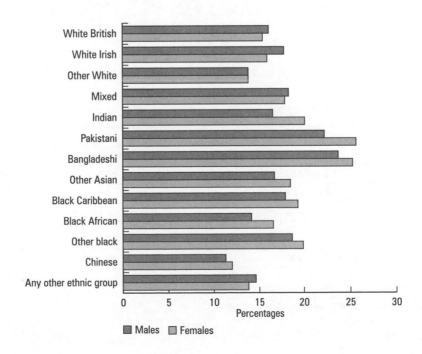

rates too. *Health Statistics Quarterly* 33 (ONS) published in Spring 2007 reported on alcohol-related deaths in the UK. The report showed that alcohol-related deaths in the UK almost doubled between 1991 and 2004. In 2004, they accounted for 1.5% of all deaths in the UK compared with 0.9% in 1991. The death rate for males was 17.6 of 100,000 population compared to 8.3 deaths per 100,000 for females. In the period 1991–2004, in relation to age the death rate for men aged 55–74 years was the highest. The largest increase in death rates for women was for those in the 35–54 age group which was almost doubled (7.2 to 14.2 per 100,000 population). Locality was also a significant factor with the highest number of deaths occurring in Scotland (15 of the localities in the top 20 localities with the highest death rates were in Scotland, 3 in England and 2 in Northern Ireland).

case study 7.3 — Infant mortality

Births, stillbirths and infant deaths by mother's country of origin, 2005

England and Wales	Numbers						Rates[1]				
Country of birth	Births		Deaths								
	Live briths	Still-briths	Early neonatal	Neonatal	Post-neonatal	Infants	Still briths	Perinatal	Neonatal	Post-neonatal	Infant
All	645,881	3,484	1,676	2,193	995	3,188	5.4	7.9	3.4	1.5	4.9
United Kingdom	511,648	2,606	1,283	1,692	760	2,452	5.1	7.6	3.3	1.5	4.8
England and Wales	501,732	2,554	1,256	1,656	739	2,395	5.1	7.6	3.3	1.5	4.8
Scotland	7,321	34	21	28	16	44	4.6	7.5	3.8	2.2	6.0
Northern Ireland	2,290	14	5	7	5	12	6.1	8.2	3.1	2.2	5.2
Elsewhere	305	4	1	1	0	1	12.9	16.2	3.3	–	3.3
Outside the United Kingdom	134,233	878	393	501	235	736	6.5	9.4	3.7	1.8	5.5
Irish Republic	3,461	23	9	14	9	23	6.6	9.2	4.0	2.6	6.6
Other European Union	20.421	100	57	68	25	93	4.9	7.7	3.3	1.2	4.6
Rest of Europe	6,947	31	14	16	9	25	4.4	6.4	2.3	1.3	3.6
Commonwealth Australia, Canada and New Zealand	4,221	10	10	12	3	15	2.4	4.7	2.8	0.7	3.6
New Commonwealth	65,135	509	222	282	133	415	7.8	11.1	4.3	2.0	6.4
Asia											
Bangladesh	8,220	59	16	20	16	36	7.1	9.1	2.4	1.9	4.4
India	10,074	69	22	26	20	46	6.8	9.0	2.6	2.0	4.6
Pakistan	16,480	175	66	91	51	142	10.5	14.5	5.5	3.1	8.6
East Africa	4,046	23	18	23	4	27	5.7	10.1	5.7	1.0	6.7
Southern Africa	4,125	16	14	15	5	20	3.9	7.2	3.6	1.2	4.8
Rest of Africa	13,761	100	51	61	26	87	7.2	10.9	4.4	1.9	6.3
Far East	1,343	4	4	4	1	5	3.0	5.9	3.0	0.7	3.7
Carribean	3,723	38	25	35	5	40	10.1	16.8	9.4	1.3	10.7
Rest of the New Commonwealth	3,363	25	6	7	5	12	7.4	9.1	2.1	1.5	3.6
Rest of World and not stated	34,048	205	81	109	56	165	6.0	8.3	3.2	1.6	4.8

1 Stillbirths and perinatal deaths per 1,000 live births and stillbirths.
Neonatal, postneonatal and infant deaths per 1,000 live births.
Source: www.statistics.gov.uk/STATBASE/Expodata/Spreadsheets/D9516.xls

activity
GROUP WORK

1 Which group has the highest infant mortality rates?
2 Which group has the lowest infant mortality rates?
3 What are the differences between women from the UK and the New Commonwealth counties?
4 What conclusions can you draw with regard to ethnicity and health inequalities from this data?

Fig 7.11 Alcohol-related death rates

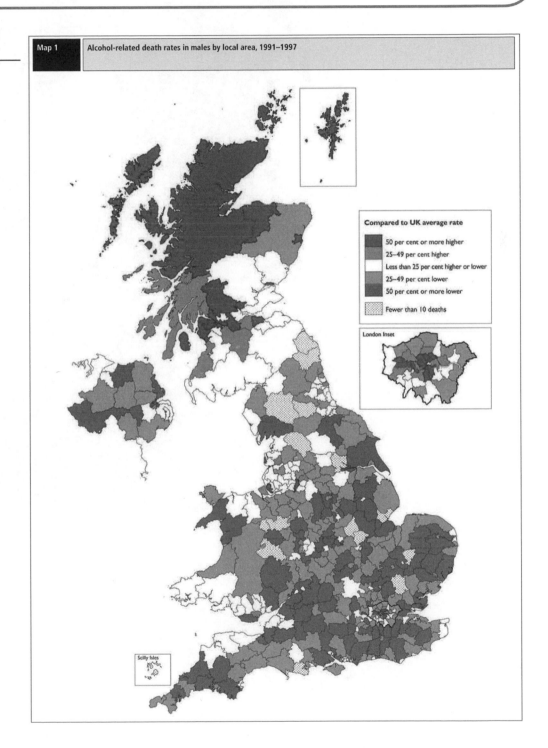

Fig 7.11 Alcohol-related
death rates (continued)

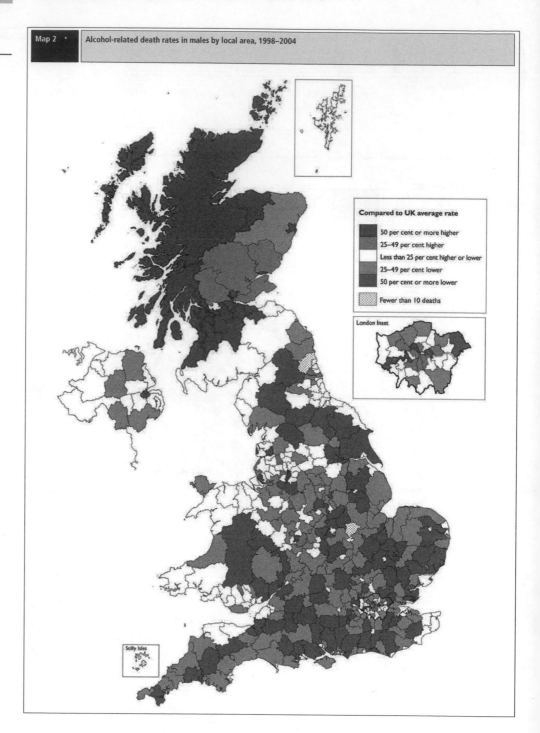

Map 2 ·   Alcohol-related death rates in males by local area, 1998–2004

Compared to UK average rate

- 50 per cent or more higher
- 25–49 per cent higher
- Less than 25 per cent higher or lower
- 25–49 per cent lower
- 50 per cent or more lower
- Fewer than 10 deaths

London Inset

Scilly Isles

Fig 7.11 Alcohol-related
death rates (continued)

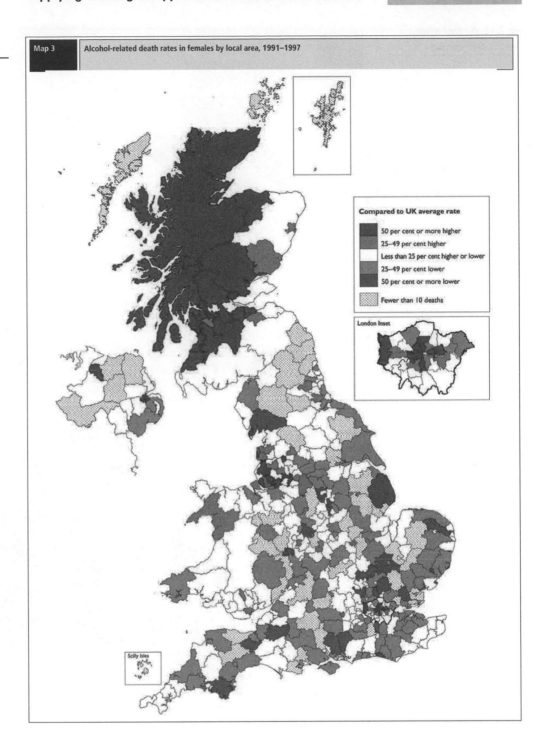

Map 3   Alcohol-related death rates in females by local area, 1991–1997

Compared to UK average rate

50 per cent or more higher
25–49 per cent higher
Less than 25 per cent higher or lower
25–49 per cent lower
50 per cent or more lower
Fewer than 10 deaths

London Inset

Scilly Isles

Fig 7.11 Alcohol-related
death rates (continued)

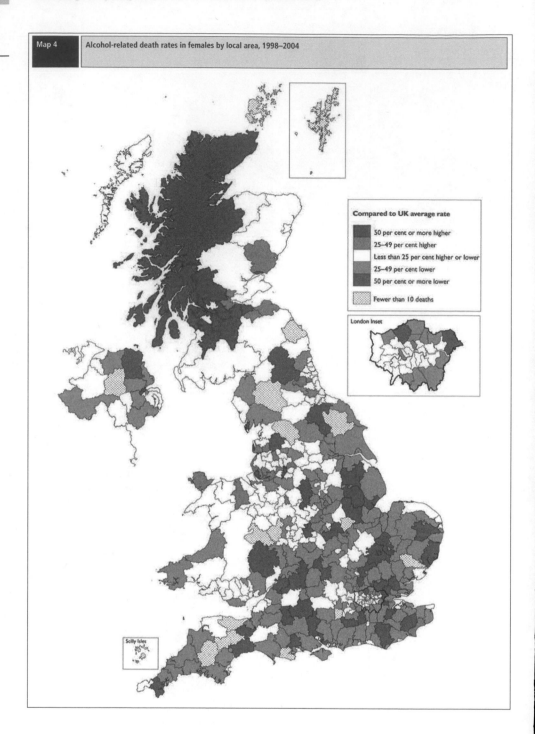

Map 4   Alcohol-related death rates in females by local area, 1998–2004

Compared to UK average rate

- 50 per cent or more higher
- 25–49 per cent higher
- Less than 25 per cent higher or lower
- 25–49 per cent lower
- 50 per cent or more lower
- Fewer than 10 deaths

London Inset

Scilly Isles

The government guidelines concerning safe limits for alcohol consumption are 21 units for adult males and 14 units for adult women. The Scottish Health Survey 2003 found that these recommendations were being exceeded by 27% of men and 7% of women.

Sociological explanations

There is considerable evidence that health inequalities remain a feature of life in the UK. Sociology seeks to apply different perspectives in order to provide an explanation for why inequalities arise and persist within the population. By understanding the underlying causes, potential solutions can be arrived at in theory. However, a number of different explanations have been presented to explain this phenomenon and all have different priorities in terms of appropriate responses.

Fig 7.12 Binge drinking

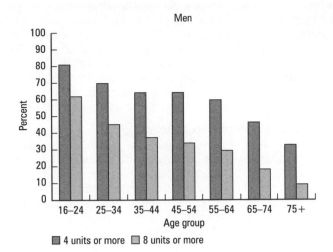

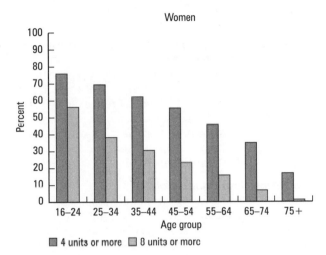

activity **GROUP WORK 7.6** **P5**

Using statistical data, compare and contrast the patterns and trends of health and illness (for example, lung cancer rates in the UK) between three different social groups, such as different social classes or minority ethnic groups.

Artefact explanation

This explanation essentially questions the methodology used in measuring health and inequalities. It questions the artificial nature of the variables used in comparison and in particular the relationship between health and social class. The artefact explanation suggests that the continued pattern of health inequality is more a result of the changing face of occupation in the UK than any direct causal link between social class and health. The changing occupational structure (the decline of the traditional un-skilled, manual labour heavy industries, such as coal mining, dock work, steel and ship-building industries) has meant a reduction in job opportunities in these occupations and, therefore, those who remain in these industries are generally older than the average labour force. As a consequence, the size of the unskilled manual labour social class V has diminished. In addition, the implication is that it is the changes in the proportion of the population within the lower social classes that have lead to a continuation of health inequalities. The assumption is also made that those moving upwards into the middle social classes in line with job opportunities in semi-skilled and skilled work, such as the electronics and technology industries, were either already healthier or their health will improve.

However, statistics continue to demonstrate that around 20% of the labour force remains in the lower social classes and a relationship remains between health inequalities and social class regardless of how this is measured. In 2007, UNICEF published a report which revealed that 35.3% of 15-year olds in the UK aspire to low-skilled work. This presents a different future of occupational and social class structure than that suggested by the artefact explanation which suggested that unskilled and low-skilled occupations would diminish as the economy developed thus devaluing the casual relationship of social class and health inequality. It would seem therefore that the artefact explanation does not provide an adequate explanation.

Natural/social selection explanation

In this explanation, it is health not social class that is the cause of inequality. The idea is based on natural selection where social class acts as a filter with health a basis for selection in terms of physical strength, robustness and vitality. Statistics show that those in the higher social classes are less likely to die early. The natural selection assumption is that this social group contains people who are the fittest and strongest in the population. The weakest in the population are therefore to be found in the lower social classes. If people have poor health, they will be less able to undertake those occupations that define the higher social classes. This explanation suggests that even if people start in a higher social class, ill health will mean they drift downwards as their health deteriorates and they either take less skilled jobs or become unemployed.

This explanation however is unable to adequately explain regional variations and the argument that those with more resources (those in the higher social classes) are more able and likely to access early intervention to prevent ill health or cope with its implications in terms of employment. Another argument is that those in social classes IV and V may be working in occupations with high levels of risk and indeed that which require considerable strength and vitality. A comparison of death rates therefore is misleading as the high levels in social classes IV–V may be more to do with the occupational hazards encountered than with fitness, such as high incidences of industrial accidents, injuries and diseases, for example, mesothelioma due to asbestos inhalation.

Cultural/behavioural explanation

This explanation emphasises the way that individuals choose to lead their lives and the differences in social groups in those behavioural and lifestyle choices. In this explanation, health inequalities are the result of people in lower social groups choosing higher risk behaviours and lifestyles than those in higher social classes who are more likely to see health as a commodity to be bought and through this ill health prevented. The proposition is that people are the problem with the emphasis on individual responsibility. People choose to smoke, drink alcohol in excess of recommended levels, eat a poor diet in terms of quantity and quality of food and do not undertake exercise in their leisure time. In addition, they do not make use of preventative health care, such as antenatal checks, child immunisation, contraception, cancer screening and general heath care advice. These behaviours are repeated through generations through the processes of socialisation and cultural influence, thus increasing the potential for inequalities to persist within this group. It is also suggested that these choices are often due to a lack of education as well as unthinking action, so that the individual is unaware of the danger they put themselves and their family in by their choices.

The evidence to support this has been the consistently higher rates of smoking among people in lower social classes, for example, statistics from GHS 1998–1999 show that 22% of males and 38% of females from social classes I & II were smokers while 83% of males and 67% of females in social classes IV & V were smokers. Given that smoking is the largest single cause of preventable death in the UK, accounting for one in five of all deaths and is the main avoidable risk factor for coronary heart disease and cancer, this has considerable implications for the health of those in lower social classes. In addition, the effects of passive smoking also have health implications for families and those around smokers. Other factors cited as evidencing similar patterns are alcohol use, diet (both quantity and nutritional value of foods) and exercise in leisure time. Research and information drawn from the GHS have consistently demonstrated a higher level of alcohol use in the lower socio-economic groups particularly in men.

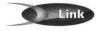

Refer back to page 265 to remind yourself about the evidence to support a locality and cultural influence in excessive alcohol use.

The problem with this approach is the assumption that lifestyle choices such as smoking are simplistic. Sociological research has however, uncovered that this is far from the reality. Health policy that results from a cultural/behavioural explanation of health inequalities focuses on social control through initiatives designed to change individual behaviour and choices, such as health promotion activities, legislation to stop tobacco and alcohol advertising, legal age limits and no smoking in public places.

Materialist/structuralist explanation

This explanation emphasises the important role the environment plays in health inequalities. It is the environment that individuals live and work in and the influence that has on their behaviour and lifestyle choices that creates inequalities. Within this explanation, it is the structure of society as a whole that is implicated as the cause. The material causes of ill health, such as unhealthy living conditions, poor access to education, stress and limited employment opportunities including more dangerous manual occupations, and the limited resources that all of these create, are the reason for higher levels of deprivation, poverty and health inequality. Poverty and deprivation are viewed as relative in terms of the ability to obtain those resources valued within society and participating fully in society. The focus is on the way society is structured so that people have problems due to the inherent inequalities that exist within a capitalist society.

> **remember**
>
> Social control means strategies used to try and regulate and control human behaviour to ensure compliance and conformity to the rules of society.

Link

See page 58 in Unit 2 for more information about the inequalities in society in terms of access to education and the impact this has on employment opportunities and as a result access to material resources such as income.

A materialist/structuralist explanation would consider, for example, the dietary choices made as being a consequence of low income rather than entirely individual choice. People on low incomes often live in poor housing (sometimes in hostel or bed and breakfast accommodation with limited facilities), in less accessible areas of a town (on the outskirts). These areas are often areas of deprivation where transport links are limited or expensive in relation to income, therefore there is limited access to larger supermarkets with more competitive prices and a wider choice. This means that individuals have little choice but to shop locally where the prices are higher with less choice especially in fruit and vegetables. People on low incomes generally shop more frequently to ensure they manage their limited resources well (fuel as well as food). Dietary choices are based on what can be bought to satisfy hunger and so diet is likely to be high in carbohydrates, low in fibre, fruit and vegetables. Limited income will also require consideration of fuel costs and this may limit cooking. Poor education both within the home and in formal education in terms of household management skills including cooking may also limit an individual's ability to produce nutritious meals that are cost effective and satisfying.

In terms of other lifestyle choices, such as smoking, research by Graham (1987) showed that young women caring for young children smoked as it was something they could do for themselves and it was a way to release the stress they felt as a result of living with poverty and deprivation where there was no sense of being able to escape their situation. Whereas the cultural/behavioural explanation views poor dietary choices and smoking as an almost wilful and irresponsible lifestyle choices (given all that is known about the harm these choices do to health), the materialist/structuralist explanation emphasises that it is inappropriate to try and understand individual behaviour out of the social context of the individual's life experience and environment. Health policy that results from a materialist/structuralist explanation of health inequalities focuses on social justice through changing the structures within society in order to reverse the inequalities that exist and achieve greater equity for all members of society. For example, access to education for all at all levels was improved by Sure Start, the government programme which began in 2001, aiming to deliver the best start in life for every child through early education, childcare, health and family support.

Sure Start   http://www.surestart.gov.uk/

Considering the Black Report and The Health Divide were published in the 1980s and 1990s and the numerous government social justice and social control initiatives aimed at creating a greater level of equity in the UK, health inequalities and unacceptable levels of poverty continue to be major concerns in the UK in the early twenty-first century. The United Nations Children's Fund (UNICEF) study published in February 2007 reported 16.2% of British children living below the poverty line. The report which considered 21 economically advanced countries stated that:

'The evidence from many countries persistently shows that children who grow up in poverty are more vulnerable; specifically, they are more likely to be in poor health, to have learning and behavioural difficulties, to underachieve at school, to become pregnant at too early an age, to have lower skills and aspirations, to be low-paid, unemployed and welfare-dependent.'

[Permission 7.19]

It appears that no one approach is adequate in explaining the reasons for the persistence of health inequalities in the UK and this is borne out by the mix of approaches used in health policy to try and address this issue.

activity
INDIVIDUAL WORK
7.7

M3

With reference to activity 7.6 (page 271), use the following sociological explanations for health inequalities to explain the patterns and trends of health and illness in the three different social groups:

■ Artefact explanation

■ Natural/social selection explanation

■ Cultural/behaviourist explanation

■ Materialist/structural explanation

activity
INDIVIDUAL WORK
7.8

D2

With reference to activities 7.6 and 7.7, examine and determine the value of each of the four sociological explanations for health inequalities in helping to explain the patterns and trends of health and illness in the three different social groups.

Scottish Executive	www.scotland.gov.uk/Home
Welsh Assembly	www.new.wales.gov.uk
Northern Ireland Assembly	www.niassembly.gov.uk/
London Health Observatory	www.lho.org.uk

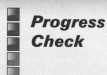

Progress Check

1   What is meant by the term *norm*?

2   How do role and status influence behaviour and interaction?

3   What is the fundamental belief of collectivism?

4   Describe what is meant by a holistic concept of health.

5   How do the socio-medical and biomedical models of health differ from one another?

6   What is *iatrogensis*?

7   How are infant mortality rates used as an indicator of health?

8   What are the difficulties in measuring health?

9   Give two examples of health inequalities in relation to gender.

10 Explain how the materialist/structuralist explanation is applied in relation to health inequalities and ethnicity.

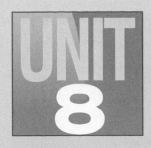

UNIT 8

Psychological perspectives for health and social care

This unit covers:

- Psychological approaches to study
- Applying psychological approaches to health and social care

An understanding of the different psychological perspectives and how these are applied is fundamental to the study of health and social care. This unit is an introduction to different psychological perspectives. It will consider what is meant by theories in the context of psychology and the diverse range of psychological theories that can be applied. The principle psychological perspectives will be examined and applied to health and social care sectors in order to determine the value of psychology to these. The unit will encourage reflection in those involved or planning to be involved in supporting others within health and social care work.

To achieve a **Pass** grade the evidence must show that the learner is able to:	To achieve a **Merit** grade the evidence must show that, in addition to the pass criteria, the learner is able to:	To achieve a **Distinction** grade the evidence must show that, in addition to the pass and merit criteria, the learner is able to:
P1 describe the application of behaviourist perspectives in health and social care Pg 291		
P2 explain the value of the social learning approach to health and social care service provision Pg 293		
P3 describe the application of psychodynamic perspectives in health and social care Pg 296	**M1** analyse the contribution of different psychological perspectives to the understanding and management of challenging behaviour Pg 300	

grading criteria

grading criteria

Psychological approaches to study

Psychology is the scientific study of the mind and its processes, such as thoughts, feelings and behaviour. There are a number of different views or perspectives which try to explain the meanings of these processes.

Principle psychological perspectives

This unit will examine six different **psychological** perspectives:

- Behaviourist
- Social learning
- Psychodynamic
- Humanistic
- Cognitive
- Biological

Behaviourist perspectives

This perspective was founded by J B Watson in 1915. It proposes that individuals learn to behave in response to their environment, either as a result of a factor that stimulates (increases interest or activity in) the individual leading to a response, or through a process of **reinforcement**. The **stimulus**–response theory is that individuals learn or are **conditioned** to behave in the way they do. Human behaviour is learned as a result of associating different stimuli with different responses. For example, the telephone rings and we associate this with someone wanting to talk to us, so we answer it.

Pavlov

Ivan Pavlov (1849–1936) conducted a series of experiments that demonstrated conditioning. Pavlov fed a group of dogs at the same time as they could hear a church bell. The experiments showed how the stimulus of the church bell (a conditioned stimulus) when paired or associated with the arrival of food (an unconditioned stimulus) as it was rung would make his dogs salivate so they were ready to eat (the unconditioned response). Over a period of time, whenever the dogs heard any bell ring (a conditioned stimulus), they began to salivate regardless of whether they were fed or not (a conditioned response).

A factor in the conditioning process is reinforcement which will embed the learned response so that it becomes internalised and so the individual behaves in that way without thinking

Fig 8.1 Pavlov's dogs

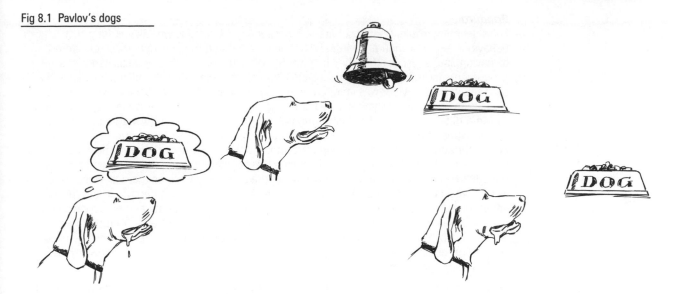

about it. However, Pavlov found that after a time the dogs stopped salivating to the bell alone and so he had to go back to the beginning to recreate the association between the stimuli, the ringing bell (conditioned stimulus) plus the food (unconditioned stimulus), in order to get the unconditioned response of salivation. This is an important point to understand and remember, as often people think that once a conditioned response is learned it will not be forgotten. In fact, it requires reinforcement and possibly returning to the conditioning process.

Nobel Prize Information   http://nobelprize.org

Pavlov's 1904 Nobel Prize winning lecture concerning conditioned responses

Skinner

The work of American behavioural psychologist Burrhus Frederic Skinner (1905–1990) developed the idea of conditioning by exploring the effect of rewards or incentives on this learning process. Skinner experimented with rats and pigeons and, whereas Pavlov would feed his dogs whether or not they salivated when he rang the bell, Skinner only fed his rats or pigeons when they did what he had conditioned them to do (press a lever to release the food). This was positive reinforcement, as the behaviour Skinner desired them to demonstrate was rewarded with food. If the rats or pigeons did not behave in the way Skinner wanted, this undesirable behaviour would be negatively reinforced through the absence of food. In other experiments using a maze, the undesirable behaviour (going to one area of the maze) resulted in the subjects being given an electric shock (negative reinforcement). This resulted in a change in behaviour so they avoided this area (the desired behaviour) and this change was rewarded with no electric shock. This type of conditioning, where learning is influenced by reward (positive reinforcement) or an unpleasant consequence (negative reinforcement), is called operant conditioning. The reward or positive reinforcement should encourage the behaviour to be repeated and the association of unpleasant consequences generally makes it less likely that the undesired behaviour is repeated.

Skinner continued his experiments to find out how often desired behaviour happened until reinforcement was necessary. He found that reward could be given after a fixed number of positive responses (desired behaviour), for example a fixed ratio of one reward for every ten examples of desired behaviour or within ten minutes. However, this led to uneven behavioural responses and the desired behaviour soon lapsed disappearing altogether once the reward was removed.

Social learning perspectives

The idea that other individuals, group, culture and society all influence behaviour and thinking has been discussed in other units in relation to the processes of **socialisation**. The social learning that takes place through these processes helps individuals to make sense of the world they live in and also helps them to understand the expected norms of behaviour as well as the taboos and consequences of behaving in ways that challenges these. Individuals' sense of identity is bound up with social learning processes and with that, self-esteem and self-worth.

Bandura

Social learning results from observing the behaviour of others as well as imitating that behaviour. Arthur Bandura identified that children imitated those people they considered as having status, especially if they had warm, powerful personalities as well. Bandura's experiments including showing groups of children a film scenario with different endings to then see what behaviour was imitated. In his experiments, Bandura showed three groups of children a film which showed an adult hitting a doll and shouting at it. Each group were shown a different ending. The first group were shown the adult being rewarded for hitting and shouting at the doll. The second group were shown the adult being punished for this behaviour and finally the third group were shown an ending where there was no consequence for the adult. When the children were given a doll to play with later, the children who saw the adult being rewarded tended to behave in the same way towards the doll. Bandura's work suggests the powerful influence that adults have on children's behaviour and this has implications for the way in which primary care givers, such as parents and nursery workers, behave towards other people as well as children, since children will learn from them and imitate this behaviour. For example, if a child is given comfort when they cry they learn to comfort others, if they receive explanations in response to their questions they will try and explain things to others.

One of the things children enjoy doing as part of growing up is playing imaginative pretend games such as role play or dressing up. Here they get to play adults and, to an extent, try out what being adult is like. They generally role play those roles they see as having high status and importance, such as parental roles, doctors and nurses, teachers and students. Observing children playing pretend games and testing out on other children behaviours imitated from their observation of adult interactions can reveal a great deal about the roles they see people in their lives playing. Children learn about the different roles that individuals occupy in society and this can have a considerable impact on their **perception** and expectations for themselves and others. For example, if children grow up with defined gender roles that are stereotypical then this may limit expectations for their own potential as well contribute to stereotyping. Children are influenced by other children and will behave in ways that gain their approval, and this may also be reinforced by observed adult behaviour. They are also influenced by the media, TV, films, games, books and toys, so a gender balance is essential to avoid reinforcing negative stereotypes.

Considerable discussion has taken place in the last thirty years about the influences that roles have on behaviour and how behaviour is affected by being within a role and by status of roles. Uniforms are a useful way to signify a particular role and with that a status and authority. Early socialisation teaches individuals about these roles and how to respond and behave in relation to these. However, even if society presents a particular role as having status and authority, if this is not reinforced through the actions of those who influence children and young people, that is primary care givers and other children, there is no guarantee the child will grow up to acknowledge this role. For example, if a child sees their parent being disrespectful of or disregarding authority, such as the law as represented by police and judicial system, then the child is likely to grow up with those same attitudes, even though the consequences of disrespect and disregard are unpleasant.

See page 246 in Unit 7 for more information about the importance of roles in society.

The self-fulfilling prophesy is a good example of how social learning impacts on individuals' lives.

Psychodynamic perspectives

When many people think of psychology, they will think of Sigmund Freud (1856–1939) and Erik Erikson (1902–1994) and the psychodynamic perspective applied in order to understand human behaviour. Psychodynamic perspectives adopt the nature approach, that it is biology that determines the individual, as opposed to the nurture approach adopted by behaviourists, socialisation and social learning theories, that it is the influence of environment that determines the individual. More recent theories believe that both are important factors in psychological development.

Fig 8.2 The self-fulfilling prophecy

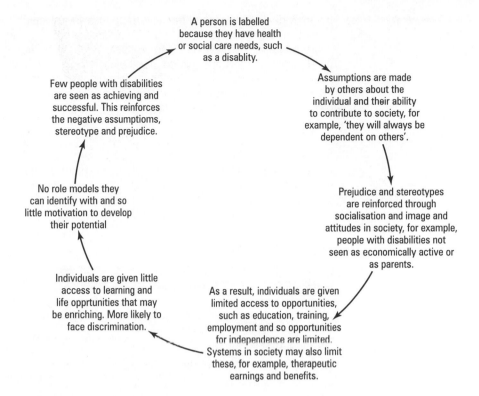

Freud

Freud, as the founding father of psychodynamic theory, believed that the unconscious mind and feelings direct behaviour and so individuals are unaware of the motivations (reasons) for their behaviour. Freud also believed that early childhood experiences were important as these have a deep and lasting influence on individuals into their adult life. Freud believed that human behaviour has two main motives: the pursuit of pleasure and the avoidance of pain. These two motives are often in conflict, such as the pain of waiting for a birthday to arrive in order to experience the pleasure of receiving birthday gifts. In addition, some pleasures, such as drinking too much alcohol, can lead to pain (a hangover). The unconscious is related more to those things the mind blocks in order to prevent remembering rather than those things that are simply forgotten. The 'Freudian slip' is a term used to describe a situation when the unconscious mind lets slip what the person is really thinking as opposed to their measured response or what the other person is expecting to hear.

Freud considered that people went through psychosexual stages of development: the oral, anal, phallic, latency and genital stages. He used this as a basis for understanding human feelings and behaviours. According to Freud, each of these, except latency, is associated with an erogenous or sexually arousing area of the body, and the pleasure, or lack of it, derived from stimulating these areas influences adult personality. Freud felt that if individuals failed to reconcile the conflicts associated with a particular stage, as adults they would develop fixations related to that stage, for example, oral fixation may be demonstrated through the individual always putting things into their mouth or having their tongue pierced. If the individual feels stressed, they may play with the tongue piercing, for example by rubbing it against the roof or their mouth or against their teeth.

Freud divided the demands of the individual's mind into three parts: the id, the ego and the superego. He believed that individuals are born with an 'id' which is responsible for the 'I' demands, such as 'I want …. The 'ego' develops as the child grows and is responsible for trying to resolve the inner conflicts between the individualist demands made by the id and the superego. The superego develops at around six years of age and tries to conform to the demands made by others, such as the expectations of parents and moral, ethical and cultural norms of society to conform and do the right thing. Personality is psychodynamic as it is made up of these three aspects which at different times lead. Sometimes it is the id with the attitude and behaviour that says 'just go for it and hang the consequences'. Sometimes it is the superego which listens to conscious thought before acting. Sometimes it is the ego attempting to satisfy the id's wants while appeasing the moral principles of the superego. There is a dynamic (constantly changing) relationship between these three within a normal personality. Freud in effect considered the mind to have a social aspect that tried to reconcile the individualism of self and the need to fit into society and be approved by people who are important to the individual, such as parents and peers. It is the ego that is aware of the world and through which individuals learn, influence and are influenced. The superego is deeply unconscious and the site of internalised early images and influences. It is not the same as the adult conscience that is able to engage in moral arguments and judgements, it is more the 'rules' and 'moral codes' learned through growing up that the individual only becomes aware of when in danger of breaking them, for example by stepping over the boundary of what is socially acceptable behaviour and arousing feelings of guilt which then stop the individual.

Freud also believed that individuals develop defence mechanisms in order to protect themselves from feelings of anxiety or guilt when they feel threatened or the demands of the id or superego become overwhelming. These normal defence mechanisms are not within conscious control and, if a stressful situation occurs, the ego will use one or more to self-protect. When defence mechanisms are out of proportion to the stress, they may become a problem as they are experienced as anxiety states, phobias, obsessions or hysteria.

Freud's eight defence mechanisms

Defence mechanism	Explanation
Repression	Putting stressful or traumatic situations into the unconscious mind. May lead to inner conflict and have a negative impact on mental health
Sublimation	Redirecting those impulses (usually sexual) considered unacceptable within society into more acceptable forms, such as creative or altruistic (selfless) acts
Regression	Returning to behaviour more in keeping with a younger more immature age or stage, such as thumb-sucking or bed-wetting
Denial	Refusing to accept the reality of the situation. Acceptable within the short term but likely to impact on mental well-being if not resolved, for example denial of medical diagnosis
Projection	Transferring feelings or thoughts (especially if undesirable or unacceptable) on to others, for example feeling angry but accusing others of behaving in this way
Reaction formation	Behaving in the opposite way to instinctive urges
Rationalisation	Having a less acceptable reason for behaviour than the more socially acceptable explanation given
Escape	Leaving the situation which is creating distress or is traumatic for the individual

Erikson

Erik Erickson built on Freud's work about psychosexual theories to develop his theory which considered the impact of biological, cultural and social influences on human development and personality. Erickson did not believe that the ego was present at birth or in childhood. Although the elements to create this were present, the personality was shaped in response to dealing with the different challenges or 'crises' that occurred through life that required the individual to resolve in order to develop. Although not all stages have to be fully resolved, failure to do so may result in psychological damage, such as lack of development or lack of self-esteem which could be overcome with help. Erickson was interested in the superego and its influence of society and how it naturally equipped human beings for dealing with world crises, such as war.

Erickson's theories are built around his belief that there are eight phases of psychosexual development during an individual's life, five during childhood and three during adulthood. Within each phase, the individual encounters particular problems which they will need to resolve in order to progress. Although Erickson's eight phases are not based on clinical or scientific evidence, they do describe some of the dilemmas and concerns faced by human beings through the course of their lifetime. As a result, his work continues to be used in relation to understanding adolescence and older age.

Erickson's eight phases of psychosexual development

Age	Stage	Development
0–1 year	Infant	The individual works out whether to be hopeful, optimistic or not, in other words whether to be trusting or mistrusting
1–6 yrs	Early childhood	The individual needs to work out if they are able to do things on their own and have a sense of autonomy (being in control) or whether they doubt their own ability. This phase is about developing self-confidence in own abilities
6–8 yrs	Play age	The individual needs to work out if they have a sense of purpose, are able to take the initiative and lead an active life without feeling too concerned about what other people may think
10–14 yrs	School age	The individual needs to work out if they will work to become skilled and competent (e.g. in social, intellectual and physical skills) or if they will doubt their ability and not try in case they fail (feelings of inferiority)
14–20 yrs	Adolescence	The individual needs to work out if they have a sense of their own identity and faith in themselves as a unique human being or they are not sure who they are
20–35 yrs	Young adulthood	The individual needs to decide if they want to be involved in society and, as part of this, are able to form close relationships and make commitments to others (love) or are only able to consider themselves and so become isolated
35–65 yrs	Maturity	The individual needs decide if they want to be concerned and care about what happens to family and other members of society (such as future generations) or whether this is of no concern to them
65 yrs +	Old age	The age of wisdom, where the individual either has a sense of fulfilment and satisfaction about their life and a willingness to face death or a sense of despair and disgust about younger generations and change and fear of death, feeling that their life has been unfulfilled

Humanistic perspectives

This psychological perspective is sometimes referred to as the Third Force as it follows the behaviourist and psychoanalytical perspectives. The founders of this perspective are Abraham Maslow (1908–1970) and Carl Rogers (1902–1987). The basic tenets (principles) of the humanistic perspective are that individuals are inherently good and that human personality and behaviour can be understood in relation to the individual's own interpretation of their life experiences. This perspective focuses on what it means to be human and proposes that individuals have an in-built (biological) drive which is the motivation to achieve personal development to achieve their potential, and that how individuals see themselves as a person(self-concept or self-image) is of great importance.

Maslow

Maslow developed a framework of human needs, Maslow's Hierarchy of Needs, which describes the reasons why humans are motivated towards psychological well-being.

Classics in the History of Psychology http://psychclassics.yorku.ca
Maslow's work on the theory of motivation

Humans must first satisfy deficiency needs, that is physiological, safety, love and belongingness and self-esteem needs, before personal growth can be achieved, that is knowledge and understanding and finally self-actualisation. If needs are not met, the individual is motivated to do something to meet them, for example, if individuals feel hungry or thirsty they will find food and water to satisfy those needs. The theory is that each level of need once met will alert the individual to the next level that is unmet. So, for example, if the overriding need is to satisfy hunger, safety needs would be of little concern at that time. However, once biological needs have been met the individual becomes aware of their need for shelter and a safe place to live. In essence, the theory is that the type of need an individual experiences at any time will be dependant on which other needs have been met. Personal growth and self-actualisation cannot be met until the other needs have been satisfied. For example, students find it difficult to concentrate and learn if they are uncomfortable, hungry, thirsty, concerned for their safety (such as if they are being bullied), do not feel they belong in the group or find themselves in a situation where they may be asked to do something they are unsure of.

remember

Self-esteem means having a sense of your own worth and value.

 Link See page 66 in Unit 2 for more information about self-esteem.

Maslow's work has been developed and extended by other psychologists to include three additional stages. In the 1970s, the model was extended to include stage five for cognitive needs (knowledge and meaning) and stage six for aesthetic needs (the search and appreciation of beauty, balance and form) with self-actualisation at stage seven. The model was further extended in the 1990s to include a stage eight of transcendence needs (going beyond self and helping others to achieve self-actualisation). Self-actualisation can be thought of as becoming the person you want to be or everything you are capable of being. Self-actualisation is within everyone's grasp and is achieved when an individual has faced a personal challenge, risen to it and achieved a personal triumph in adversity or against the odds. Things that really challenge a person are individual and usually mean the individual gains an insight into their personality, their strengths and capabilities that they were previously unaware of. As a result, the individual has greater insight into what it means to be human and is, from the humanistic perspective, considered to be a fully functioning person as they have reached the peak of their psychological well-being.

Maslow's theory has been questioned as experience has shown that some individuals are able to achieve transcendence in terms of selflessly helping others achieve their potential while they themselves are not able to achieve their own potential. For example, helping other people may be used as a way of helping individuals with mental health issues, such as depression to improve. In this way, the person with depression may meet their own needs in terms of belongingness and self-esteem.

Rogers

Carl Rogers applied humanistic principles into clinical practice in psychotherapy and developed client- or person-centred therapy. Rogers' aim was to create a situation that would enable the client to overcome the constraints that resulted from the impact and internalisation of negative and damaging experiences (i.e. all the negative things an individual believed about themselves that damaged or distorted their self-concept and self-esteem) and as a result of this to achieve personal growth. Positive self-regard and self-esteem was essential, as without this individuals were unable to trust their innate abilities and resourcefulness and take control in their lives, for example, in terms of decision-making and exercising choice. Rogers believed that individuals were in the best position to deal with personal problems because they knew themselves better than anyone else. To overcome problems, however, the individual must first be free of all the negativity that results from life experiences, such as fear of punishment, social pressures and coercion. Roger felt the therapist's role was to create the conditions that would enable individuals to navigate their way to a new self-concept and self-regard so they could solve their problems and through

Fig 8.3 Maslow's hierarchy of needs

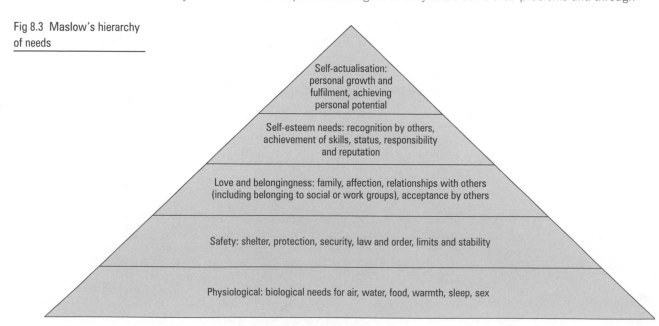

Self-actualisation: personal growth and fulfilment, achieving personal potential

Self-esteem needs: recognition by others, achievement of skills, status, responsibility and reputation

Love and belongingness: family, affection, relationships with others (including belonging to social or work groups), acceptance by others

Safety: shelter, protection, security, law and order, limits and stability

Physiological: biological needs for air, water, food, warmth, sleep, sex

this achieve personal growth. The conditions Rogers spoke about involved the relationship between practitioner and client and this required three factors to be present if the practitioner was to understand the individual's subjective experience.

The three factors Roger felt were essential for 'facilitative conditions' are:

- congruence: being genuine and authentic, being oneself and acting in a human way not hiding behind a persona or role. Rogers felt that the way people behave with others will have a powerful influence on whether or not people respond to them positively. Genuineness is likely to influence the level of trust achieved in a relationship with others. Without this, it is unlikely that anyone will respond with positive motivation or confidence.

- unconditional positive regard: respecting an individual, demonstrating non-possessive warmth and an accepting and non-judgemental attitude (neither condoning nor approving of actions). Acceptance requires the separation of the person and their worth, from their behaviour, and getting this across to them clearly and unambiguously in all forms of communication.

- empathy: caring and warmth and entering the other person's world in order to understand it from their perspective. This includes understanding the significance for the other person of their situation, their interpretation of it and the expectations that it leads to, how it meshes with or conflicts with their values or self-image, feelings triggered, past events echoed and old emotions reawakened.

Cognitive or information processing perspectives

This perspective explores how human beings process information and how these processes influence thoughts and behaviour. The cognitive perspective takes the view that humans are not passive learners but are actively involved in the processing of information about their world and that learning is achieved through active engagement with the world. Unlike behaviourists' theory of the stimulus– response relationship, the cognitive perspective considers that humans process the information received (i.e. stimuli via senses) before the appropriate response is initiated making learning an active process.

The five information processes are:

- perception: how humans use their senses to understand (perceive) things
- attention: how humans concentrate on one thing at a time (focus attention) or several different things at one time (divided attention)
- language: the ability to communicate
- memory: how to organise, store, retrieve and recognise information about the world that surrounds human beings
- thinking: problem solving, reasoning, reflecting, forming ideas and making decisions and judgements.

According to cognitive perspectives, perception can be understood as an individual's senses working together with innate abilities called **gestalten** and past experiences. Gestalten are abilities to tidy up a stimulus, making it seem whole, so that it can be understood better which helps to make sense of the world. Past experiences impact on perception, as two individuals may see the same thing but perceive it differently depending on whether they had a positive or negative past experience or no previous experience, or whether there are any social or cultural factors in their experience. According to cognitive perspectives, these factors also affect memory, as what two people remember of the same event will be different based on what each perceived as important. Memory is also crucial to day-to-day functioning as well as thinking and problem solving. Although cognitive abilities are individually important, the different information processes work together to enable individuals to function in the world.

Piaget

Investigating children's cognitive development, Jean Piaget (1896–1980) theorised that children think differently to adults because their brains are biologically immature in comparison to adult brains. Piaget believed that cognitive development occurred in stages and it was not until a child reaches 11 years of age that they demonstrate more sophisticated ways of thinking and problem solving and this is due to the biological maturation of the brain. Piaget identified four stages of cognitive development in childhood.

- Sensorimotor stage (birth to 2 years old): During this time much of the baby's behaviour is reflexive, for example, a finger stokes baby's cheek and its reflex action is to turn its head towards the sensation. Babies are concerned only with their own needs and are egocentric. Piaget believed that the first ideas babies have to help them deal with the world are through action schemas (mental representation or ideas about what things are in order to understand how to deal with things). In the first two years, babies are assimilating (gathering information about different things) and accommodating (extending and modifying schemas). Babies develop ideas about objects around them based on what they can do with them. They also develop understanding about how one thing can impact on another as well as ideas about time and space. They show they are capable of intelligent thinking, for example when they use one object to get another which is out of their reach. Babies behave as if an object does not exist if it out of sight until about 8 to 12 months when they continue to look for something even when it is no longer visible (object permanence).

■ Preoperational stage (2 to7 years old): Piaget believed that children combine schemas to organise them into logical sequences as well as modify them in response to new experiences. The main features of this stage are symbolisation, egocentrism, animism and moral realisation. Symbolisation is where the child has the ability to understand how something can represent something else, for example, that a red traffic light means stop. Words are also symbols and during this stage vocabulary increases. These together enable the child to use their imagination, for example when playing. Egocentrism is where the child can only see things from their point of view and believe theirs is the only possible view others could hold. Other psychologists such as Martin Hughes disagreed with Piaget and found that children of this age could imagine other points of view and so were capable of decentring (shifting their focus from themselves to another perspective). Animism is when the child believes that everything that exists has a consciousness and feelings or experiences the same things as humans, for example, if a child walks into a chair and hurts themselves, they may smack the chair and call it 'a naughty chair for hurting them'. Moral realism relates to egocentrism and is where the child thinks that what they believe to be right and wrong will be shared by everyone else. As the child is egocentric they can only focus on one aspect of a situation and so, for example, rules will have to be obeyed at all times regardless of circumstance or motive.

■ Concrete operations (7 to 11 years old): At this stage of development, thinking becomes more rational and adult-like. During this stage, children develop their ability to think logically and are capable of manipulating their thoughts without needed a physical object. Egocentrism and animism decline during this stage and gradually children learn that objects are not always what they appear to be. Children are able to reverse a process or sequence of events and see that they would return to how they started. Children also learn to conserve things like volume, number, length, mass and area, that is they can think about different features of an object at the same time so that just because one aspect changes not all aspects change.

Fig 8.4 Understanding conservation of volume

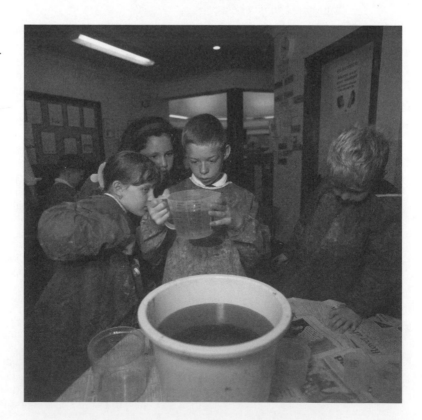

- Formal operations (11 to 15 years old): Thinking becomes increasingly adult-like and children are also able to work more with concepts, abstract ideas and thoughts, not just concrete objects. Moral and philosophical issues also form part of their thinking, such as honesty, morality, ethical issues, justice and freedom. They are able to see things from a number of different perspectives and argue from different points of view, take motives and reasons into account as well as identify the moral dilemmas in life. Research indicates that some people never make the transition from concrete to formal operations and so struggle with these aspects of thinking and learning.

Kelly

Steve Kelly has more recently conducted research into implicit learning and how knowledge of patterns or regularities is learned without conscious awareness that learning was taking place. Examples given relate to how people learn the grammatical rules within their native language without conscious awareness of the rules. Kelly's research with people who have dyslexia identified how implicit sequence learning occurred even when individuals were unaware of the sequence structure.

Biological perspectives

The biological perspective believes that behaviour is a result of inherited characteristics, genetics and physiology (the way human body systems function). It is the only psychological perspective that considers thoughts, emotions and actions from a medical and biological physical standpoint. Psychologically, humans are the result of biology, that is of genetics and the actions of the central nervous system. Therefore, from a biological perspective, physical or psychological illness results from genetic or physiological damage, disease or accident. As a result, skills such as acquiring language are inevitable as the cerebral cortex and Broca's area in the brain are responsible for the articulation of speech and Wernicke's area is responsible for understanding speech and language while other part of the brain receive other information to assist in recognition, memory and sensory input, all of which help with interpretation.

> **remember**
>
> Chromosomes are rod-shaped structures in cell nucleus carrying the genetic material that determines sex and other characteristics an organism inherits from its parents.

Maturational theory

The maturational theory of language from the biological perspective believes that human beings cannot help but develop language unless they are in exceptional circumstances, such as lacking human contact. If a child is in an environment where they are exposed to language, their language skills including comprehension will develop gradually as a result of biological pre-programming and consequently all children will demonstrate particular sounds at around the same age.

Importance of genetic influences on behaviour

The inherited characteristics carried in chromosomes and genes are responsible for the individual's personality and well-being as their genes hold all the information regarding their potential in all aspects of their life including their potential to develop certain illness or susceptibility to particular types of disease. The existence of too few or too many chromosomes is known to create genetically inherited conditions which have a detrimental effect on development. For example, trisomy (three instead of two chromosomes) 13 causes Patau's Syndrome, a condition where the individual has multiple abnormalities and where 80 to 90% do not survive infancy due to the severity of these, and those who do have a learning disability. Turner's Syndrome, which affects girls, is an example of a missing chromosome. In this case, instead of having the normal sex chromosome 46XX the girl has 46XO. With Turner's Syndrome, although mental development may be normal heart defects are common and the girl is short in stature and infertile due to underdevelopment of the ovaries.

Developmental delay or deficit will impact on behaviour if this is considered to be a maturation process and one which requires all body systems to be working to their potential. Children and adults with a learning disability progress slower and often have a limited potential. However, evidence and experience has shown that although an individual may genetically have the make up that suggests their mental capabilities are limited, the influence of their environment has a significant part to play in assisting or obstructing them in achieving their potential. In the past many children and young people with Down's Syndrome (trisomy 21) were able to achieve very little and grew up dependent on others with no or limited education and life skills. The belief being that their potential was solely determined by their genetics and therefore their limited potential inevitable. In reality, a person with Down's Syndrome, given access to appropriate education and life skills teaching, is capable of a great deal more than dependence with an increasing number of people living independent lives and achieving the same goals as their non-disabled peers. The nature-nurture nature debate is particularly relevant to discussions regarding the genetic influence on behaviour.

See page 130 in Unit 4 for more information about the nature-nurture debate.

Some conditions have been found to be genetically influenced but are not genetically inherited because no single gene is responsible, rather a number of genes have an influence. One such example is schizophrenia, a psychiatric disorder that affects coherence of the personality and includes detachment from reality and emotional instability. Research into behavioural genetics has been searching for associations between specific genes or groups of genes and particular behaviours, for example, addictive behaviours, alcoholism, smoking, as well as anti-social and criminal behaviours. Research has found the existence of a genetic influence on alcoholism, smoking and addictive behaviours, but the extent to which genetics plays a part in initiating the behaviour and in the persistence of that behaviour is unclear. Debates about the influence of environment on addiction and on anti-social behaviour are dependent on the research group. For example, the mental health perspective would be different to that of criminologists. In relation to anti-social behaviour, correlations have been demonstrated between genetic influence and behaviour. However, it is important to also consider that this may be due to concentrations of genes within families as men and women tend to mate on the basis of similarity (assortative mating). This creates families that are different from the norm within the population and, in addition, there is a tendency for antisocial parents to have more children than the norm. The nurture debate would also indicate that growing up in an environment when the norm is antisocial behaviour would perpetuate this personality type.

Influence of the nervous and endocrine systems on behaviour

In considering the biological perspective, it is important also to consider the influence of the nervous and endocrine systems on behaviour. The body is maintained in a state of equilibrium through homeostasis however, even minor changes in chemical balances can have significant effects on the body.

See page 178 in Unit 5 for more information about homeostasis.

For example, the neurotransmitter dopamine is produced in excess to the body's requirements if an individual has schizophrenia, and depression is found to occur when the production of serotonin is suppressed. The over- or under-production of sex hormones will affect sex drive and sexual behaviour. An over-production of androgens is likely to increase sex drive and this will impact on the individual's behaviour as they seek to satisfy the body's demands. This may lead to behaviour which others find unacceptable. Under-production of the hormone thyroxin by the thyroid gland while the brain is developing will lead to the individual having learning disabilities. Under-production of thyroxin in adults will result in slowed metabolism, weight gain, slowing of mental activity and often depression. All of these affect an individual's behaviour as will hyperthyroidism, when too much thyroxin is being produced. In this case, behaviour changes include excessive tiredness, restlessness and nervousness (which also may lead to other behaviour changes if undiagnosed). Conditions that affect the nervous system, including damage or destruction through diseases, such as multiple sclerosis or dementia, or through accidents, such as a brain haemorrhage or trauma, will result in parts of the brain and related functions being affected. If the areas associated with personality are affected, behaviour will also be affected and changes from that individual's norm will be apparent. For example, if an individual develops dementia such as Alzheimer's disease, this will affect their behaviour as their memory (in particular their short-term memory) deteriorates. The loss of short-term memory makes daily living activities that are generally taken for granted once learned increasingly difficult, for example recognition skills, sequencing, understanding concepts and abstract thoughts including consequences of actions. So much of day-to-day living requires individuals to use their memory and this along with the loss of abstract thought can lead to the individual behaving without due care for their safety or that of others. For example, walking in the road as they lose awareness of the potential danger from traffic and the need to take precautions, such as following safe crossing strategies that have been learned through life.

See page 160 in Unit 5 for more information about the nervous and endocrine systems.

Gesell

Arnold Gesell was an American developmental psychologist who conducted experiments with children aged 2½ years to 9 years old during the 1920s and 1930s. Gesell believed that normal development progressed according to a predetermined sequence. He created a series of tests, measuring procedures and observations through which he hoped to develop normative scales that could be used to assess a child's development. The resultant scales considered motor skills, adaptive behaviour, language development and personal-social development. The tests that were carried out included building towers with bricks, answering a series of questions, writing, copying shapes, puzzles, eye-hand coordination and memory tests. The Gesell Developmental Assessment has three different levels that could overlap as it is the child's developmental age and not their chronological age that is the stronger indicator of their ability to learn within a formal educational environment. This can be useful in determining if a child is in the correct environment for learning, for example, being placed in the appropriate class. The 'normal' is determined in relation to other children rather than to a fixed external standard. The purpose of the Gesell Developmental Assessment is to observe a child's overall behaviour and compare this to their chronological age so as to understand the child's overall growth pattern, and through comparison over time. It can also help to identify atypical behaviour which would warrant intervention to enable development within normal limits.

Applying psychological approaches to health and social care

Application of psychological perspectives to health and social care practice

Psychological perspectives provide insights into human behaviour and motivation. These can be applied to health and social care work settings to develop appropriate strategies and work practices which enable the individuals being supported to manage their lives and personal growth and development.

Behaviourist

Pavlov and Skinner's behaviourist perspectives concerning conditioning and the impact of positive and negative reinforcement can be used to view the way behaviour is shaped from an early age.

Refer back to pages 276–277 to remind yourself about Pavlov and Skinner's theories.

The realisation that behaving in a certain way produces a response from others is something babies learn early in their lives. Early childhood games like peek-a-boo demonstrate that if the child reacts in a particular way, for example, smiles or laughs, this is likely to result in the other person smiling or laughing and continuing the game. This is an example of positive reinforcement, as the child learns that this behaviour results in a pleasurable outcome (the other person learns this too and so is likely to repeat it). A negative reinforcement will result when the child behaves in a particular way in reaction to something unpleasant happening. For example, when a baby is uncomfortable, for example, in pain or has a wet or dirty nappy, they will cry. The baby's cry alerts the parent or care giver to the baby's needs and they will respond by meeting those needs.

If a child has a tantrum and the parent or care giver pacifies the child by giving them something they like, such as a sweet, or by letting them have what they want, this acts as a positive reinforcement, as they are being rewarded for their behaviour. The child learns that their behaviour (a tantrum), gets them what they want (a sweet) ,and so they will repeat the behaviour. The use of bribery (using something like sweets or a treat to pacify) in an attempt to change behaviour will not result in behaviour change or modification. When bribery is used, all that is learned is what to do to please the person who holds the rewards, not the preferred behaviour.

If changing or modifying behaviour is the desired outcome, there is no mention of reward at the time and this only comes after the desired behaviour has been demonstrated and linked to the behaviour. For example, if an adult asks a child to tidy their toys up, praise should be given telling them how well they did this and how helpful it is only after they have completed the task. On the other hand, when shaping behaviour is the desired outcome, the reward could be indicated when the request for desired behaviour is made. For example, 'When you have tidied all the toys up we can go for a walk to the park and play on the swings.' It is important that the desired outcome is clear and that positive reinforcement is not confused with bribery or that punishment is seen as negative reinforcement. Ignoring undesired behaviour and rewarding desired behaviour is more effective than punishing someone. However, so often it is the undesired behaviour which is given the greatest attention, for example, the person is told off or punished which ensures attention from others, while desirable behaviour is overlooked or taken for granted and not rewarded through, for example, recognition or praise.

One of the problems with behaviourist perspectives and behaviour modification is the uncertainty of exactly what is being learned. An individual may only learn to behave in the desirable way if they are likely to get caught and suffer the consequences. However, if they think the risk of being caught is low they may behave in an undesirable way. For example, if an individual living in a residential care home shouts or hits another resident and this is seen by a member of staff they will be told this is unacceptable behaviour and to not do it again. Following this incident, no further incidents are reported. Staff may feel the individual has learned from this incident and modified their behaviour. However, the individual may continue to behave in an aggressive manner towards other residents but do so in a part of the home less visible to staff. What the individual learned was not to behave in that way when others could see them, not that their behaviour was unacceptable and needed to change. If behaviour is to be modified, the individual needs to understand what needs to change and how to achieve this as well as the benefits to them that making the change would bring. If they do not see any benefits to them, they are unlikely to change.

Changing and shaping behaviour using conditioning and positive and negative reinforcement also helps individuals to learn about the social norms in society as part of their socialisation. Behaviourist perspectives can be applied to health and social care in relation to health promotion advice which usually requires individuals to change their behaviour in order to manage their illness, condition or disease or to maintain their health and well-being. A token economy approach may also be used to change or shape behaviour. Tokens are given in response to desired behaviour and these tokens can be collected and exchanged for something the individual values. This type of behaviour modification is used in many different ways. For example, parents may use star charts to record incidents of agreed behaviour being demonstrated and the reward may be a treat. It is also used in some health and social care settings as part of learning or to encourage individuals to manage their behaviour positively.

Understanding challenging behaviour

Remember that 55 per cent of communication between individuals is through body language, that is behaviour, so when individuals present behaviours that challenge, they are in fact trying to communicate something to those around them. Challenging behaviour is behaviour that challenges someone or something, for example the health or social care service being provided. What may be viewed as challenging behaviour in a health and social care setting may be viewed as normal behaviour if it occurred within the individual's own home. For example, if a person goes home after they have had a frustrating day, to release these feelings they may slam the door or shout. This would only be considered as challenging if it infringed on others and they were distressed (or challenged) by it.

An individual may use behaviour to try and convey a number of different emotions, such as feelings of insecurity, fear, dislike, pain, anxiety, distress, or concerns, for example about their environment, or to exert some control. The behaviourist perspective states that if the appropriate responses are made, behaviour can be changed, but to do this effectively it is important to understand what the individual is trying to convey through their behaviour, as conditioning and reinforcement can modify behaviour so that undesirable behaviour disappears.

When an individual behaves in a way that challenges others they are likely to become emotionally aroused and understanding this can help to work out an appropriate strategy to diffuse the situation and modify behaviour. If the behaviour gains the attention of others, this may be the purpose of the behaviour for the individual. If the response from health and social care workers is one which positively reinforces this, for example, giving the individual attention with no unpleasant consequences, they are likely to repeat this behaviour. If the worker response is one that appears to be a negative reinforcement, such as removing the individual from the situation and reprimanding them, this may be effective if the situation was not the cause of the behaviour in the first place, that is if the individual was doing something they enjoyed. In this situation, the individual learns that challenging behaviour = undesirable outcome and therefore the behaviour will be less likely to be repeated. If, however, behaving in a challenging manner means the individual gets lots of attention as others come to see what is going on and then a worker spends individual time with them on a one-to-one basis, this may be exactly the outcome the individual wanted and so reacting to this by intervention produces in effect a positive reinforcement for the individual and they may repeat the behaviour. Also, if the situation was the cause of the behaviour, that is if the individual was finding the situation itself distressing, and the worker response was to remove the individual and find out the reasons for the behaviour and how the situation can be avoided or managed in future, then this is a good outcome for the individual. They therefore learn that challenging behaviour leads to being removed and being understood and having needs met, so challenging behaviour = desirable outcome from their point of view, and so they may repeat that behaviour.

The health and social care workers response is crucial here if they are to effect the desired outcome for all involved. In order to achieve this, they need to understand the communication underlying the behaviour. Emphasising the individual's strengths and praising desired behaviour are ways in which workers can use the behaviourist perspective to modify behaviour and minimise challenging behaviour.

Professional Practice

Health and social care workers can support the individual more effectively to manage behaviour through:

- improving communication systems, structures and methods within the setting and with relevant others
- using multimedia profiling to empower an individual with communication differences to communicate effectively
- providing appropriate and safe opportunities for individuals to express their emotions
- providing more choice and control in the individual's life
- understanding individual needs and potential triggers and developing appropriate strategies to support them
- responding consistently, personally and as a team
- acting as a positive role model for others (service users and colleagues).

Changing or shaping behaviour

There are a number of different types of behaviour therapy using behaviourist psychology that aim to change stimulus–response associations that an individual has made which is impacting on their behaviour and life. For example, aversion therapy is used to help an individual to learn how to avoid things that are harmful to them and so the pleasant response associated with the harm is replaced with an unpleasant response. Desensitisation programmes aim to gradually change dysfunction responses, such as fear, to function responses, such as relaxation, and are often used when an individual has a phobia (irrational fear of something).

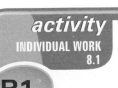

activity
INDIVIDUAL WORK 8.1

P1

Describe how behaviourist perspectives can be applied in health and social care work in areas such as health promotion and supporting changes from negative to positive behaviour.

Social learning perspective

A social learning perspective is used within health and social care work to promote anti-discriminatory behaviour and practices through reversing the self-fulfilling prophesy and changing the systems and structures in society that work to reinforce the attitudes and behaviour that can lead to discrimination.

case study 8.1

Slip, Slop, Slap!

The 'Slip, Slop, Slap' health promotion campaign that began in Australia before being adopted in the UK is an example of how behaviourist psychology is used to try and change behaviour. In this case, the campaign attempts to teach people how they can still enjoy the sunshine while avoiding the unpleasant and life-threatening consequences of skin cancer which is increasing in incidence.

Fig 8.5 Safe Sun campaign poster

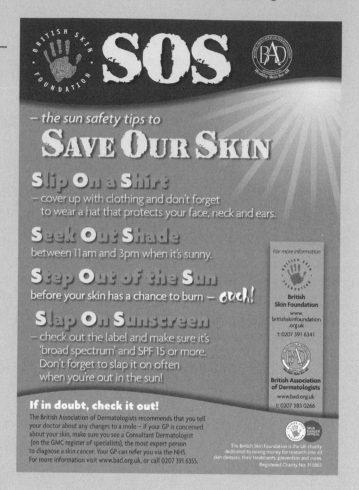

activity
GROUP WORK

1 What type of reinforcement is being used?
2 What other examples can you think of that use behaviourist psychology to change or modify behaviour?

 Link

Refer back to page 279 to remind yourself about the self-fulfilling prophesy. See page 54 in Unit 2 and page 372 in Unit 11 for more information about promoting anti-discriminatory practice.

Promotion of anti-discriminatory behaviours and practices
Promoting anti-discriminatory practice requires an understanding of those factors within society that influence attitudes and behaviour. These factors include assumptions, prejudice and stereotypes that relate to diversity, disability, age, gender, sexuality, race, ethnicity, religion, culture, nationality, and so on, as well as how these are perpetuated. These discriminatory attitudes and behaviours can be challenged through positive representations of diversity within all aspects of life and, in particular, within those early influences such as primary care givers, education and the media. Children are not born being aware

of difference, they learn this as they grow up through socialisation. Promoting anti-discriminatory behaviour and practices requires the use of positive and diverse role models and on an individual, organisational and societal basis discrimination to be constructively challenged.

Use of positive role models in health education campaigns

The use of positive role models in particular in health education campaigns is based on Bandura's work and the fact that people respond well to those held in high status as well as having warmth and a powerful personality.

Refer back to page 278 to remind yourself about Bandura's work.

The individuals will need to have credence with the target group, for example, a younger person if the health education is targeted at young people. Other health education campaigns such as National Blood Service have used a number of people who are well known to the general public to advertise the difference blood donation can make to someone's life and the range of uses blood has in saving lives.

Fig 8.6 National Blood Service campaign

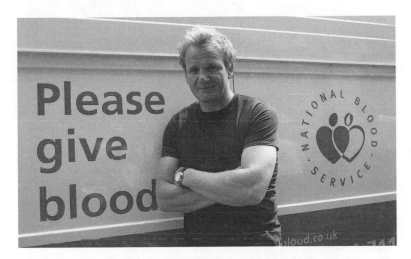

activity
INDIVIDUAL WORK
8.2

P2

Explain the value of applying a social learning approach when implementing policies to promote anti-discriminatory practice within health and social care service provision.

Psychodynamic perspectives

This perspective provides insights into the long term impact that influences and experiences in the early years of an individual's life may have on adult behaviours. Freud's belief that there is an inner struggle between the selfishness of 'id' and the selflessness of ego and superego presents a potential explanation for behaviour that challenges others (remembering that this is a potentially wide range of behaviours).

Understanding challenging behaviour

If Freud's theory is applied then challenging behaviour could be understood with reference to the psychodynamic relationship of id, ego and superego.

Refer back to page 279 to remind yourself about Freud's work.

case study 8.2 — Rethink media campaign

In March 2006, Rethink piloted an anti-stigma campaign in Norwich, England. This led to positive and measurable changes in public awareness of mental health problems and attitudes towards people living with mental illness. Now Rethink is mounting a larger anti-stigma and mental health awareness campaign across Northern Ireland.

Fig 8.7 Rethink posters

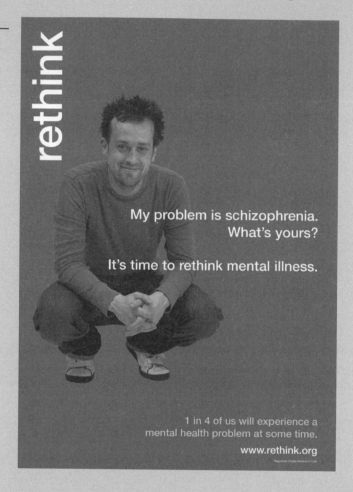

From January 15th to February 12th 2007 the campaign featured TV, outdoor and bus advertising combined with extensive PR, lots of local activities and events. An important feature of the campaign is the involvement of mental health service users and carers. A number of service users have trained as media volunteers and are willing to share their stories and experiences through the media. There are also opportunities for the public to get involved and to support the campaign.

 www.rethink.org/how_we_can_help/campaigning_for_change/index.html

activity
GROUP WORK

1 How do these adverts present positive role models?
2 How do you think these challenge negative assumptions, prejudices and discrimination?
3 How do you think this type of health education campaign may influence individuals to change their attitudes towards mental health issues?

Someone whose behaviour challenges others may have an 'id personality' and their libido (the free-floating psychosexual energy at the centre of id) is demanding to be satisfied. The individual is either unwilling or unable to manage or control these demands. They are concerned only that their needs are met with the minimum pain to them and will do anything to achieve this. This may result in them making repetitive demands for whatever it is they consider will meet their needs. This repetitive behaviour may present as challenging to others. Another expression of the overwhelming demands of id may be regression in the individual's behaviour so they become immature or child-like, such as having a tantrum, stamping their feet, shouting or physically hitting out at others in an effort to get their own way. Another type of behaviour that challenges others is when an individual becomes fixated or obsessed with something, such as an object or an action. Personalities that are led by id can also be impulsive and because the motivation is unconscious they are often unable to adequately explain why they did something. For example, if an individual did something illegal the reasons they would give for their action was purely because they 'felt like it'. In these situations, the dynamic nature of their personality means there is an imbalance as the three aspects are not balanced and so able to keep the individual's behaviour within socially and morally acceptable limits.

Distraction can be used to manage the behaviour but understanding what the individual is trying to communicate is fundamental to providing active support to enable the individual to understand and manage their own behaviour. A lack of insight into what is or is not socially acceptable may be at the root of such behaviour. This behaviour may also be defensive in nature as a way of managing stress or maintaining some level of control within the situation.

If someone's superego is overdeveloped, Freud believed they would have an overwhelming sense of guilt and as personalities this may make them very anxious which may lead to irrational behaviour. For some people, this type of behaviour may be challenging as it is difficult to rationalise and help individuals to change their behaviour.

If Erickson's theories are applied, they too can provide insights as if particular stages and the associated crises or dilemmas are unresolved then it is likely the individual will have difficulty in managing certain situations or aspects of their life.

Link   Refer back to page 280 to remind yourself about Erickson's work.

If Erickson's ideas are applied it would follow that if a child's basic physical needs were not met they are likely to mistrust rather than trust others. If relationships are poor, this too will impact on their ability to form positive relationships. If a number of significant factors combine, such as lack or trust, lack of self-esteem both of which will also impact on the ability to form relationships this will have a considerable impact on the individual's life. If Freud's ideas about coping or defence mechanisms is applied, it provides scope for understanding motivations that appear self-destructive, for example, projection of feelings (anger, resentment, fear) on to others as well as regression or repression (especially if there is associated past trauma or abuse). However, that is not to say that the individual cannot change and learn to trust or develop a more robust self-esteem, and so on, or that once successfully achieved these states cannot be shaken by experience, but Erickson believed that fundamentally the individual could recover from this and any damage repaired.

Understanding and managing anxiety

Psychodynamic perspectives can also be applied in order to try and understand and manage anxiety. As discussed previously, anxiety states, phobias and obsessions can arise as a result of excessive deployment of defence mechanisms. Understanding the underlying reason for the anxiety is the first step to managing it. Sometimes the anxiety is related to a past trauma that has been repressed and forgotten or the memory distorted. If the memory is distorted, it can be difficult to understand the reality in order to confront the anxiety, phobia or obsession. Sometimes the trigger may be incorrect, for example, someone who has an obsession about cleanliness may believe this is to prevent contamination or infection which they link to being sick, which may be a coincidence rather than root cause. Over-development of the superego may also create anxiety states as a result of excessive feelings of moral responsibility and guilt. Specialists, such as psychotherapists, would work with the individual to break down the behaviours in an attempt to help the individual to understand the unconscious intentions behind their actions. This requires careful and sensitive handling as well as a trusting relationship and time as inexpert handling could lead to the individual deploying more defence mechanisms which pushes the individual further away from locating a solution.

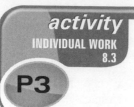

activity
INDIVIDUAL WORK
8.3

P3

Describe how psychodynamic perspectives can be applied to understand the effect that being subjected to abuse is likely to have on an individual.

Humanistic perspectives

The work of Maslow and Rogers and the humanist approach is applied extensively within health and social care work with current practice underpinned by the principles of promoting independence, rights and choices.

Refer back to pages 281–2 to remind yourself about Maslow and Rogers' work.

The humanist belief that people have an innate motivation to grow and develop their capabilities and potential as human beings is acknowledged though approaches to communication, building effective practitioner-client relationships and non-directive interventions. A non-directive approach to working with individuals is used within health and social care work to enable an individual to facilitate change in their life at their own pace as the outcome is more likely to be positive and enduring. The humanistic perspective underpins good practice guidance about establishing, developing and sustaining professional relationships with individuals being supported.

Developing empathy and an understanding of the individual's needs and circumstances as well as what it important to them in terms of their values, beliefs, culture, interests and priorities is an essential first step in determining how to assist and support an individual. Person-centred approaches to assessment and care planning emphasise the need for practitioners to work with the person as an equal and to understand the situation from the person's perspective and not make assumptions or judgements about their needs, wishes or expectations. Demonstrating respect for other people is considered to be fundamental in establishing and sustaining a constructive and supportive relationship, as without this the relationship will falter or be problematic or, involve conflict and resentment. The codes of practice for both health and social care emphasise the importance of respecting other people and having a non-judgemental approach.

See page 372 in Unit 11 for more information about codes of practice.

Empathy

To achieve empathy (to enter imaginatively into someone else's life) is difficult as, in reality, knowing what another person is experiencing is beyond our understanding. Even if the experience is a shared one, such as an event, each individual's subjective experiences and interpretations will be different as they will be imbued with their individual values, beliefs, culture, gender, age, race, ethnicity, past experiences, knowledge, understanding and interpretation making it unique to them. However, striving to achieve a level of empathy is desirable, as research has shown that receiving empathy builds an individual's self-esteem as they realise that they are 'understandable' and that the worker believes they are sufficiently important to try to understand them. Empathy is a powerful influence when working with an individual who is expressing resistance to support or change, as it enables the individual to become more aware of their feelings and a first step to taking responsibility for those feelings.

Understanding

Understanding also needs to be conveyed to the individuals being supported and this can be achieved through using effective communication skills. As a health and social care worker, giving the person a feeling that you are 'with them' means not only using non-verbal signals but also being able to filter out and feed back to them the key themes in their communication with you. Individuals often present their problems in a state of confusion, distress or a loss of direction or motivation. The health and social care worker's role is to facilitate a person-centred approach to assessment and care planning. In effect, this means being able to support individuals to identify their problems, their resulting needs, their strengths as well as exploring with them the available options to resolve, change or manage the situation.

Active listening

Active listening skills include not just hearing what the individual is saying but also the intention behind their words and showing them that you are attentive and interested. Ways of demonstrating active listening include maintaining eye contact (if culturally appropriate) with the individual, nodding and smiling to show encouragement, interjecting with 'I see...' as well as reflecting what they have said back to them to check out your understanding of what they have said, paraphrasing and summarising the main points they have made. Active listening also involves giving the individual space and time to express their thoughts and feelings, not interrupting or finishing their sentences or making assumptions about what they want to say, and asking open and probing questions to encourage them to express their concerns. Active listening is an example of how the humanistic approach and the belief that humans have the answers to their problems within their own resources is applied in practice, as it is non-directive but it does enable the individual to make sense of their situation and draw some conclusions before they progress to solutions. To achieve effective active listening, the individual needs to be aware of their non-verbal communication (body language) as this can create incongruence (conflict between what is being thought and said) which will compromise the trust within the relationship. Active listening is to an extent the practical demonstration of Rogers three principles of congruence (genuineness), unconditional positive regard and empathy.

Non-judgemental approach

A non-judgemental approach is the cornerstone of anti-discriminatory practice and, if the health and social care worker wants the individual to work with them, they need to show that, while not condoning behaviour, it does not interfere with their desire to work effectively with the individual to facilitate change in their circumstances. In practice, taking a non-judgemental approach is vital when supporting individuals with substance use problems to change their behaviour, supporting smoking cessation interventions and supporting an individual with a terminal illness when they have refused treatment. Although on a personal level some of these behaviours are difficult for health and social care workers to understand, they must think through their reasons for their discomfort or disagreement and accept these and recognise the conflicts that exist in being human, so that they can work with others who share different ideas. It is essential that workers do not become part of the problem but remain part of the solution and this can only be achieved if they have self-awareness which enables them to take a non-judgemental approach.

Government guidance for health and social care, such as 'Independence, Well-being and Choice' and the 'Expert Patient', increasingly emphasises the need for health and social care workers to work with individuals in a way that recognises them as their own experts with regards to their needs and circumstances. In practice, this has meant that organisations need to ensure that individuals have access to greater control over decision making and planning services to meet their needs. This is being achieved through person-centred approaches as well as initiatives such as direct payments and being in control of individual budgets. For example, there are seven ethical principles underpinning self-directed support. These are:

- right to independent living
- right to an individual budget
- right to self determination
- right to accessibility
- right to flexible funding
- accountability principle
- capacity principle.

Humanistic interventions also include those that help individuals to understand their self-concept and how this may differ from their ideal self (who they want to be) and consider how to achieve their ambitions and goals and become more like their ideal self. The ideal self changes as an individual goes through life and their priorities change as well as their skills, knowledge and understanding. Being able to reach self-understanding is considered vital to enable a greater level of psychological well-being.

case study 8.3 — Laura's Story

Laura's mum and dad supported her to tell her own story of how she now has her own personal assistants and is living life her way, attending college and leading a varied life following her many interests.

'Twenty years ago I was born in Liverpool on the 8th February 1985. My mum and dad called me Laura Jane Hughes. At this time, my dad, Tom, and mum, Elaine, did not know how special I was. At 12 years old, I was diagnosed with Rothmund Thompson Syndrome. This is a rare genetic condition. I have learning difficulties with challenging health needs and limited communication skills.

I attended Hope Special School from the age of three until I was nineteen. When I turned fourteen, at my transitional review my mum and dad were advised to look around local day centres which they said would be the only suitable place to meet my needs, as they didn't think I would cope with a college environment.

After looking around the day centres, my mum and dad knew they were not right for me. The problem was that my local college didn't offer non-foundation courses for people with learning disabilities.

So I started to access ten hours support a week through direct payments to enable me to have a more independent social life without my mum and dad always there. I now employ six personal assistants (PAs) with the help of my parents. They work with me and help me do things that would have otherwise been impossible. With the help of my PAs, I attend Skelmersdale college four days a week. I hope the teachers and social workers who said I was not suitable for college are reading this.

I have a job with Scope collecting and counting the money from the charity boxes with help from PAs. More recently, I have started in a young person's centre which is something new for the 16 to25 age group. I am very busy in the evenings and at weekends, I enjoy line dancing, going out for meals and drinking Smirnoff Ice in my local pub, where I am well known. I also enjoy swimming and bowling at every opportunity.'

[Permission 8.7]

activity — INDIVIDUAL WORK

1 Explain how the humanist perspective underpins self-directed support?

2 Explain how you could apply Maslow's hierarchy of needs to Laura in the case study.

3 Where do you think Laura would be in Maslow's hierarchy of needs if she was not able to access self-directed support?

activity — INDIVIDUAL WORK 8.4

P4

Describe how the humanistic approach underpins effective health and social care practice and the value this has to the quality of service provision.

Cognitive perspectives

This perspective can be applied into a number of different types of therapeutic intervention as well as being combined with other approaches, such as cognitive-behavioural therapy. Cognitive therapy uses the power of the mind to influence emotions and behaviour based on the theory that previous experiences influence the sense of self and condition attitudes, emotions and the ability to deal with situations. It arose from the idea that individuals could become disturbed not just by what they see but as a result of how they interpret what they have seen, that is, feelings are not just automatic reactions to events but are created by the thoughts we have about them. For example, during the night the hook holding a framed picture comes out of the wall causing the picture to fall and the glass to break making a loud crashing noise. The feelings of the person woken by the noise are influenced by how they think about the situation. If they thought the sound may be due to something falling then they may feel concerned about possible damage or annoyed at being woken. If they think the noise may be intruders then their feelings would be quite different as they may be frightened and anxious. Individuals are able to construct their thoughts and these can be irrational and keep hold of negative emotions and unsuitable or inappropriate behaviour or they can be reconstructed into more positive thoughts, appropriate behaviour or affirmations about themselves. Cognitive therapy is a way for individuals to talk about the connections between how they think, feel and behave so that they can begin a process of reconstruction to achieve more positive behaviours that nurture rather than damage psychological well-being. In other words, the way an individual thinks about life events (cognition) impacts on how they feel about those events (emotions). Cognitive therapy is used in a wide range of situations including supporting individuals who have emotional problems or who have depression.

Cognitive therapy particularly concentrates on an individual's unrealistic ideas that can undermine self-confidence and have a detrimental affect on psychological well-being and lead to mental health issues, such as depression and anxiety. Cognitive therapy also looks at individuals' rules for living or personality style, that is their schema (how they think, feel, act, relate to others and understand the world).

Individuals process information quickly and this can result in both appropriate and inappropriate behaviours becoming embedded as they are also subject to other influences (social and cultural) which reinforce assumptions about acceptable norms. Individuals therefore experience psychological and emotional distress when they encounter situations which they interpret as threatening and as a result their perceptions and interpretations can become selective, egocentric and rigid and a consequence of this is that they make systematic errors in reasoning (cognitive distortions). An example of this is when an individual becomes fixed on a single negative detail rather than being able to put it into the context of a whole situation. They can be rigid in their thinking, seeing things as only clear-cut and definitive even when they are part of a continuum or making rigid and absolute demands of themselves, others or the world, such as, 'I must/should/ought/have to' or catastrophising situations (making them appear more grave than they are in reality). In general, the individual makes negative, blaming statements about themselves and is unable to recognise or acknowledge anything positive about themselves.

Cognitive therapy is also used to support individuals with post-traumatic stress disorder (PTSD). PTSD occurs as the result of an individual being exposed to a traumatic event in which they experience, witness or are confronted with actual or threatened death or serious injury or the threat of physical injury to them or others, and where the individual's response involved intense fear, helplessness or horror. PTSD can become apparent through the individual experiencing other psychological or emotional symptoms such as anxiety disorders, depression, phobias, and substance misuse or relationships problems. The individual will utilise a range of defence mechanisms to cope with the psychological and emotional effects of the trauma, such as rationalisation. However, their schemas that relate to that event will have become wounded or damaged and this will make it difficult for them to make sense of the world on its previous terms. Old belief systems will be resurrected as they try and make sense of what they have experienced and their own identity as a result of events.

Following traumatic events, individuals should be given the opportunity to debrief (talk through the event, their feelings and actions). If this does not occur, the likelihood that they will develop PTSD is increased. Critical incident debriefing enables the individual to bring the unconscious memories into the conscious so they can process the information and then relocate it into a safer place, having dealt with their emotions. Individuals who may be exposed to critical incidents (any event which is extraordinary and which produces significant reactions in any person) as part of their work, such as emergency workers, health and social care workers, armed forces personnel should have access to learning opportunities which provide both information and experiential learning (such as simulation activities) to enable them to prepare for and deal with critical incidents, as well as recognise the signs of PTSD. In the event of a critical incident, there should be on-scene support available and then a critical incident debriefing (both team and individual as appropriate). Debriefing involves talking through the events and acknowledging what has been experienced and then an opportunity to discuss events so as to normalise emotions and responses. This is achieved through a structured and sequential process facilitated by a specially trained individual. Cognitive therapy involves helping the individual to restructure the memories associated with the event and enabling them to take control of them and achieve a perspective through setting

remember

Schemas are not within the conscious mind and help to determine how to interpret the world and how to respond in different situations.

goals which help the individual to unlearn their unwanted reactions and to gradually learn new responses. Therapy is usually short term as once the individual understands how and why they do what they do they can begin to take control so they can maintain the changes made. The therapist is likely to use a humanistic approach (based on the work of Carl Rogers) working in partnership with the individual in order to engage with them, understand the situation from their perspective, provide encouragement and support to agree goals together that will achieve the change desired by the individual.

Refer back to page 282 to remind yourself about Rogers' work.

Professional Practice

Health and social care workers often find themselves in situations that are critical incidents, such as traumatic events, assault or threatening behaviour from others, and so should ensure for their psychological and emotional well-being that they are:

■ given learning opportunities which equip them to prepare and deal with critical incidents

■ able to access support from others at the time and following

■ able to recognise that asking for help is a strength not a failure; it is about being professional

■ active in maintaining their own mental well-being, for example through having a good life-work balance, interests and activities.

Cognitive-behaviour therapy combines cognitive and behavioural therapies and is designed to help relieve the symptoms an individual is experiencing as well as resolve problems and help the individual to acquire coping skills and strategies. These will then help them to modify the underlying cognitive structures so they can manage or change their behaviour or responses. The focus is often on the practical effects a problem has on an individual and finding better ways of dealing with these. Both cognitive and cognitive-behaviour techniques can be used in supporting individuals with a learning disability who may have difficulties in managing their emotions and consequently their behaviour. Changing thoughts and expectations through teaching, for example, relaxation techniques may be used to manage feelings of anger or fear. Cognitive therapy may also be used to deal with recurring negative patterns of thought which, if the individual is unable to manage them, can lead to behaviour which others find challenging. Cognitive-behaviour therapy tries to help the individual to understand more about their thoughts, beliefs and ideas and how these relate to feelings and actions towards themselves and others. Adults with learning difficulties may not have moved successfully from the concrete operations stage to the formal operations stage and this may make it difficult for them to manage aspects of their life in terms of abstract thought, understanding others' motivations, and so on. They may also remain quite egocentric and so cognitive therapy may also help them to begin to understand the impact their behaviour has on others. It may also be useful in restructuring responses if the individual believes that when things happen they are due solely to their actions (egocentric response) and this may result in anxiety, challenging behaviour patterns and fixations.

Refer back to page 283 to remind yourself about Piaget's four stages of cognitive development.

---

activity
INDIVIDUAL WORK 8.5

P5

M1

1 Explain how being able to apply the cognitive perspective to aid understanding about an individual's behaviour and motivation is valuable in providing appropriate and effective health and social care support and intervention.

2 Analyse how being able to apply different psychological perspectives contributes to greater understanding of challenging behaviour and its consequent management.

Biological perspectives

Understanding developmental norms

Understanding developmental norms is one of the principle ways in which the biological perspective can be applied to health and social care. The work of psychologists such as Piaget and Gesell has produced frameworks that describe child development in language and motor skills. Mary Sheridan's work on developmental sequences produced more detailed information on the prescribed stages that children move through linked to the child's age. However, not all children conform to these milestones and some variation is natural, for example, not all children crawl before they walk, some will 'bottom-shuffle' (moving along in a sitting position) and then walk. In reality, children may achieve milestones at different times making more advances in one area, such as motor skills, while fewer in another, such as language skills. More recent child development research has suggested that it is not a linear process and more a holistic web of learning and development which increases in complexity as the child matures. Developmental norms, however, are useful in identifying learning and developmental delay which can occur due to a number of different conditions, for example, deafness, blindness, autism or learning disabilities. Early intervention will have a significant impact on enabling the child to catch up or receive additional support which may be physical, such as hearing or sight aids, so that their learning needs can be met and their further development is not hindered, thus enabling them to achieve their potential. Past experience has shown that lack of access to appropriate learning and support will reduce the individual's potential not necessarily because it is limited but because it is not nurtured and supported appropriately.

Mary Sheridan's child development scales

Age range	Gross motor skills	Fine motor skills and vision
1 month	*Prone (lying face down)* The baby lies with its head to one side but can now lift its head to change position. The legs are bent, no longer tucked under the body. *Supine (lying on the back)* The head is on one side. The arm and leg on the side the head is facing will stretch out. *Sitting* The back is a complete curve when the baby is held in sitting position.	The baby gazes attentively at carer's face while being fed, spoken to or during any caring routines. The baby grasps a finger or other object placed in the hand. The hands are usually closed.
3 months	*Prone* The baby can now lift up the head and chest supported on the elbows, forearms and hands. *Supine* The baby usually lies with the head in a central position. There are smooth, continuous movements of the arms and legs. The baby waves the arms symmetrically and brings hands together over the body. *Sitting* There should be little or no head lag. When held in a sitting position the back should be straight, except for a curve in the base of the spine. *Standing* The baby will sag at the knees when held in a standing position. The placing and walking reflexes should have disappeared.	Finger-play – the baby has discovered its hands and moves them around in front of the face, watching the movements and the pattern they make in the light. The baby holds a rattle or similar object for a short time if placed in the hand. Frequently hits itself in the face before dropping it! The baby is now very alert and aware of what is going on around. The baby moves its head to look around and follows adult movements.

Age range	Gross motor skills·	Fine motor skills and vision
6 months	*Prone* Lifts the head and chest well clear of the floor by supporting on outstretched arms. The hands are flat on the floor. The baby can roll over from front to back. *Supine* The baby will lift its head to look at its feet. The baby may lift its arms, requesting to be lifted and may roll over from back to front. *Sitting* If pulled to sit, the baby can now grab the adult's hands and pull itself into a sitting position; the head is now fully controlled with strong neck muscles. The baby can sit for long periods with support. The back is straight. Standing Held standing the baby will enjoy weight bearing and bouncing up and down.	Bright and alert, looking around constantly to absorb all the visual information on offer. Fascinated by small toys within reaching distance, grabbing them with the whole hand, using a **palmar grasp**. Transfers toys from hand to hand.
9 months	*Prone* The baby may be able to support its body on knees and outstretched arms. May rock backwards and forwards and try to crawl. *Supine* The baby rolls from back to front and may crawl away. *Sitting* The baby is now a secure and stable sitter – may sit unsupported for 15 minutes or more. *Standing* The baby can pull itself to a standing position. When supported by an adult it will step forward on alternate feet. The baby supports its body in the standing position by holding on to a firm object and may begin to side-step around furniture.	Uses the inferior **pincer grasp** with index finger and thumb. Looks for fallen objects out of sight – is now beginning to realise that they have not disappeared for ever. Grasps objects, usually with one hand, inspects with the eyes and transfers to the other hand. May hold one object in each hand and bang them together. Uses the index finger to poke and point.
12 months	*Sitting* Can sit alone indefinitely. Can get into sitting position from lying down. *Standing* Pulls itself to stand and walks around the furniture. Returns to sitting without falling. May stand alone for a short period.	Looks for objects hidden and out of sight. Uses a mature pincer grasp and releases objects. Throws toys deliberately and watches them fall. Likes to look at picture books and points at familiar objects. **Pincer grasp** using the thumb and first finger.

Age range	Gross motor skills	Fine motor skills and vision	
15 months	Walks alone, feet wide apart. Sits from standing. Crawls upstairs.	Points at pictures and familiar objects. Builds with two bricks. Enjoys books; turns several pages at once.	
18 months	Walks confidently. Tries to kick a ball. Walks upstairs with hand held.	Uses delicate pincer grasp. Scribbles on paper. Builds a tower with three bricks.	
2 years	Runs safely. Walks up and downstairs holding on. Rides a trike, pushing it along with the feet.	Holds a pencil and attempts to draw circles, lines and dots. Uses fine pincer grasp with both hands to do complicated tasks. Builds a tower of six bricks.	
3 years	Can stand, walk and run on tiptoe. Walks upstairs one foot on each step. Rides a tricycle and uses the pedals.	Can thread large wooden beads onto a lace. Controls a pencil in the preferred hand. Builds a tower of nine bricks.	
4 years	Climbs play equipment. Walks up and downstairs, one foot on each step. Can stand, walk and run on tiptoe.	Builds a tower of 10 or more bricks. Grasps a pencil maturely. Beginning to do up buttons and fasten zips.	
5 years	Can hop. Plays ball games well. Can walk along on the balancing beam.	Can draw a person with head, trunk, legs and eyes, nose and mouth. Can sew large stitches. Good control of pencils and paintbrushes.	
6 years	Rides a two-wheeled bicycle. Kicks a football well. Makes running jumps.	Can catch a ball with one hand. Writing hold is similar to the adult.	
7 years	Can climb and balance well on the apparatus. Hops easily on either foot, keeping well balanced.	Writes well. Can sew neatly with a large needle.	

Understanding genetic predisposition to certain illness or health-related behaviours

Refer back to page 286 to remind yourself about the importance of genetic influences on certain illness and health-related behaviours.

An individual may have a predisposition due to genetic influences to become addicted to alcohol, smoking or other factors and so knowledge of this can help them and others to plan strategies to avoid addiction. A person may have the predisposition to depression and if they are aware of this can identity those factors which may trigger depression, such as excess stress. Alternatively, they could plan strategies to deal with life events that are know to be stressful, such as moving house, relationship problems or the death of a loved one. Genetic research has identified where disease or the predisposition to certain diseases is inherited and it can be attributed to a specific chromosome, gene or group of genes, such as cystic fibrosis, muscular dystrophy, Huntington's disease and breast cancer. In addition, research has indicated a number of diseases where the actual link is less specific but nonetheless inherited predisposition has been demonstrated, such as bipolar disease (manic depression), schizophrenia, diabetes mellitus, multiple sclerosis, early onset Alzheimer's disease as well as a number of cancers.

If a genetic link can be isolated, prenatal screening can be offered to parents whose unborn child is at risk of developing the disease or carrying the faulty gene. Parents would be counselled regarding the risks, their options and the likelihood of the child developing the disease. This is not without its moral and ethical dilemmas, not least the value attributed to people with a disability. In addition, accessing early treatment or taking steps to monitor health if a predisposition exists are also options, such as regular mammograms for a woman who has a familial history of breast cancer or the option to have a bilateral mastectomy to avoid the possibility of developing breast cancer. However, bearing in mind that genetics are not the whole story, an individual may have the predisposition and never develop the condition while equally they may have the predisposition, take reasonable precautions to avoid potential triggers and environmental factors and still develop the condition or disease. The interaction of genetics and environment and the power of each in the outcome are still unclear.

Understanding the effects of shift work on individuals

Biological perspectives can also be applied to understand the effects of shift work on individuals. The normal body rhythm or circadian rhythm is the daily pattern of activity which involves sleeping at night and being awake during the day. Working night shifts disturbs this normal rhythm and so it becomes desynchronised. In other words, the internal body clock is out of phase or step with the environmental stimuli of sunrise and sunset.

This lack of synchronisation disrupts many normal biological functions such as gastrointestinal action, the sleep-wake cycle and attention levels. This is thought to be due to the fact that although the individual's working pattern has changed their internal body clock is so established in its rhythm that it does not change. The normal environmental stimuli which help to maintain the circadian rhythm, such as daylight, continue to stimulate the individual with the effect that they may become fatigued as they cannot sleep during the day even though they are tired. Normal body functions become disrupted which can lead to a number of problems, such as irregular eating habits, which can lead to indigestion, weight loss or more likely weight gain. Research has also shown potential links between shift work, especially night work, and irregular heart rhythms and increased risk in developing breast cancer. If an individual works shifts, this can create not only stress to their body systems but stress within their life as they seek to manage activities, such as family life, household activities, and so on, and so it is not easy to determine the exact cause of such ill health in a shift worker. Trying to sleep during the day is problematic and the quality of sleep is not that experienced during night-time sleep. Lack of sleep has been shown to be detrimental to the performance of tasks especially those involved with precision and higher thinking skills, such as decision making, which are likely to be part of a health and social care workers role.

Understanding the biological impact of shift work can help individuals to take steps to minimise the ill effects. For example, to avoid gastrointestinal problems such as indigestion and weight gain, the advice would be to eat small portions of food and to avoid spicy food when working nights.

case study 8.4

Turning things around

Gap year volunteer Charlotte Ashton spent a month with a charity that helps former drug users get back to work.

Thursday March 9, 2006

I didn't know anything about drugs, addiction or rehabilitation when I started volunteering at Transition, a charity based just off the Royal Mile in Edinburgh that helps recovered and recovering drug addicts and alcoholics back into further education or work.

It was a steep learning curve and on the way I discovered some pretty shocking things about addiction and the struggle to recovery, not least that I am addicted to one of the country's most widely used drugs. I've been using it regularly since I started university and I would find the demands of day-to-day life almost unbearable without it. I get tired and irritable if I can't get a regular fix, but fortunately maintaining my addiction isn't expensive and it does not make me behave noticeably different. Giving up would be tough: I've tried twice now but relapsed after a couple of days – the headaches and fatigue were unbearable.

I may only be addicted to caffeine, but the difficulties of giving up are the same, in principle, to those faced by a Class A drug addict. The difference is that Class A drug addicts and alcoholics are battling against far more than physical dependency on a harmful substance. The students at Transition have come through the physical discomfort of withdrawal (unlike millions of coffee lovers worldwide) and are now having to establish a sustainable, substance-free lifestyle.

There is no middle road. For heroin addicts, methadone is only a route out of crime and the dangers of needle sharing. It won't get you a job. As Craig, a recovering cocaine addict, pointed out: 'You can turn a recreational user into an addict, but not the other way round.'

Transition's students are having to start from scratch rebuilding their lives. In the course of the month, I learned that the basic discipline of a daily routine is fundamental to successful rehabilitation. Transition offers the emotional and practical support that allows students to get used to a normal routine. They pay bus fares and lunch expenses and the key workers offer emotional support and encouragement. But they do not let the students get too comfortable; the purpose of them being there is to move on to a job or further education.

Addiction is a full-time occupation and Transition fills the hole left after the drug is given up. 'As an addict, you spend all day figuring out how you're going to get the money for your next fix and then you go and get it,' one of the students explains. 'When you get clean, you don't have a reason to get out of bed anymore so you just sit around at home watching daytime TV, letting the world pass you by. Transition gave me stability and routine – and that helps you build up your confidence again.'

In one Personal Development class, the students had to explain why they started at Transition and what they hope to achieve during their time there. All of them want to get qualifications and feel they have no time to lose. 'I've wasted enough of my life already,' was a common theme in their answers, which is why it is so crucial that Transition offers a rolling educational programme that addicts can join as soon as they are out of detox or rehab. The wait until the start of a new term could be a dangerously empty time.

Many of the lessons, particularly Personal Development and Communications, involve a lot of group discussion and the students told me how refreshing it is to talk about something other than drugs and addiction with people outside of the

▶

increasingly narrow circles they were moving in. Most of them have already been through a considerable amount of counselling and therapy and are quite simply bored of it.

'The problem is that it normalises your problem. I've been telling the same shit to different people for years and years. I've been over everything so much I can talk about it without even getting emotional,' Craig told me.

The students seem to respond well to the concrete goals, tangible results and clear boundaries afforded by the prospect of qualifications and a work placement. The more they put in, the more they get out, so the relationship between staff and students is contractual and mature. Their learning plans are reviewed at least monthly and they are expected to treat the lessons like a job: persistent absenteeism or poor behaviour result in an official warning. Three warnings and you are out for two months to gather the resolve to be more dedicated should you chose to start again.

Success stories

The results are impressive – in the last two years Transition has moved 33 former addicts into work and 103 of them have got qualifications. This month's success story is Derek, who completed a work placement with M&S and was invited back for interview. He did well and has been offered a job as soon as a vacancy becomes available. He is over the moon. 'Transition has turned my life around. I didn't think any of this would be possible when I started here in November but they've brought the best out of me and built up my confidence.'

Another student, Angie, who works one day a week at a local media company agrees that jobs and qualifications, not counselling and therapy, are the true confidence builders. 'I'm out and about meeting people now and I take my son places. Before Transition I was just taking things as they came, but now I'm hoping to go to university.'

These are the success stories, but many of the students will lapse and relapse and fall off the Transition programme only to return months later to start all over again. On average there are nine students in each class – a lot compared to some of the local mainstream colleges – but attendance can be erratic and the staff have no idea who will arrive each morning.

It is not surprising that the climb back to a steady routine is long and steep; normality poses challenges to recovering users that had not even occurred to me. One of the students, who has returned to work a number of times but has always relapsed, told me he is not ready to have a job because he can not handle having money. This seemed strange; surely the comfort and freedom wealth allows is nothing but positive? Not for this student. For him, it is too much of a temptation. For him, it buys drugs, the ultimate loss of freedom.

And that's not all. For some of the students, sustaining a drug-free existence demands rejection of friends from their past life, so the reality can be quite lonely. Persistent relapse has cost many of them the support of other friends and family who have run out of patience and their efforts are often met with scepticism.

Nature or nurture?

To insure they do not relapse, alcoholics and drug addicts alike have to address the problems that drove them to substance abuse in the first place.

Some of the more candid students described these problems and class discussions would often turn into a nature-nurture debate. The fact that hundreds of thousands of people are addicted to caffeine points to a natural predisposition, but there was general consensus among the students that where you come from determines the likelihood of you developing a habit.

Addiction is natural, but nurture may determine whether you become a junkie or not. As one student pointed out, you are more likely to take drugs if the streets you played in as a child were littered with syringes and you were using before you had even thought about Standard Grades (GCSE equivalents). Transition's referral figures are testament to this: over 70% of students who started the programme live in so-called SIP (Social Inclusion Partnership) areas – Edinburgh's worst council estates.

True rehabilitation is not just about addressing the addiction itself, but all the problems that drive people to addiction in the first place or are brought about while they were under the influence, such as single parenthood or the struggle for access to children, no family support, or despairing parents, no qualifications, job prospects or work that is badly paid and unfulfilling.

The main battle against addiction isn't fought during detox. It only starts once addicts and alcoholics are clean and dry.

As Phil, one of the Transition key-workers explained, 'Drugs are only a small part of addiction – they're just the medium people use to escape all the other issues in their lives. They're a chemical buffer against the rest of the world.'

---

activity
GROUP WORK

1   What factors were identified within the article as being contributory to problems of addiction?

2   How does the nature-nurture debate relate to other psychological perspectives?

3   How can different psychological perspectives be applied to address the problems of addiction?

---

activity
INDIVIDUAL WORK
8.6

P6

Use examples to describe how biological perspectives are applied within heath and social care.

---

activity
INDIVIDUAL WORK
8.7

M2

D1

1   Reflect on the examples from activity 8.6 to describe how different psychological perspectives are applied to health and social care in practice. Analyse the value and contribution each makes to health and social care service provision.

2   Weigh up the value of each psychological perspective in terms of its role and contribution in providing effective health and social care interventions.

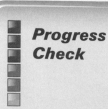

Progress Check

1 What is meant by *positive reinforcement*?

2 What is the self-fulfilling prophesy?

3 According to Freud, what are the three parts of an individual?

4 What are the three factors that describe Roger's humanistic approach to working with individuals?

5 Give an example of how genetic inheritance can influence behaviour.

6 According to the behaviourist perspective how can behaviour be shaped?

7 How does social learning influence health behaviour?

8 How can humanistic approaches be applied to developing practitioner – service user relationships?

9 How can cognitive techniques be applied to working with individuals with emotional problems?

10 How can the biological perspective be related to pre natal health screening?

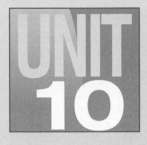

Caring for children and young people

This unit covers:

- Why children and young people may need to be looked after
- How care is provided for children and young people
- The risks to children and young people of abusive and exploitative behaviour
- Strategies to minimise the risk to children and young people of abusive and exploitative behaviour

Children and young people from birth to 18 years old may need to be looked after for a variety of reasons. There are a variety of settings where this care may be provided. This unit will explore these reasons and consider the different types of care available. The risks to children and young people of abusive and exploitative behaviour will be examined alongside strategies to minimise risks.

<table>
<tr>
<td rowspan="8" style="writing-mode: vertical-lr;">grading criteria</td>
<td>To achieve a Pass grade the evidence must show that the learner is able to:</td>
<td>To achieve a Merit grade the evidence must show that, in addition to the pass criteria, the learner is able to:</td>
<td>To achieve a Distinction grade the evidence must show that, in addition to the pass and merit criteria, the learner is able to:</td>
</tr>
<tr>
<td>P1
describe the main reasons why children and young people may need to be looked after away from their families
Pg 310</td>
<td></td>
<td></td>
</tr>
<tr>
<td>P2
identify the current relevant legislation affecting the care of children and young people
Pg 313</td>
<td>M1
analyse how policies and procedures help children/ young people and their families whilst the child is being looked after
Pg 313</td>
<td>D1
evaluate the legislative rights of the child/young person and the rights of their families, bearing in mind that the needs of the child/young person are paramount
Pg 314</td>
</tr>
<tr>
<td>P3
describe health and social care service provision for looked-after children and young people   Pg 319</td>
<td>M2
compare the care provided by at least two different organisations offering care to children and young people
Pg 319</td>
<td></td>
</tr>
</table>

grading criteria

To achieve a **Pass** grade the evidence must show that the learner is able to:	To achieve a **Merit** grade the evidence must show that, in addition to the pass criteria, the learner is able to:	To achieve a **Distinction** grade the evidence must show that, in addition to the pass and merit criteria, the learner is able to:
P4 describe signs and symptoms of child abuse Pg 332		
P5 describe appropriate responses where child abuse is suspected or confirmed, making reference to current legislation and policies Pg 337		
P6 identify the strategies and methods of supporting children, young people and their families where abuse is suspected or confirmed Pg 343	**M3** explain strategies and methods to minimise the risk to children and young people where abuse is suspected or confirmed Pg 343	**D2** evaluate a range of strategies and methods to support children/young people and their families where abuse is suspected or confirmed Pg 343

Why children and young people may need to be looked after

Looked-after children

Following imposition of a care order

A **care order** is a court order that places a child under the care of a local authority. The local authority will share parental responsibility for the child with the parents, and will make most of the important decisions about the upbringing of the child or young person, such as where they live and how they are educated. A court will only make a care order if it is sure that a child is suffering, or likely to suffer significant harm by their parents, if it is likely that harm will be caused due to insufficient care being given to the child by the parents in the future or if the child or young person is likely to suffer harm because they are beyond parental control. A care order can only be made for a child under 17. It would stop if a child or young person was adopted and can only last until their 18th birthday. A care order may result in temporary or permanent care.

With the agreement of the parents

The social services department's primary duty is to work with parents and the child or young person to prevent the child or young person being made the subject of a care order. If the local authority has decided to investigate the child or young person's circumstances, it will work with the family by providing support services. At this point, the local authority will discuss with the family and child or young person the possibility of accommodating the child for a limited period, until the problems can be resolved. Where possible, a **voluntary arrangement** with the parents' consent will be reached.

According to Childline, approximately three out of five children in care are under a care order.

Potential reasons

Family-related reasons

Bereavement

When a parent or main carer dies, often children and young people are cared for by their extended family. However, as society changes and families become more mobile, not every child or young person has an extended family. It may be necessary to organise a short-term emergency placement while a long-term plan is made, with the child's views and wishes taken into account.

Parental illness or incapacity

When a parent or main carer is ill, physically or mentally, or has had an accident, a child or young person may need an emergency placement or a period of short-term care. Where possible, placement would be sought within the extended family, or with close friends. Where this is not possible, the child or young person may be placed with a foster family. In households where parents or carers are dependent upon substances such as alcohol or drugs, this is likely to result in an inability to fulfil major obligations, such as ensuring children and young people have adequate food, are encouraged to go to school, are cared for and given emotional and practical support. If **substance abuse** is left unaddressed, the quality of parenting is likely to decline further, with children and young people having to take on the role of parent. Children and young people living with substance abusing parents are more likely to experience **socio-economic disadvantage** and social isolation.

Child- or young person-related reasons

Health problems

For children and young people with major health problems, in particular a **terminal illness**, hospices offer **palliative** care that provides a service to improve the quality of life for the child or young person and his or her family. This arrangement is likely to be a voluntary arrangement between parents, social services and the health authority.

Behavioural problems

When children and young people repeatedly misbehave in a way considered much worse than one would normally expect for their age, it can lead to family breakdown. For younger children, displays of constant temper tantrums, hitting or kicking other people, destroying property and possessions and frequent lying can result in parents feeling unable to cope and continue to care for their child. Young people may begin to bully others, fight, display cruelty to people and animals, be involved in mugging and frequent truanting. These factors can lead to the child or young person needing to be looked after by the local authority.

Learning difficulties

Children who have a significant impairment in their ability to learn are described as having learning difficulties. Some children and young people with learning difficulties may attend a special placement which can be a long way from the family home. The need for children with learning difficulties to be looked after are often complex. Family circumstances, parents' ability to cope long term with conditions that may require 24-hour care and lack of local specialist provision may all contribute to the need for children and young people to be looked after.

Disabilities

Some children or young people who require intensive care due to the nature of their disability may be looked after for short periods by the local authority. Short breaks allow the family to recharge their batteries and give the child or young person access to wider leisure opportunities and to develop new friendships. These breaks may be in a residential setting, or with approved families and are known as **respite care**.

Every Child Matters   www.everychildmatters.gov.uk
There are around 13,300 disabled children in long-term residential placements.

remember

According to the Department for Education and Skills (DfES), less than 2% of children in care are there because of things they have done.

As a result of committing an offence

A disproportionate number of crimes are committed by children and young people between the ages of 10 and 17. According to the Audit Commission, there are many factors associated with offending behaviour, such as inadequate parenting, aggressive and hyperactive behaviour in early childhood and unstable living conditions, and boys are more likely to offend than girls. Young people who offend, who may be on a final warning or appearing before a court are likely to be supported by the Youth Offending Service.

case study 10.1 — Clem

Theresa and Andy have a son, Clem, who has severe learning disabilities and a profound communication disorder. Theresa has given up work to care for Clem, meaning that Andy is having to do overtime to support the household financially. When Theresa had to go into hospital, both parents agreed voluntarily that Clem should spend time with foster carers until Theresa was fully recuperated. Clem spent six weeks with a family nearby. The family continue to offer short-term care to allow Clem's parents some respite from caring and to broaden Clem's social network.

activity — INDIVIDUAL WORK

1   There are a range of national organisations providing short-term care for children with disabilities. Use the internet service at your college learning resource centre to identify an organisation. Describe the aims of the organisation.

2   Produce a leaflet for parents giving information about the organisation, its philosophy and contact details.

activity — INDIVIDUAL WORK 10.1

P1

In the UK today, many children and young people live in a setting other than their family. This can be within a foster family, small residential setting or special school. It can be short term or long term.

Describe the main reasons why children and young people may be looked after away from their families.

Professional Practice

- There are approximately 78,500 looked-after children in the UK.

- In England, Wales and Northern Ireland, approximately one in every 200 children and young people are looked after by a local authority. In Scotland, the figure is one in every 100.

- Around two thirds of children in care live in foster homes.

- Approximately 12% of looked-after children live in residential care homes.

- In England, 62% of children and young people in care are there because of abuse or neglect.

- Throughout the UK, 55% of children and young people in care are boys.

- A disproportionately high number of children in care are disabled.

- Approximately 2,400 unaccompanied asylum seekers under the age of 16 are in care. 70% of these are in London.

- Over a quarter of prisoners were in care as children.

- Between a quarter and third of rough sleepers were in care as children.

National statistics bulletin	www.dfes.gov.uk/rsgateway
Social Services statistics Wales	www.lgdu-wales.gov.uk/eng/project
Children Order statistics	www.dhsspsni.gov.uk/publications/2003
Voice for the child in care	www.vcc-uk.org
The Who Cares Trust	www.thewhocarestrust.org.uk
Care zone	www.carezone.org.uk
British Association for Adoption and Fostering	www.baaf.org.uk
National Youth Advocacy Service	www.nyas.net

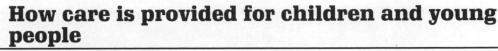

How care is provided for children and young people

Legislation/legal framework

Relevant to home country

An overview of the law affecting children under the care or supervision of local authorities was commissioned in 2001. In Scotland, the Children (Scotland) Act (1995) is the key legislation concerning the care and welfare of children. Part I describes the legal rights and responsibilities of parents for their children and makes provision for resolving disputes about children between family members. Part II sets out the arrangements for public services for children in need of protection and support, including arrangements for dealing with children who offend. Part III amends aspects of the Adoption (Scotland) Act (1978). In England, the General Social Care Council (GSCC) regulates the social services workforce and their education and training. In Wales, the equivalent body is the Care Council for Wales (CCW), while in Northern Ireland, the Northern Ireland Social Care Council (NISSC) performs this role.

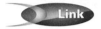

See page 54 in Unit 2 for more information about national initiatives in promoting anti-discriminatory practice in health and social care.

United Nations Convention on the Rights of the Child (1989)

Convention on the Rights of the Child	www.unicef.org/crc

The United Nations (UN) Convention on the Rights of the Child is a universally agreed set of standards and obligations. In 1989, world leaders decided that children needed a special convention just for them because people under 18 years often need special care and protection that adults do not.

Article 4, the protection of rights, places a responsibility on governments to ensure that children's rights are respected, protected and fulfilled. When countries join the Convention of the Rights of the Child, they agree to assess their social services, legal, health and education systems, as well as levels of funding for these services. They are obliged to take steps to ensure that the minimum standards set by the convention in these areas are being met.

Article 20, children deprived of family environment, states that children who cannot be looked after by their own families have a right to special care and must be looked after properly by people who respect their ethnic group, religion, culture and language.

See page 69 in Unit 2 for more information about equality, diversity and rights.

Article 25 of the Convention on the Rights of the Child also states that children who are looked after by the local authority, rather than their parents, should have their situation reviewed regularly.

The Children Act (1989)

Children and young people may be subject to a care order made by the court under section 31 of the Children Act. The Court would need to be satisfied that the child or young person is suffering, or would suffer, significant harm without one.

Children and young people who are accommodated by the local authority on a voluntary basis come under section 20 of the Children Act. This section covers approximately one third of all looked-after children.

The Children Act (2004)

A series of documents have been published which provide guidance under the Act to support local authorities in implementing new statutory duties. For looked-after children and young people, the Department for Education and Skills (DfES), working with the Department of Health (DoH) is supporting the development of standardised contracts, which can be used by all local authorities when purchasing placements in the private and voluntary sector, due to be launched in April 2007.

> **remember**
> About 65% of all looked-after children are subject to a care order under The Children Act (1989).

Liam's story

Liam lived at home with his mother. He regularly missed school and often would appear with fading bruises on his arms. The teacher with responsibility for child protection began to log these incidents. On one occasion, Liam appeared with a fading black eye. He said he had slipped but appeared agitated when questioned. His mother was asked to come into school to enable the school to discuss concerns. She refused and Liam did not attend for five days. The concerns were referred to social services and a social worker wrote to Liam's mother, asking to visit. When no reply was made, a social worker attempted to visit but was refused entry to the home.

activity
INDIVIDUAL WORK

1   Obtain a copy of the child protection policy at your placement setting. Describe the role of the designated child protection officer at your setting.

2   Describe your own role in your setting when raising concerns about children's well being.

Human Rights Act (1998)

The Human Rights Act (1998) incorporates most of the rights in the European Convention on Human Rights into domestic law in the United Kingdom. It has long been recognised that there may be tensions between the Children Act (1989), whereby children and young people may be looked after by a public authority, and the Human Rights Act which makes unlawful any action by a public authority to intervene in family life (Article 8). The implications for professionals is the need to consider human rights issues at each stage of assessment, planning, implementation and review.

Data Protection Act (1998)

The Data Protection Act (1998) is designed to ensure that personal data held by a local authority is looked after properly. While a person is entitled to see personal data held by a local authority, there are rules about how data may be accessed. Parents of children under 12 can apply to see data held about them, but do not have a legal right to see all data, apart from educational records held by school.

Link   See page 71 in unit 2 for more information about the Data Protection Act (1998)

Professional Practice

To access data:

■ apply in writing (Emails are acceptable)

■ give your full name and address

■ supply proof of identity with a photo.

Framework for the Assessment of Children in Need and their Parents (2000)

The Framework for the Assessment of Children in Need and their Families was jointly issued by the DoH, the DfES and the Home Office in 2000. The purpose of the framework is to provide a systematic way of understanding, analysing and recording what is happening to children and young people within their families and the wider context of their home community.

Every Child Matters (2003)

The Children Act (2004) provides the legal underpinning for Every Child Matters – Change for Children (2003). The overall aim of Every Child Matters is to improve outcomes for all children. To date, outcomes achieved by looked-after children have been unacceptably poor and the government is committed to addressing this disparity. 45% of the 8,100 children leaving care aged 16 or over during 2005 to 2006 had at least one GCSE or GNVQ on leaving care. This was an increase of 2% since the previous year.

One of the key objectives of Every Child Matters is to improve the early support available to families in the hope that more children can be supported safely in their families. The government's priorities for looked-after children are to improve the stability of placements and to improve their educational achievement.

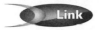

Professional Practice

The five critical components in direct work with children during assessment of need are:

- seeing
- observing
- talking
- doing
- engaging.

Other relevant local policies

In the Schools White Paper (2006), the government announced its intention to consult on wide ranging proposals for improving outcomes for looked-after children. Achieving a major change in life chances for this group is a continuing theme in Every Child Matters, prioritising improvements in residential and foster care.

Link

See page 73 in Unit 2 for more information on improving standards in health and social care settings.

In 2006, the government produced a guidance document entitled 'Supporting Looked-After Learners – A Practical Guide for School Governors' designed to help school governing bodies ensure that their school policies and practices are fully inclusive of the needs of looked-after children.

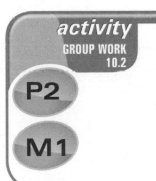

activity
GROUP WORK 10.2

P2

M1

1. As a practitioner in the field of care, you must work within a legal framework that protects the children and young people that you care for, and protects you.

   With reference to practical workplace experience, show your awareness of the current laws that affect your daily practice.

2. Children and young people in the looked-after system are often considered to be one of the most vulnerable groups in society. It is important that you are clear about the policies and procedures within your setting. With close reference to the principles of **confidentiality**, use a vocational practice example to illustrate how clear policies and procedures support children, young people and families in the looked-after system.

Care
Temporary and permanent

Care can be organised on a temporary or permanent basis. Most children and young people will go home but some will go to live with other families and others may live independently. Temporary care may take the form of shared care, where a child who has a disability or long-term illness may have a break away from home for a few days. This is also known as **respite care**.

Link

See page 314 for more information about respite care.

Temporary care can help alleviate pressure on families during short-term periods of crisis. Long-term or permanent care is sometimes needed for children and young people with severe physical and learning difficulties who require 24-hour specialist care.

Foster care

Foster care is where local people provide a safe and caring environment in their own homes for children and young people with different levels of care needs. This can be on a full- or part-time basis, ranging from one day to several months or even years. Foster carers are of all ages, come from different social and cultural backgrounds and may be single, married or living together, including gay or lesbian families.

case study 10.3

Profile of a foster carer

When my children were younger, I worked as a childminder. I was asked to consider fostering after the mother of one of the children I cared for became ill and had to spend time in hospital. In the last 16 years, over 30 children have stayed with us. The youngest was just 20 days old and the oldest were 16-year old twins. Some children stay for a very short period, although two have been with us for eight years. Both have learning difficulties and need lots of time and care.

Sometimes we have to cope with difficult behaviour. So I am grateful for the training we have undertaken. We also had to go through a strict approval process and know where to go for advice and support.

I think our main role is to make the children feel safe and welcome, to keep information about the children and young people confidential and never pass judgement on their past.

activity
INDIVIDUAL WORK

1. Describe the process a prospective foster carer will need to undertake to become a registered foster carer.
2. The Children Act (1989) requires foster carers to be aware of cultural and religious needs of the children and young people that they care for. Identify how this may be put into practice in the home.

activity
INDIVIDUAL WORK 10.3
D1

The Children Act (1989) established the 'paramountcy principle' whereby the needs of the child or young person are paramount. With awareness of this principle, evaluate the legislative rights of the child or young person and their family.

Respite care

Many local authorities offer respite care to children with disabilities and their families. Often the scheme is offered by a local voluntary organisation. For parents of a child with a disability, a break is very important, as everyday things, such as shopping, taking another child swimming or having an evening out, can be difficult to organise. Host families who receive payment and training, are often referred to as link families.

Adoption

Adoption provides the legal basis for the assumption of parental responsibilities in respect of a child by a single person or a couple, who need not be married and can be heterosexual or gay or lesbian. Nowadays, adoption is used to provide permanent families to children of all ages, from infants to teenagers.

Adoption Line Information   www.adoption.org.uk
up-to-date statistics on the number of children adopted in the UK

Professional Practice

Why is respite care important?

For the child or young person:

■ it provides opportunities to make new friends

■ it provides a chance to widen their experience by spending time away from home

■ they can build up a secure relationship with carers over time.

For the child or young person's family:

■ it provides an opportunity to spend time together and give time to another member of the family

■ it provides time to enjoy a break

■ they can relax knowing that their child is being cared for by someone who is an approved carer and who can meet the needs of the child.

For the link family:

■ they can use some of their free time to help another family

■ they can make rewarding new friendships

■ they can help their own family understand the special needs of others.

case study 10.4 — Luanne

Luanne was a recently divorced parent with four children aged between 7 and 18. Following a difficult divorce, she enrolled on a childcare course at a local college. As part of the course, she needed to undertake work experience in various childcare settings but the demands of college work and bringing up four children were stressful. A parent living nearby had two children, Ralph and Rosie. Ralph had autistic spectrum disorder. Luanne's tutor suggested that she apply to become a link family as part of gaining experience in the field of childcare. Luanne applied to a local voluntary agency and was accepted as a link parent after satisfying a range of procedures, including an enhanced Criminal Records Bureau check. Ralph and his mother went to Luanne's house every Wednesday and, when Ralph was settled, he stayed one weekend in four to give his parents a break and provide him with new opportunities. Ralph's parents owned a holiday home in the New Forest and invited Luanne and her children to join them on weekends.

It has been a beneficial experience for both families. Ralph, Rosie and their parents have enjoyed expanding their network and Luanne and her children regard Ralph and Rosie as brother and sister.

activity
GROUP WORK

1 In your group, discuss the benefits for both families of the arrangement.

2 Using the facilities in your college learning resource centre, identify which organisations locally are providing respite care for children with disabilities and their families.

3 Design a leaflet for children and their families, outlining what is available locally.

Residential childcare

In July 2000, the Children Matter Task Force established several principles which underpin developments in residential childcare policy.

Residential childcare is an integral part of the child welfare system. There is an underlying commitment from the health and social services trusts to place children locally, unless the need for specialist services dictates otherwise. There is also an intention that homes should be small and domestic in nature, and that campus sites and sites providing for other users are deemed unsuitable.

Provision of residential childcare can be from three sources:

- Statutory provision
- Voluntary provision
- Private sector provision

Residential childcare can provide for short-, medium- and long-term placements and often will accommodate children and young people on emergency arrangements.

Planning for care in partnership with child or young person, parents and other agencies as relevant

Every young person looked after by the local authority has a care plan that prevents unnecessary time spent away from their family. Care plans usually concern creating changes in order to provide a speedy return home. Under the Children Act (1989), a young person's care plan must be reviewed:

- at four weeks
- at three months
- every six months
- until a court order is made or a young person is discharged from local authority care.

See page 69 in Unit 2 for more information about the legislative framework for service planning.

Local authorities have a duty to safeguard and promote the welfare of children in need within their area and so far as it is consistent with that duty, to promote the upbringing of children within their families, by providing a range and level of services appropriate to the child's needs. When a court considers any question relating to the upbringing of a child under the Children Act (1989), it must have regard to the **Welfare Checklist** set out in section 1 of the Act.

Professional Practice

The Welfare Checklist requires the court to consider:

- the ascertainable wishes and feelings of the child concerned (considered in light of his age and understanding)
- the child's physical, emotional or educational needs
- the likely effect on the child of any change in circumstances
- the child's age, sex, background, and any characteristic of the child which the court considers relevant
- any harm which the child has suffered or is at risk of suffering
- how capable each of the child's parents and any person in relation to whom the court considers the question to be relevant, is of meeting his needs
- the range of powers available to the court under The Children Act 1989 in the proceedings in question.

Organisation of care provision

Central government:

To improve the life chances of the poorest and most disadvantaged families and break the cycle of poverty and inequality, the government has identified five key outcomes for children and young people.

Department of Health

Raising the attainment of looked-after children is a key priority for the Department of Health. The continued cycle of poor performance of looked-after children in education compared to their peers has led to national policy makers placing this at the top of their agenda. Statistics show that looked-after children fall well behind their peers at all key stage levels and only 1% go on to university.

Fig 10.1 The government's five key outcomes for children and young people

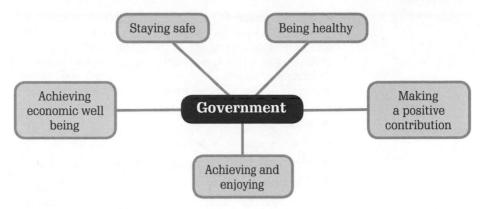

National Health Service

The National Health Service (NHS) was set up in 1948 and is now the largest organisation in Europe. It is recognised as one of the best health services in the world by the World Health Organisation but is having to change to cope with 21st century demands. An NHS plan, published in July 2000, launched a full-scale modernisation programme designed to totally transform the NHS and the way it cares for patients. Locally, NHS providers and organisations work in partnership with social care services to look after the health and welfare of the population.

The founding principles of the NHS can be summed up as the provision of quality care that:

■ meets the needs of everyone

■ is free at the point of need

■ is based on a patient's clinical need, not their ability to pay.

National Service Framework for Children, Young People and Maternity Services

In April 2006, the Department of Health published 'Emerging Findings', a document setting out some of the early thinking in the development of the National Service Frameworks for Children, Young People and Maternity Services. The National Service Framework will set standards across health and social care partnerships. Its objectives are:

■ to put children and families at the centre of care

■ to develop effective partnership working so that the needs of the child are always considered

■ to develop needs-led services.

Standard 8 of the National Service Framework for Children, Young People and Maternity Services relates to disabled children and young people and those with complex health needs.

Local government

Integrated services

Policy directives in both health and social care promote the delivery of more co-ordinated (integrated) services developed through partnership and joint working. Proposals for integrated children's services were passed in to law with the Children Act (2004).

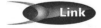

See page 54 in Unit 2 for more information about the active promotion of anti-discriminatory practice.

Integrated children's services will move away from the traditional structuring of services around professional disciplines. This system will create joined up services, centred around the needs of children, young people and their families and focus upon how services are planned, commissioned and delivered. This will integrate all services provided for children and young people from birth to 19, or with some vulnerable groups, up to 25.

Children's services

After the publication of 'Every Child Matters: Next Steps', which formed the heart of the Children Act (2004), many local authorities created children's services authorities to improve the co-ordination of services to children and young people.

Children's trusts

Children's trusts bring together all services for children and young people in an area and focus upon improving outcomes. The Children's trusts support those who work with children, young people and their families to deliver more integrated and responsive services. Professionals work in effective multi-disciplinary teams having undertaken radical training across disciplines to address cultural and professional divides. For children and young people in the looked-after system, this should mean:

- a joint needs assessment
- shared decisions on priorities
- identification of all available resources
- joint plans to deploy resources.

This joint commissioning, underpinned by pooled resources will make sure that the right packages of services are provided by those trained to do so.

| Every Child Matters | www.everychildmatters.gov.uk |

more information about children's trusts

---

case study 10.5   My way

At 17 years old, Louie had lived at home with his mother all his life. Louie has severe learning difficulties and, although he had spent short breaks in respite care, his mother's ill health made the home situation unsustainable in the long term. A place was available at a college for young people with high support needs and Louie's mother persuaded the local authority to fund the placement. Aware that this placement could only cater for Louie until he was 19, his mother got in touch with a national charity, Macintyre Care, who were piloting a scheme to help ensure that young people with high support needs had an individual package of care, based on their unique needs. The 'My Way' project is all about supporting young people with learning disabilities to take control of their lives through individualised funding.

A meeting was held with Louie's mother, an individualised funding manager from the 'My Way' project, a representative from the adult services division of social services and a connexions adviser. Louie was able to contribute using symbols and a multi-media profile outlining his likes and dislikes. In this way, a circle of support involving all the significant people in Louie's life and Louie has begun to be created.

| MacIntyre | www.macintyrecharity.org |

'My Way' project

---

activity
INDIVIDUAL WORK

Using the facilities at your college learning resource centre, carry out some research into the use of 'Unified Assessments' and describe how their use helps children and their families to contribute to their care planning.

See page 320 for more information about connexions advisers. See page 73 in Unit 2 for more information about putting the service user at the heart of service provision.

Children's centres

Children's centres, often under the umbrella of Sure Start, are places where children under five and their families can access seamless, integrated services and information. They also provide a focal point for help from a multi-disciplinary team. Sure Start children's centres are at the heart of the government's strategy for early years, which makes a commitment to provide a Sure Start children's centre for every community by 2010. They form part of the government's 10-year childcare strategy to enable all families with children to have access to an affordable, flexible childcare place, combining choice for parents and the best start in life for children. The Department for Education and Skills have commissioned a public/private partnership called Together for Children to support local authorities in planning the location and development of centres.

activity
INDIVIDUAL WORK 10.4

P3

M2

In 2004, the government set out a ten-year strategy of key themes to support local authorities in providing services for children and young people. There have been long-standing concerns regarding the achievement of children and young people in the looked-after system.

1   Using the facilities at your college learning resource centre, describe what health and social care provision is available, with particular reference to children and young people in the looked-after system.

2   Identify two organisations offering a service to children and young people and compare the care provided.

Together for Children   www.togetherforchildren.co.uk

information about children's centres

Early Years Foundation Stage

Improvements in early education is a national target for the government and one of the main provisions set out in the Education Act (2002). In England, the **Early Years Foundation Stage** forms part of the National Curriculum, covering education for children aged three until the end of their reception year.

The Foundation Stage Profile is a single national scheme that provides for the effective monitoring of a young child's progress. Early learning goals have been identified within some areas of learning, with stepping stones of progress towards those targets.

Sure Start programmes

The government is committed to promoting the welfare and development of all children and young people. Good quality care, education and play for all children, particularly in the early years, raise educational standards and opportunities and enhance children's social development. Ensuring that childcare services provide secure and safe environments for children and young people can alleviate pressure on families who are economically and socially disadvantaged, which in turn may prevent the admission of children and young people into care.

The Children Act (1989) set out a legal framework for registering and inspecting day care and childminding. Fourteen national standards cover a number of areas including child protection, special needs and care, learning and play.

> **remember**
>
> Registered providers have to meet required ratios of adults to children within settings. There are also requirements for staff qualifications.

Nursery provision

All three-year-olds are entitled to six terms of free nursery education from the term following their third birthday. From 1999, this was introduced for three-year-olds from families considered to have social and economic disadvantage, but became a universal right in April 2004. Local authorities are allocated funding for the provision of free care and can decide how this should be spent according to local needs. While the local authority has a legal duty to provide for all three- and four-year-olds, the rights do not extend to parents being able to choose the facility of their choice.

Extended schools

In June 2005, the Extended Schools Prospectus set out a core offer of services that should be accessible to all children by 2010:

■   A variety of study support activities, for example, homework, sports and music clubs

■   High-quality childcare provided on primary school sites or through local providers, with supervised transfer arrangements where appropriate, available from 8.00 a.m. to 6.00 p.m. all year round

- Parenting support, including information sessions for parents at key transition points, parenting programmes run with the support of other children's services and family learning sessions to allow children to learn with their parents

- Identification of children with particular needs to ensure swift and easy referral to a wide range of specialist support services, such as speech therapy, child and adolescent mental health services, family support services, intensive behavioural support and sexual health services

- ICT, sports and arts facilities and adult learning for the wider community

Every Child Matters   www.everychildmatters.gov.uk

Professional Practice

Many local authorities are running language projects to help parents learn the skills to promote language development of young children. In the Vale of Glamorgan, the language programme deliverers from the Language and Play programme work with local college students to train them. They in turn undertake placements in local playgroups working alongside parents to develop the language skills of their children.

Connexions partnerships

For young people aged 13 to 19, or 25 for young people with learning difficulties or a disability, connexions partnerships provide advice and information about a range of everyday matters.

Fig 10.2 Connexions partnerships

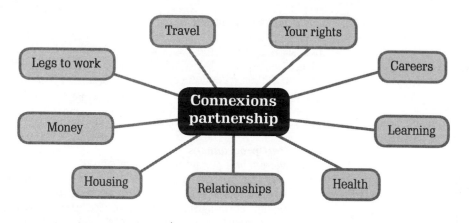

The Connexions service   www.connexions-direct.com.

Voluntary sector

The voluntary sector plays an important role in enabling the government to meet its targets in respect of providing good quality childcare, learning and play opportunities for all young children. The Preschool Learning Alliance is the largest voluntary sector provider of early years education and childcare. The Preschool Learning Alliance has been at the forefront of developing guidance for schools wishing to develop childcare provision, in line with the government's extended schools initiative. The Preschool Learning Alliance has 15,000 members who look after 500,000 young children in England every year.

Preschool Learning Alliance   www.preschool.org.uk

Private providers

In many local authorities, private sector providers are included in the plans to meet the aims of the Sure Start initiative. Private day nurseries are registered with OFSTED and inspected annually. Most nurseries provide care for children up to five and are open from 7.30 a.m. to 6.00 p.m. from Monday to Friday.

Advantages of using private day care nurseries are:

- children can mix socially
- they are geared towards the needs of working parents
- staff are experienced
- they are open all year
- they provide out-of-school care
- they provide opportunities for outdoor play
- they provide opportunities to participate in outings

Young offenders

A **young offender** is a young person who is found guilty of committing a crime. Often, custody is the last resort and when young people get into trouble for committing minor offences or anti-social behaviour, they can be dealt with outside the courts.

Local authority secure children's homes focus on attending to the physical, emotional and behavioural needs of the young people they accommodate. Generally, young offenders aged 12 to 14, girls up to 16 and 15- to 16-year old boys who are considered vulnerable are accommodated in local authority secure children's homes. They are run by the local authority social services department and overseen by the DOH and the DfES. The aims of this provision are to prevent youth crime and to promote the welfare of young people.

Young offenders institutions replaced borstals and detention centres in the 1980s. A sentenced prisoner under the age of 21 years will be placed in one of two types of secure accommodation:

- Secure training centres which are run by a private operator and house vulnerable young people who are sentenced to custody in a secure environment. They will receive education and rehabilitation
- Youth offending institutions which are run by the prison service and accommodate 15- to 21-year-olds. They have lower ratios of staff to young people and generally accommodate large numbers.

Job roles

Director of Children's Services
The Children Act (2004) required every unitary local authority (in England) to appoint a Director of Children's Services, who is professionally accountable for the delivery of education and social service functions for children, and for any health function delegated to the local authority by a NHS body.

Social workers
Social workers help people with their lives in a variety of contexts. They can work with families where there is domestic abuse, in situations of child abuse, with children and people with disabilities, assist with fostering or adoption and work with young people who misuse substances such as drugs or alcohol.

Foster parents
Foster parents offer children and young people a home while their own parents are unable to look after them. Foster parents can be all ages and backgrounds, living in all kinds of homes. They can be married, single, working, unemployed or retired but what they have in common is a desire to make a difference to a young person's life.

Support workers
Support workers can work in a variety of settings helping children and young people with a range of everyday living tasks. This can include helping people with personal care, supporting them during a college day or on an outing, for example, a trip using public transport.

MacIntyre   www.macintyrecharity.org.uk

Details of the role of a support worker

Residential care staff
Staff in children's residential care work closely with children and young people, parents, other family members, foster carers and other agencies to promote better lives for children and young people.

Tutors

Tutors are qualified professional teachers who take responsibility for managing a course and providing pastoral support for students on the course.

Lecturers

Lecturers are qualified to teach post-16 and will have an industrial or professional background in the subject area they are delivering.

Nurses

Registered nurses make up the largest health care occupation with 2.4 million jobs. Three of every five are working in a hospital setting but nurses can also work in the community and in specialist settings, such as MacMillan nurses who care for people with terminal cancer. They perform basic duties that include treating patients, educating patients and the public about medical conditions and providing advice and emotional support to patients' family members.

Health visitors

Every family who has a child under five will come into contact with a health visitor, who will commence a child health promotion programme 14 days after the birth of a baby. The role of the health visitor is to give advice to families and carers on a range of issues around the needs of the developing child.

Educational psychologists

Educational psychologists play a key role in the statutory assessment and **statementing** process for children with special educational needs. Their role is to work alongside all those involved with a child to find a solution to problems relating to behaviour, communication, learning, and so on.

Counsellors

Counsellors work with children and young people who may have had a bereavement, have low self-esteem or have suffered abuse. They are trained in different styles and approaches to counselling. They aim to work with the child and young person to help them:

- see their situation more clearly
- understand what is making them unhappy
- develop the best course of action
- come to the right decision for them.

Nursing, health care and social care assistants

Nursing, health care and social care assistants work with children and young people with a disability or **learning difficulty** to support independence and help access leisure and play opportunities.

Education welfare officers

The Education Welfare Act (2000) set up a National Education Welfare Board which appoints education welfare officers to work with schools, teachers, parents and community or voluntary bodies to encourage regular school attendance and develop strategies to reduce absenteeism.

Learning mentors

Learning mentors came about after the Excellence in Cities (EiC) initiative and work in primary, secondary and college settings. They work with pupils and students to help them address barriers to learning. EiC is a government initiative to address the under achievement in education and the low aspirations of young people from disadvantaged backgrounds. It aims to drive up educational standards in major cities.

The Standards Site   www.standards.dfes.gov.uk

Play therapists

A play therapist is trained to use play to understand and communicate with children about feelings, thoughts and behaviour. An important aspect of **play therapy** is to develop a therapeutic (healing) relationship between the child and play therapist to help the child feel safe and understood.

Play workers

A play worker's role is to plan, organise and supervise play activities for children and young people aged 5 to 15. This can include team games and sports, arts and crafts, drama, dance, music and cooking. Their role includes supervising children and ensuring health and safety procedures are followed.

Connexions advisers
Connexions is a support service for young people aged 13 to 19. The idea is that the young person will have a personal advisor to offer support in areas such as learning and work choices, housing, family matters, health and other matters.

Fig 10.3 Connexions adviser

Connexions	www.connexions.gov.uk

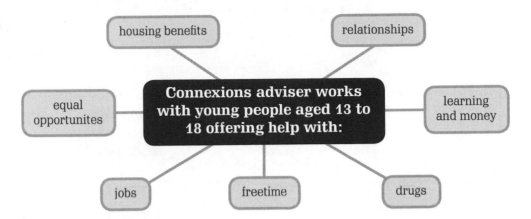

Early years workers
Early years workers work in a variety of settings. They may work alongside qualified teachers in state nursery or reception classes, in private nurseries with children aged between six weeks and five years old, in hospital settings with children with health problems, in voluntary organisations or Sure Start settings. All share a common responsibility to provide a safe, secure and stimulating environment.

Youth workers
Youth workers work in a range of settings including youth centres, youth clubs, schools, churches and youth offending teams using a variety of methods such as organising leisure activities to providing guidance and counselling.

Youth justice workers
Youth justice workers work with children and young people aged 10 to 17 who have either offended or are at risk of offending. The majority of young people who have offended more than once will be put in touch with a youth justice worker whose role is to supervise them in the community.

Prison officers
Prison officers work within prison settings with responsibility for security, enforcing the rules, calming tension and dealing with difficult and challenging behaviour.

Fig 10.4 Roles and responsibilities of a prison officer

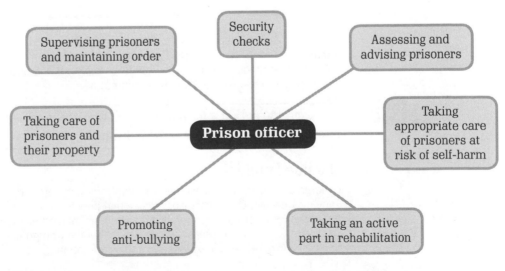

The risks to children and young people of abusive and exploitative behaviour

Risk of abuse

Within family

While many families under great stress manage to raise their children in a warm, loving and secure environment, where their needs are met and they are safe from harm, sources of stress within a family can have a negative impact upon child development. This may be because it affects the capacity of parents to respond to their child's needs.

Fig 10.5 Sources of stress

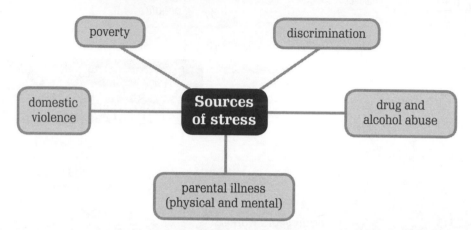

> **remember**
>
> Local Safeguarding Children's Boards (LSCB) were created under the Children Act (2004) as the statutory body responsible for protecting children at risk of significant harm.

case study 10.6

Suzanne and Rob

Suzanne had been living with Rob and their two children for eight years. When Rob lost his job as a steel worker, four years ago, he became very depressed. After months of unsuccessful job applications, he became withdrawn, spending most of the day watching television and every evening in the pub. He began to get angry with Suzanne and the children and, more recently, began to threaten Suzanne with violence. As the debt mounted and Rob became angrier, Suzanne left and went to stay with a friend several miles away. With the help of a friend, she got a job in a local café and moved into a rented flat. Although she is frightened of Rob, she is thinking of returning to him, as she is lonely living in an area where she does not have many contacts.

activity
GROUP WORK

Consider each of the sources of stress in figure 10.5. Making use of ICT facilities and publications in the college learning resource centre, carry out a short research activity to identify what is available in your area to support families under stress.

Most families who become caught up in the child protection system are at risk of **social exclusion**. The SSI report 'Child Protection: Messages from Research' shows that many have multiple problems which need careful assessment and targeted intervention by local authorities, to ensure that children are not put at risk.

See page 130 in Unit 4 for more information about how life factors and events can influence the development of the individual.

Outside family

Children and young people who go missing from home are a particularly vulnerable group. They may encounter a number of risks. Young people who sleep rough or stay with someone they have only just met are more likely to be hurt than other runaways and those who sleep rough are vulnerable to sexual assault. Young people who go missing from home or care are at risk of violence, sexual exploitation and victimisation.

In care settings

The recruitment and retention of skilled and experienced staff has a major impact upon safeguarding arrangements for children and young people who are looked after. During the 1970s and 80s, the risks to children and young people living away from home in residential homes, foster care and residential schools were seriously under-estimated. In 1997 to 98, the Department of Health received reports of 91 cases of children dying or suffering serious injury at the hands of adult abusers.

Link   See page 361 in Unit 11 for information on the potential for abuse in health and care settings.

Risks of exploitation from visual, written and electronic forms of communication and media

There have been concerns about the risks posed to children and young people, both directly and indirectly through the use of photographs on websites and other publications. Photographs, when accompanied with personal information, can be used as a means of identifying children. This information can make a child vulnerable to an individual who may wish to start to 'groom' that child for abuse. There is also the danger that the content of the photograph can be used or adapted for inappropriate use.

Professional Practice

- Consider using a model or an illustration if you are promoting an activity.
- Avoid the use of first names and surnames in a photograph to reduce the risk of unsolicited attention.
- Always obtain written consent from parents before taking photographs.

The following key principles should always be adopted in relation to the use of photographs and recorded images:

- Parents or carers and children have a right to decide whether children's images are to be taken and how those images may be used.
- Parents or carers and children must provide written consent for children's images to be taken and used.
- Care should be taken to ensure that images are not sexual or exploitative in nature and not open to obvious misinterpretation and misuse.
- All images of children should be stored securely.
- When images are used on websites, particular care must be taken to ensure that no identifying features facilitate contact with a child by a potential abuser.
- Never publish personal details of a child or young person, such as an email address or telephone number.

Family functioning

Family types and partnership arrangements

The type of family a child grows up in has a significant impact on their well-being. The quality of family interactions is the main factor affecting children's development.

Changing face of the family

During the 20th century, the family in Britain has gone through significant change. One of the most notable changes has been the rise in lone-person households. In addition, attitudes towards divorce have changed. In the past, people got married and stayed married. In part, this was due to the lack of choice faced by women, as women had limited economic power and were dependant upon a husband's income. Divorce was complicated, expensive and tended to take a lot of time. Other factors that have changed the face of family life include the rise in the number of children born to parents who are cohabiting while the average age of women giving birth has also risen.

Fig 10.6 Family types

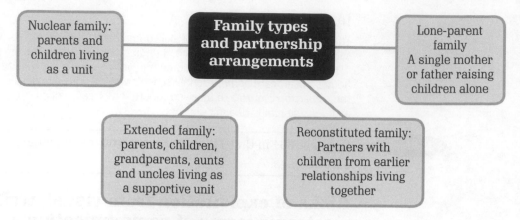

Percentage of dependant children living in different family types

Family type	Percentage
Coupled families	76%
Lone-mother families	22%
Lone-father families	2%

Social disadvantage

In September 2006, the Department for Education and Skills and the Department of Health launched Reaching Out, an action plan to address the social exclusion and disadvantage still experienced by some families. Sure Start centres throughout Britain are already providing support to families who are socially disadvantaged.

Different concepts of discipline

There are different ways of ensuring that a child and young person behaves in a way that is acceptable to their family and socially acceptable. Discipline does not mean punishment and different children and young people respond to different approaches. There have been long-standing debates about smacking but professional thought is that, whilst smacking may have an instant impact upon behaviour, it does nothing to change unwanted behaviour in the long term.

Abuse within families

Child sexual abuse can take place within the family by a parent, a step-parent, sibling or other relative. The child may feel afraid to break away from the abuser due to fear of the anger or shame of other family members, or because the abuser threatens the child with violence or loss of love.

Cultural variations

In some cultures, a practice known as female circumcision is common. Supporters of the practice, which is usually carried out in western and southern Asia, the Middle East and large parts of Africa, often by untrained people, claim it is done for cultural and religious reasons. Girls as young as three can undergo the process but the age varies from country to country.

remember
While child abuse occurs in all social classes, factors such as poverty, social exclusion and poor housing can affect how a family functions and how parents are able to care for their children.

remember
A child whose mother is living with a boyfriend is 33 more times likely to be exposed to physical or sexual abuse than if he or she is in a two-parent married family.

Due to health campaigns, female circumcision has been falling in some countries in the last decade. In Kenya, in 1991, a survey found that 78% of teenagers had been circumcised compared to 100% of women over 50. (https://news.bbc.co.uk)

Predisposing factors

Predisposing factors in relation to the abuser

Substance abuse

Misuse of drugs, alcohol or solvents may affect the ability of parents to care for the emotional, physical and developmental needs of their children. Due to the fact that substance abuse is generally frowned upon in society, parents may try to hide their problems and not seek help for fear that their children may be taken away from them.

It has been estimated that the number of children who may be exposed to the consequences of drug misuse in the UK is between 250,000 and 350,000, while around two million children are affected by parent's harmful drinking.

Social Care Institute for Excellence   www.scie.org.uk

Lack of knowledge about children's needs

Many of the more recent initiatives in social policy recognise the importance of good parenting as a key factor in addressing social inequality. For some parents or carers, their own experience of childhood has lacked an awareness of what children need to thrive and flourish. Parents may feel that experts, such as teachers, should be responsible for their children's learning or GPs responsible for their children's health.

---

case study 10.7

Lindsay and May

At 15, Lindsay had a baby daughter, May. She had been doing well at school but the pregnancy had disrupted her education during her GCSE year. After the baby's birth, Lindsay started attending the young parents group co-run by Sure Start and the local college, attending classes in key skills and taster sessions in craft, design, parenting and nutrition. May was placed in the college nursery. At 16, Lindsay and May moved into a flat provided through a local housing association. May was a calm, placid baby who usually slept through the night. One weekend, Lindsay was invited to a party at a friend's house. She decided to leave May in her cot and join the party for a few hours.

activity
INDIVIDUAL WORK

1   Can Lindsay's action be considered to be neglect?
2   What are the possible indicators of abuse in this case study?

Lack of attachment

The bonding process begins even before a child is born. During the nine months in the womb, a child requires good nutrition and careful avoidance of substances such as alcohol. During the child's first three years, he or she will be exposed, in a healthy situation, to love, nurturing and care which will enable the child to bond with parents or carers. If this bonding cycle is interrupted, problems can occur. A child born into an environment of neglect and abuse may fail to bond with his parents or carers and is likely to suffer from a range of problems. Through careful observation, early years workers should be able to identify when babies and children have made attachments.

Four broad indicators of attachment are:

■   actively seeking to be near the other person

■   crying or showing visible distress when that person leaves or, for babies, is no longer visible

■   showing joy or relief when that person appears

■   acute awareness of that person's presence, for example, looking up at them from time to time, responding to their voices, following their movements.

Fig 10.7 Bonding cycle

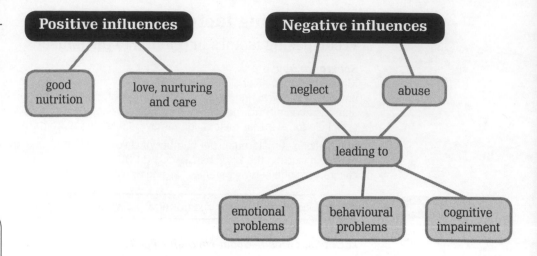

What is attachment?
A special enduring form of emotional relationship with a specific person (www.childtrauma. org.uk)

Lack of role models

The idea of role models has long been recognised by social learning theorists. Bandura (1969) was a proponent of the idea that much of the learning that occurs in child development is acquired through observation and imitation. Parents who have not had good role models to follow themselves may not be able to find strategies to manage children's behaviour positively.

Social problems

Factors such as poverty, poor housing, unemployment, social exclusion are all stress factors which can affect parent's ability to properly care for their children.

Mental illness

Many children will grow up in a family where a parent has a mental illness. Short-lived illnesses can usually be treated by the GP, but for some children, they may be living with a parent who has a long-term debilitating mental illness, such as manic depression. According to the Royal College of Psychiatrists, in long-term situations like these, children may:

- be separated from parents if they require regular admission to hospital for treatment
- not be looked after properly
- be hurt or mistreated
- have to care for siblings
- be upset or afraid of their parent's behaviour

Personality

If parents have lacked a good role model of parenting, this can impact upon their parenting skills. No consistent personality traits have been linked to parents or carers who mistreat children, but characteristics which can impact upon child abuse include:

- low self-esteem
- feelings of lack of control over one's life
- depression
- anxiety

Predisposing factors in relation to the child or young person

Prematurity

One in ten babies are born prematurely in Britain each year. Many are so tiny that they cannot be held and this can interrupt the bonding process in the early stages.

See page 327 for more information about the importance of bonding.

Disability

For many families, raising a child with a disability can trigger stress factors which may affect their ability to parent. These include a sense of loss for the child they thought they had, accompanied by a shift in hopes and expectations. The strain of caring for someone around the clock accompanied by lack of sleep can also affect the ability to parent well. Families raising children with a disability are often socially isolated, having to attend lots of specialist appointments and losing out on the natural network of support that many parents find at the school gate.

Types of abuse and neglect

Abuse

Physical

Physical abuse is intentional physical harm to a child or young person. Growing children often have minor accidents resulting in bruises and grazes so it is important that the early years practitioner is able to distinguish between accidental and non-accidental injuries.
In the 1960s, American paediatrician Dr Henry Kempe coined the phrase 'battered child syndrome', a term that engaged public sympathy for the phenomenon of abuse.

Emotional

When a person they love or trust abuses them, children understandably become distressed and confused. Emotional abuse is present in all other types of abuse and leads to low self-esteem and lack of self-worth.

Intellectual abuse

The notion of intellectual abuse has been recently introduced although this category is not widely recognised within social care and welfare. It refers to situations when a child's thinking, or ideas are belittled or disregarded. Parents or carers may leave little scope for children to think things through for themselves, limiting their ability to problem solve.

Sexual abuse

Kempe defined sexual abuse as 'the involvement of dependent, developmentally immature children and adolescent in sexual activities they do not truly comprehend, to which they are unable to give informed consent, or that violate the social taboos of the family roles'. Kempe applied theories around attachment to child abuse and neglect, concluding that mothers who abused their children suffered from poor attachment experiences in their own childhood.

Neglect

Physical neglect

The physical effects of neglect can have significant impact upon a child's development. In 1990, Kempe defined neglect as 'a very insidious form of maltreatment which can go on for a long time. It implies the failure of the parents to act properly on safe-guarding the health, safety and well-being of the child. It includes nutritional neglect, failure to provide care or to protect a child from physical and social danger'.

Emotional neglect

Emotional neglect can include acts such as belittling a child, causing a child to view himself or herself in a way that is consistent with their parents' or carer's words. Being cold towards a child deprives a child of the confidence to explore and learn their social environment and will inevitably lead to an impairment in adult relationships.

Intellectual neglect

Failing to teach a child the moral rights expected in a democratic society, or encouraging children or young people to engage in lawless or anti-social behaviour impairs their ability to function in normal society.

Bullying and harassment

Bullying can mean different things. Childline has complied a list of bullying experiences as documented by children and young people who have contacted them:

- Being called names
- Being teased
- Being pushed or pulled about
- Being hit or attacked
- Having your bag and other possessions taken and thrown around
- Being ignored or left out
- Being forced to hand over money or possessions
- Being attacked or teased or called names because of your religion or colour
- Being attacked or teased or called names because of your sexuality

Harassment, sometimes called 'hate crime' can include damage to property, unprovoked assault, abusive correspondence and oral abuse.

Indicators of abuse

Physical indicators

- Bruises on soft areas of the body (inner arms, thighs, buttocks)
- Fingertip bruising on the face (maybe caused by forced bottle-feeding)
- Unusual shaped bruises
- Thumb and fingertip bruises on sides of torso
- Unexplained injuries, including bruises, burns, scalds, black eyes and fractures
- Pain or itching in the genital area (but this could be due to threadworm or thrush)
- Bite marks
- Underweight (can be a sign that a child's nutritional needs are not being met, indicating neglect)
- Poor personal hygiene (children may appear to be dirty and unkempt)
- Frequent minor infections, mainly due to inappropriate nutrition and being run down
- Failure to thrive (no obvious medical problem but failure to gain weight can indicate neglect)
- Pinpoint haemorrhage in the ears can be caused by shaking

remember

A dog bite will look very different to a human bite. Small children sometimes bite but an adult bite is much larger than a child's.

Link

See page 356 in Unit 11 for more information about the different types of abuse and indicators of abuse in health and social care settings.

Behaviour indicators

- The child may withdraw from forming relationships with their peers, avoiding inviting them home to tea or to play.
- Changes in behaviour, such as aggression or hostility, may indicate physical abuse.
- Children who have been subjected to abuse may show distress at being with a particular adult or may become upset when undressing for PE.
- Behaviours such as rocking or head banging are perceived as self-comforting behaviour by children who may have suffered neglect.
- A possible sign of neglect is a hungry child who may constantly be looking for extra food and who may scavenge.
- Children may show reluctance to leave with a particular adult/s and display distress at home time.
- Children who have suffered neglect and a lack of parental interest in their development may lack confidence and have a low opinion of their worth.
- If a child has not had access to common childhood experiences, such as being read to or sung to, or access to creative play, such as cooking and playdough, they are likely to struggle in nursery or school.

case study 10.8

Matthew's falls

Matthew is four years old and has been attending the nursery class in which you are the classroom assistant for just over half a term. He has had a variety of minor injuries during this time, all occurring outside of nursery hours. They include a black eye, a broken tooth and cut lip and other less obvious bruising (a large bruise on his shoulder and marks on his back). Matthew says he keeps falling out of his bunk bed.

Matthew has been away from the nursery for three days. When he arrives today, he has another bruise under his eye. He says he fell out of bed. He becomes quite aggressive towards staff members when this explanation was queried by a staff member.

activity
GROUP WORK

Why might staff be concerned about Matthew?

Consequences of abuse

Emotional

Fig 10.8 Emotional effects

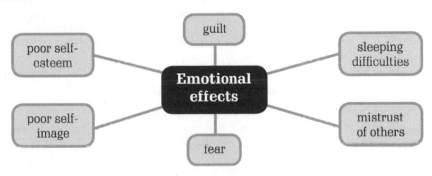

Social

Fig 10.9 Social effects

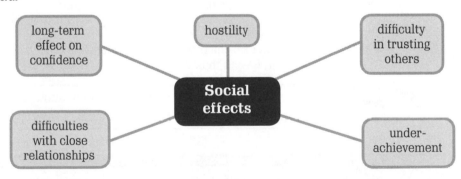

Physical

Fig 10.10 Physical effects

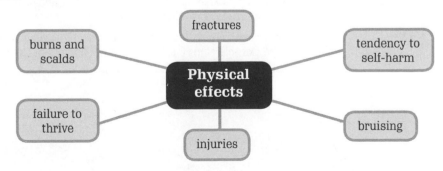

Models of abuse

There are many factors that contribute to abuse and neglect of children but one thing is very clear, abuse is not restricted to any class, culture, race or religion.

Medical model

Early researchers coined the phrase ' battered child syndrome' which led to the causes of child abuse being viewed as a disease with specific signs and symptoms. By presenting child abuse in this way, it led people to believe it was preventable and curable.

Sociological model

Sociological research has concentrated on the changing patterns of society and how this has affected family functioning. Unemployment, poverty, poor housing, poor health care and social exclusion are all cited as reasons for people abusing their children. If this were the case, one could expect all child abuse to occur in families who are classed as social class 5 on the Registrar General's Social Scale. However, statistics show that child abuse occurs across all social classes.

Psychological model

Psychologists have suggested theories which relate to the way a family functions as a family and refers to the breakdown of these relationships as 'family dysfunction'. This theory, or model, suggests that family therapy can repair poor relationships and thus prevent child abuse.

Feminist model

These theories are based mainly on sexual politics and examine the power relationship between men and women. Feminists argue that a patriarchal (male-dominated) society regards children as possessions at the disposal of male members of the family. This model ignores the fact that many abusers are women.

Recognition of abuse where children or young people cannot communicate

Babies and very young children

Most babies and young children are cared for and protected by loving and caring parents. According to the NSPCC, statistically, children under one year are most at risk of abuse and neglect. A baby crying constantly can trigger a tired parent to hit out or shake them. Bruising in babies under one year is usually considered a sign of abuse.

Children with alternative forms of communication

There are many children who are not able to express themselves through spoken language. There are a range of augmentative communication strategies used to help these children to communicate, such as the Pictorial Exchange Communication System (PECS) or objects of reference. It is important that there is a member of the multi-disciplinary team who can communicate with the child using their preferred method.

> **remember**
>
> Never shake a baby: it is dangerous. Babies cry because it is their way of communicating their needs such as hunger or discomfort. A parent responding to a baby crying is demonstrating a nurturing and protective role.

Link See page 55 in Unit 2 for more information about alternative methods of communication, such as PECS or objects of reference.

---

activity
INDIVIDUAL WORK
10.5

P4

According to the NSPCC, 'child abuse is the term used when an adult harms a child or young person under the age of 18'. While it is generally held that child abuse can take four forms (physical abuse, emotional abuse, neglect and sexual abuse), bullying and domestic violence are also forms of child abuse.

Visit www.nspcc.org.uk and using bullet points, produce a checklist for a new employee to show the possible signs and symptoms of all forms of child abuse.

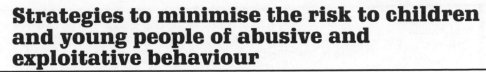

Strategies to minimise the risk to children and young people of abusive and exploitative behaviour

Strategies with children and young people

Person-centred approach

The Framework for Assessment of Children in Need and their Families recommends that all agencies adopt a **person-centred approach** to working with children and young people. National voluntary organisations such as Circles Network work in a person-centred way to support children, young people and vulnerable adults who are at risk of social exclusion.

See page 333 for more information about the Framework for Assessment of Children in Need and their Families.

Provide active support

The National Service Frameworks for Children, Young People and Maternity Services, launched in 2005 states that 'all children and young people achieve optimum health and well-being and are supported in achieving their potential'.

Refer back to page 317 for more information about the National Service Frameworks for Children, Young People and Maternity Services.

Every young person, irrespective of their needs wants:

- friends, fun, meaningful activity, a comfortable home, money, relationships, support for good health
- to be given information about what is available for their situation, in a format that is meaningful for them
- to know what their options are
- to be confident that their needs will be met without stigma
- help with development of skills to pursue meaningful employment or activity
- choice and opportunities
- to be valued for who they are and who they may become and not seen as a diagnosis or parental construct
- supported independence
- support to make difficult decisions and take risks (particularly in relation to health issues)
- a break.

Care Services Improvement Partnership   www.integratedcarenetwork.gov.uk

Importance of promoting empowerment, assertiveness, self-confidence, self-esteem and resilience

It is an important part of the role of the early years practitioner to teach children that it is acceptable to say 'no' to adults when they feel uncomfortable.

In 1993, the National Pyramid Trust (known formerly as Pyramid) was set up to help children from 5 to 12 fulfil their potential in school and in life by building self-esteem and resilience. They aim to: 'provide support within the community and educational settings to quiet, withdrawn or isolated children who are finding it difficult to integrate or make friends, helping them to develop social and emotional confidence and well-being.'

Pyramid works by organising activity clubs in primary schools for pupils who are shy, withdrawn or having difficulties making friends. Using strategies such as games, cookery, arts and crafts, they can help these children. A range of outcomes for the young people involved have been identified:

- A sense of belonging
- Increased self-esteem and confidence
- Ability to make new friendships
- Improved academic performance
- More willingness to participate
- Better relationships with peers and adults
- Improvement in self concept
- Better social skills

Pyramid for information on Pyramid activity clubs and parenting groups.
www.nptrust.org.uk

Sharing information and not keeping secrets

An important part of the role of the early years practitioner is to teach children about:

- good and bad secrets
- saying 'no' to adults they know as well as strangers
- that their body belongs to them
- where they can get help
- good and bad touching
- privacy

Some strategies that can be used to promote self protection include the 'Private Triangle' and 'Colour in the personal space'.

Fig 10.11 Sharing information

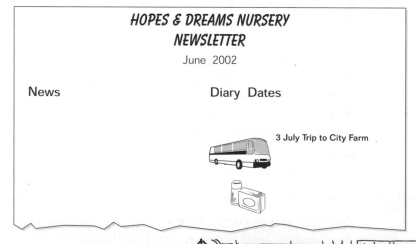

HOPES & DREAMS NURSERY NEWSLETTER

June 2002

News   **Diary Dates**

3 July Trip to City Farm

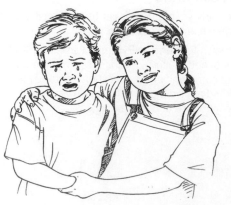

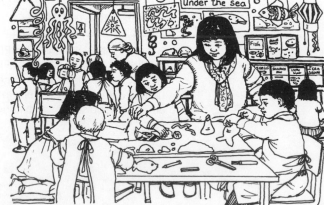

Providing information to children according to their age, needs and abilities

How to respect their bodies and keep safe

There are a number of commercial resources, such as the *Cosmo and Dibs Keeping Safe* video which features short, fun safety stories suitable for children aged 3 to 6 and available from Kidscape.

Kidscape	www.kidscape.org.uk

Making sure that children develop an awareness of body parts through games such as 'head, shoulders, knees and toes', promoting good physical care routines in dressing and undressing for PE or dance, ensuring children know their address and home telephone number, all help children to keep safe.

Transmission of disease

The best approach to avoiding transmission of disease is by **empowering** children to know that their body belongs to them. Good physical care routines as described above, openness about 'good' and 'bad' touching and 'good' and 'bad' secrets all empower children to know that it is fine to disobey adults in situations where they feel uncomfortable or unsafe.

Working with parents and families

Partnerships with parents and families

Legislation and policies over the last decade have underpinned the importance of working in partnership with parents and families. The clear message to early year's practitioners in Every Child Matters: Change for Children is that parents, carers and families should be supported in order to improve outcomes for children. In particular, the government made a commitment to ensure that specialist support was available at local levels for families. This included structured parenting groups.

Every Child Matters	www.everychildmatters.gov.uk
information on health-led parenting support groups	

Partnership legislation

The Children Act (1989)	Promotes the principles of working in partnership with parents . This includes working with parents by means of voluntary arrangements when seeking court orders
Working together to Safeguard Children (1999)	Sets out how organisations should work together to safeguard and promote children's welfare. It is a government priority delivered through the Every Child Matters: Change for Children programme that advice, information and signposting to other services should be available to all parents
Framework for Assessment of Children in Need and their Families (2000)	Focuses specifically on children in need; aims to reduce the bureaucracy in making multi-disciplinary assessment of need, further reducing the pressure upon parents

Involving parents in the assessment of children's needs

Unified assessments are considered to provide a person-centred approach to managing care. The process requires statutory agencies to work together to provide care in a joined-up manner. The needs of parents or carers must be taken into account when planning services for children and young people. The Common Assessment Framework provides a nationally standardised approach to assessment, aiming to reduce bureaucracy for families and also reduce the number of separate assessments a child and family may have to undertake.

Helping parents recognise the value and significance of their contributions

The Every Child Matters: Change for Children programme has as its central theme a recognition of the importance of parents, carers and families in influencing what happens in a child's life.

The Integrated Care Network is a national initiative with members from health and social care in both the independent and voluntary sectors. It aims to improve commissioning for health and social care services. It is independent, accounting to local health and social care providers.

The Integrated Care Network identified that parents and carers needed:

- support with their child's growing independence, decision making and risk taking
- information about options for independence, such as housing, employment and leisure
- support for their own changing role
- a break
- practical support as the physical demands of a growing child become greater
- benefits advice and financial support if the young person is leaving the family home
- advice about employment or career options and personal development

Care Services Improvement Partnership   www.integratedcarenetwork.gov.uk

Encourage the development of parenting skills

There are many strategies that can be used by the early years practitioner to promote and develop parenting skills. For example, early years workers can model good practice through their interactions with children. Many parents may have had a poor experience of childhood, with limited play opportunities. Sharing ideas, offering workshops to teach a skill, such as making playdough, inviting parents into a setting and involving them in the planned activities are all ways of developing skills.

Sure Start   www.surestart.gov.uk

more about the government's strategy for developing parenting skills

Procedures where abuse is suspected or confirmed
Policies of the setting

It is important that organisations have a proper child protection policy and procedures for dealing with issues of concern.

Professional Practice

A policy should establish the following principles:

- The welfare of the child is paramount.
- All children without exception have the right to protection from abuse.
- All suspicions and allegations of abuse will be taken seriously and responded to swiftly and appropriately.

The Children Act (2004) established Local Safeguarding Children's Boards to encourage key agencies to work together. They came into effect on April 1st 2006 and replaced Area Child Protection Committees.

Safe working practices that protect children, young people and adults who work with them

Key documents support provision in the Children Act (2004), including 'Guidance on the duty to make arrangements to safeguard and promote the welfare of children', which sets out key arrangements agencies should make to safeguard and promote the welfare of children in the course of their normal duties.

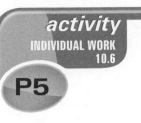

activity
**INDIVIDUAL WORK
10.6**

P5

You are employed as a nursery nurse in a Sure Start setting. There are twin girls who attend on a daily basis. They are nearly two years old. Both girls are usually tired and always hungry. They have had colds and an ear infection for nearly two weeks but, while the mother acknowledges that they are unwell, she has not visited the GP. Both children do not engage in any of the play activities, wanting to be held by a favourite member of staff and crying if she tries to put them down. Today, one child has bruises on both arms. You and your colleague are concerned about their well-being.

Describe your response to your suspicion of child abuse, referring to the procedures and policies in your current placement setting and current legislation.

Adults working with children and young people in a variety of settings are in a position of trust. It is important that employers provide detailed guidance on safe working practices.

Teaching Personnel   www.teachingpersonnel.com

detailed guidance on developing safe working practices

Professional Practice

- Adults working with children and young people should not use their position to gain access to information for their own advantage.

- Adults working with children and young people should not use their position to form relationships with children and young people which are of a sexual nature.

- Adults should treat information they receive about children and young people confidentially.

- In some circumstances where abuse is alleged or suspected, a member of staff may be expected to share information about children.

- Adults should be aware of the guidance from their employer regarding the giving or receipt of gifts.

remember

'Working together to safeguard children' defines sexual abuse as 'forcing or enticing a child or young person to take part in sexual activities whether or not the child is aware of what is happening'.

Whistle blowing

Under the Public Interest Disclosure Act (1998), each employer is required to provide a clear and accessible whistle-blowing policy.

Lines of reporting, accurate reporting and security of records

The Data Protection Act (1998) covers all personal data about children and young people. All settings working with children and young people can expect their employer to have a clear system in place for recording serious incidents. It should also be made clear to staff the means by which information about incidents can be accessed by senior management.

See page 71 in Unit 2 for more information about the Data Protection Act (1998).

Child Protection Register

remember

The Department for Education and skills provides detailed guidance to adults working with children and young people about recording data.

Following an initial concern or referral from family, friends or neighbours, an early years worker or health service professional, consideration will be given to a child's immediate safety. If a child is considered to be at immediate risk, an emergency protection order can be granted under the Children Act (1989), compelling parents to produce the child and allowing the local authority to remove him or her to a place of safety. Alternatively, the police have powers to remove a child. If a child's immediate safety is certain, details of the concern will be passed to the duty team manager and a duty team social worker will make initial enquiries. Following initial enquiries, a duty manager will decide if a child protection investigation is necessary. A full investigation will be carried out under section 47 of the Children Act. If parents or carers refuse to co-operate, a child assessment order can be obtained to compel some co-operation.

A child protection conference is the next stage in this sequence of events, bringing together the family and other relevant professionals with information to share. On the basis of this evidence, the conference decides whether to place the child on the **Child Protection Register**. A child's name will only be placed on the register if the child protection conference so decides and only when registration criteria are met.

Children can be placed on the register as early as birth or before birth. In some cases, while the child is not placed on the register, further work may still be undertaken with the family. Once a child is placed on the register, a core group, consisting of a key worker, relevant professionals, parents and the child if deemed old enough will be formed whose remit is to develop a child protection plan.

Roles and responsibilities

Following policies and procedures of the setting

Child protection procedures should be linked in with the procedures of Local Children's Safeguarding Boards or the All-Wales Child Protection Procedures, as relevant. These procedures should include giving a named person a clearly defined role and responsibility in relation to child protection.

In addition, Child Protection procedures should include:

- a code of behaviour for trustees, staff and volunteers
- safe recruitment, selection and vetting procedures including Criminal Record Bureau checks
- a well publicised complaints procedure in which adults and children can voice concerns
- systems to ensure staff are monitored and supervised.

Observation

During activities such as dance, swimming or PE, or with younger children, during nappy changing, you may notice signs that cause you concern, such as bruises. It is important that you make a written record of your concerns, which must be dated and signed. In law, such facts are not legally admissible if they are not recorded within 24 hours. You must also be aware of the child protection policy within your setting which will require you to alert your manager or the designated child protection officer of your concerns.

Appropriate recording and reporting

Procedures should include a process for recording incidents, concerns and referrals and storing these securely in compliance with relevant legislation.

Fig 10.12 Blank diagram of child to use in noting abuse

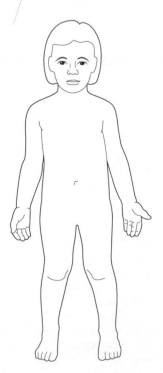
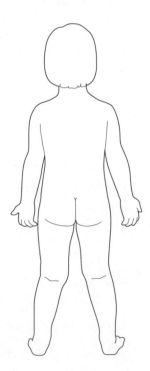

Recognising signs and symptoms of abuse
Procedures should also include a description of what child abuse is and the procedures of how to respond to concerns.

Knowing how to respond following disclosure
When a child chooses to disclose (inform about abuse), the most important thing is to listen to what is being said. A child may often choose an inconvenient moment but it is important to hear what is being said and to note the child's body language. Avoid direct questions and use reflective listening. Children usually want to please the adults around them and may agree to questions to achieve this. It is important that you do not promise to keep a secret, nor criticise the person who has hurt the child. Following the **disclosure**, you have a responsibility to make notes as soon as possible and within the same day. You also need to consult the child protection officer in your setting.

Maintaining confidentiality according to the policies of the setting
The health or social care setting should offer guidance on confidentiality and information sharing. It is the responsibility of the health and social care worker to know what these policies are.

NSPCC   www.nspcc.org.uk
Information on developing and updating safeguarding policies and procedures

Disclosure

Direct
Children may choose you as the trusted adult to disclose abuse to. In this situation, it is important to listen carefully and allow the child to share information at his or her own pace. Avoid asking direct questions and be aware of your body language. Tell the child that you believe them (young children rarely lie or imagine abuse). Any disclosure of abuse will challenge you. Make sure that you do not promise to keep what is being told a secret as you must report what you have been told.

Indirect
A child may indicate abuse through their play. You may observe a child handling dolls or teddies roughly or threatening them verbally. They may use a safe medium such as paint, clay or playdough to express their emotions. It is still important to keep an **accurate record** of your concerns and to share them with the designated child protection officer.

Listening carefully and attentively, communicating at the child or young person's own pace and without undue pressure
If you find yourself in a position where a child is disclosing abuse to you, you need to respond in a way that will support the child. Try not to fill the silences which children may use to organise their thoughts. Avoid leading questions, as younger children usually want to please an adult and may try to guess the 'right' answer.

Professional Practice

- Attempt to make the child secure and safe.
- Give reassurance that you believe what they are saying.
- Avoid looking shocked, however troubled you may feel.
- Do not express any criticism of the perpetrator.
- Do not make any promises that you may not be able to fulfil.
- Make sure the child knows that they are not to blame.

Taking the child or young person seriously, and reassuring and supporting them
It is only comparatively recently that society has listened to children seriously when they have tried to share aspects of their home life which may give cause for concern. If you think that there is any possibility of abuse, the most important skill you can use is to listen carefully.

Professional Practice

- Give the child time to talk to you, where possible in a quiet place, without distractions.
- Do not complete a child's sentence.
- Observe the child's body language.
- Note your own body language and the message you may be conveying.
- Take care not to ask any leading questions, or to jump to conclusions.

Unconditional acceptance

Unconditional acceptance, whereby the early years practitioner responds to the child or young person with empathy and gives a positive message, is at the heart of the approach adopted by Carl Rogers, an American psychologist.

See page 284 in Unit 8 for more information about the work of Carl Rogers.

Boundaries of confidentiality

The NSPCC states that for those who work with children and young people, it is vital that they are trained in recognising the signs and symptoms of abuse. They need also to understand the implications of confidentiality. The NSPCC offers training in Child Welfare and Child Protection with a range of courses reflecting National Standards in Training and Development.

Source www.nspcc,org.uk

Promptly following the correct procedures for the setting

Each setting will have a lead member of staff with responsibility for child protection. This staff member will have received specific training to support them in the role and ongoing support. He or she should be known to every member of staff. While every member of staff should take responsibility in being alert to possible signs of abuse, they should also be clear that, in the first instance, their responsibility is to report their concerns to the lead member of staff.

How to deal with own feelings and emotions

Those with lead responsibility for co-ordinating child protection have a responsibility to staff who have raised concerns about a child. This should include keeping them informed of decisions made and actions being taken. However, it is inevitable that issues around child abuse trigger a range of emotions. Useful strategies to support those who are involved in the safeguarding of children include providing regular supervision by a more experienced member of staff or referral to in-house or professional counselling services.

Support for children/young people who disclose
Empowering children and young people

The reaction of the trusted adult to disclosure will play a large part in how the child and family cope with the situation. It is important that you let the child know that you believe what they are saying. Reassuring the child about the involvement of other adults, such as the police or social services, will also be important. Families need support in these situations, as they may become over-protective. Working with them, encouraging them to stick to familiar routines will help stabilise the situation.

Kidscape have produced a 'keepsafe code' to help children and young people know their rights.

remember

In suspected cases of child abuse, the parent or carer of a child will be kept informed about what is happening at each stage of the enquiry. If another person has reported the possible abuse, it is unlikely that social services will be able to tell you about their work with the child or family, for reasons of confidentiality and the Data Protection Act.

The Keepsafe Code

1. Hugs	Hugs and kisses are nice, especially from people we like. Even hugs and kisses that feel good and that you like should never be kept secret.
2. Body	Your body belongs to you and not to anyone else. This means all of your body. If anyone harms you or tries to touch your body in a way which confuses or frightens you, say NO, if possible, and tell.
3. No	If anyone older than you, even someone you know, tries to touch you in a way you don't like or that confuses you, or which they say is supposed to be a secret, say NO in a very loud voice.
4. Run or Get Away	Don't talk to anyone you don't know when you are alone, or just with other children. You don't have to be rude, just pretend you didn't hear and keep going. If a stranger, or a bully, or even someone you know tries to harm you, get away and get help. Make sure you always go towards other people or to a shop, if you can.
5. Yell	Wherever you are, it is all right to yell if someone is trying to hurt you. Practise yelling as loud as you can in a big, deep voice by taking a deep breath and letting the yell come from your stomach, not from your throat.
6. Tell	Tell a grown-up you trust if you are worried or frightened. If the first grown-up you tell doesn't believe or help you, keep telling until someone does. It might not be easy, but even if something has already happened that you have never told before, try to tell now. Who could you tell?
7. Secrets	Secrets such as surprise birthday parties are fun. But some secrets are not good and should never be kept. No bully should ever make you keep the bullying a secret and no-one should ask you to keep a kiss, hug or touch secret. If anyone does, even if you know that person, tell a grown-up you trust.
8. Bribes	Don't accept money or sweets or a gift from anyone without first checking with your parents. Most of the time it will be all right, like when you get a present for your birthday from your grandma. But some people try to trick children into doing something by giving them sweets or money. This is called a bribe – don't ever take one! Remember, it is possible that you might have to do what a bully or older person tells you, so that you can keep yourself safe. Don't feel bad if that happens because the most important thing is for you to be safe.
9. Code	Have a code word or sign with your parents or guardians, which only you and they know. If they need to send someone to collect you, they can give that person the code. Don't tell the code to anyone else.

Keepsafe Code from www.kidscape.org.uk

Unconditional acceptance of the child or young person

By listening to the child and showing them that you believe what they are saying, you will have begun the first stage of help.

Awareness of the potential impact on the child or young person and other family members

The Children Act (1989) requires the local authority to provide services to families and, where possible, prevent family break up. It is an unfortunate myth that social workers will rush in and remove children, a far more likely outcome is that the abusing parent will be asked to leave the home. If this does not happen, the child or young person may be removed to a place of safety. This situation will inevitably provoke a range of feelings from anger to disbelief and shock.

Counteracting possible stereotyping

See page 51 in Unit 2 for more information about **stereotyping**.

The national standards regulating childcare providers require settings to be proactive in devising strategies that promote equality. This includes challenging some of the assumptions surrounding child abuse.

Professional Practice

- Reassure the child that they have done the right thing by telling you.
- Tell them that you will help them in whatever way you can.
- Explain that you understand how hard it is for them to tell you this information.
- Find an appropriate setting, or make arrangements to talk to the child somewhere else as soon as you can if you are not in a suitable place (for example, if it is very exposed to being overheard by others).
- Remain calm.
- Keep your facial expression and body language positive.
- Give the child time.
- Be a good listener.
- Be patient, the child will most likely need to stop to sort their thoughts out.
- Reassure the child that whatever the situation, they are no way to blame.
- Ensure that you do not make a promise that you cannot keep.
- Explain that there are other people that you may need to contact.
- Explain that these people will also want to help them.
- Ask the child if they have told anyone else.
- Ask them who else they think they can tell.
- Maintain strict confidentiality, working on a 'need to know' basis.
- Follow the reporting guidelines for your setting.
- Let the child know what will happen next.
- Keep the child informed until the situation is out of your hands.

[permission 10.11]

activity
GROUP WORK

Check your own practice against some of the following assumptions:

- Afro-Caribbean fathers tend to be authoritarian.
- Parents of disabled children tend to be overprotective.

Discuss your thoughts with a partner.

Alleviating the effects of abuse

Encouraging expression of feeling

For younger children, much of what should be available in a well-planned early years environment will support children who have been abused and provide an outlet for their feelings. Materials such as clay, dough, sand and water can allow children to explore their feelings. Puppets and role play also provide an opportunity to explore feelings safely. For non-verbal children, dance, music and instruments can be a powerful way of exploring feelings.

Improving self-image

Well-planned and varied play experiences and the positive images reflected in the setting through role models and images are an important tool for the early years practitioner to use to develop **self-image**. Including the child in all activities, providing lots of opportunities to succeed and giving the child small responsibilities are also helpful strategies.

Building self-esteem and confidence

Play therapy

Therapeutic play is an umbrella term that includes play therapy. A qualified therapist will use a variety of techniques such as storytelling, puppets, masks, dance and movement to provide a child with strategies to cope with the problems they encounter in everyday lives.

PTUK   www.playtherapy.org.uk
more about play therapy

Counselling

Childline, launched in 1986, and Childline Cymru launched in Wales in 1993 provide a free telephone helpline where trained counsellors can advise children and young people about bullying, abuse and family breakdown.

Role of voluntary organisations

A range of voluntary organisations exist to work alongside child victims of abuse. The Children Act (1989) requires social services to provide services to children 'in need' and many of these functions will be delivered by a voluntary organisation, such as NCH Action for Children who provide respite care for children with disabilities.

---

activity
INDIVIDUAL WORK
10.8

P6

M3

When child abuse is suspected or confirmed, there should be a twofold approach to supporting children, young people and their families. Community-based strategies that support adults in their role as parents should be available, alongside targeted work with children to develop a range of self-protection strategies.

1   Using the resources at your college learning resource centre, identify the strategies and methods of supporting children, young people and their families where abuse is suspected or confirmed.

2   Explain the strategies and methods you would then use to minimise the risk.

---

case study
10.9

Louisa and her children

Louisa had two small children, Daniel aged two and Nicole aged eight months. The health visitor was concerned about the family. They were living in damp rented accommodation with no close family nearby. Louisa was quite withdrawn after her partner had been jailed for theft. Both children were underweight and frequently unwell. Louisa rarely sought advice from the GP. Both children had a persistent nappy rash. The health visitor felt that the neglect was not deliberate but was due to Louisa's low self-esteem and isolation.

---

activity
INDIVIDUAL WORK

1   What support might an informal parenting group offer Louisa?

2   What strategies could be used to support the children in their development?

SureStart   www.surestart.gov.uk
Gingerbread   www.gingerbread.org.uk

---

activity
INDIVIDUAL WORK
10.9

D2

There are a range of strategies that can be used to support children or young people and their families when abuse is suspected or confirmed. Professionals from a range of disciplines, such as play therapists, can contribute to this. Rigorous employment practices, enhanced Criminal Records Bureau (CRB) checks and clear policies all go some way towards protecting children and young people.

Identify the strengths and weaknesses of a range of strategies that can be employed when abuse is suspected or confirmed and present your findings in a report.

Progress Check

1 What are the potential reasons why children and young people may become looked after?

2 What is the United Nations Convention on the Rights of the Child?

3 Describe the different types of alternative care for children and young people.

4 What role does the voluntary sector play in providing care?

5 What is meant by the changing face of the family?

6 Identify the different types of abuse.

7 Describe three strategies that may be used to minimise the risk of abuse to children and young people.

8 What strategies may be used to develop parenting skills?

9 Why is it necessary to have a child protection policy within a health or social care setting?

10 Why must confidentiality be maintained?

11 How should you, as a care worker, respond to disclosure?

12 What strategies can you use to empower children and young people who disclose?

13 How can the care worker improve the self-image of a child or young person who discloses?

14 What is the role of the voluntary sector in supporting children who disclose?

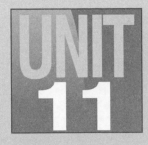

Supporting and protecting adults

This unit covers:

- Supportive relationships with adult users of health and social care services
- Types of abuse and indicators of abuse in health and social care contexts
- Potential for abuse within health and social care contexts
- Working strategies to minimise abuse

An important part of health and social care work is protecting adults who use services from potential or actual abuse. To do this effectively, health and social care workers need to understand the importance of developing supportive relationships which respect the individual's rights and choices. They also need to understand how these relationships have the potential to become abusive and the workplace policies and procedures that are used to minimise this abuse. They need to be able to recognise when those they support are vulnerable adults and are therefore at risk from abuse, as well as indications that abuse is or has taken place. They need to understand the different types of abuse and the range of working strategies, underpinned by legislation, policy and good practice guidance, used to minimise the potential for abuse within health and social care settings.

grading criteria

To achieve a **Pass** grade the evidence must show that the learner is able to:	To achieve a **Merit** grade the evidence must show that, in addition to the pass criteria, the learner is able to:	To achieve a **Distinction** grade the evidence must show that, in addition to the pass and merit criteria, the learner is able to:
P1 explain how individual rights can be respected in a supportive relationship Pg 356	**M1** explain how supportive relationships can enhance the life experiences of individuals receiving health and social care services Pg 356	**D1** use examples to evaluate the role of supportive relationships in enhancing the life experiences of individuals receiving health and social care services Pg 356
P2 describe different forms of abuse that may be experienced by vulnerable adults Pg 361		
P3 describe different indicators of abuse in vulnerable adults Pg 361		

To achieve a **Pass** grade the evidence must show that the learner is able to:	To achieve a **Merit** grade the evidence must show that, in addition to the pass criteria, the learner is able to:	To achieve a **Distinction** grade the evidence must show that, in addition to the pass and merit criteria, the learner is able to:
P4 describe the potential for abuse in health and social care contexts Pg 361	**M2** analyse the potential for abuse in four health and social care contexts Pg 369	
P5 describe strategies and working practices used to minimise abuse Pg 376		
P6 identify the legislation, policies and procedures that protect adults receiving health and social care services Pg 382	**M3** explain how legislation, policies and procedures contribute to the protection of vulnerable adults Pg 382	**D2** analyse the role of multi-agency working in minimising the risks of abuse in health and social care contexts Pg 378

Supportive relationships with adult users of health and social care services

Supportive relationships in health and social care work are different from other relationships we have in our lives. To understand these differences we will consider some of the different types of relationship individuals encounter through their lives.

Supportive relationships

One of the most interesting and rewarding things about working in health and social care is the opportunity to form supportive relationships with a diverse range of people. For these to be effective for both parties, you need to know and understand yourself. You need to understand the impact that you have on other people and align this with your role and responsibilities as a health and social care worker. That impact can be a positive and enabling one or it can be a disabling one.

Attitudes towards the worker-service user relationship have changed considerably in the past 20 years. The worker's role is to enable and **empower** the service user, with a responsibility to ensure that individuals have the same rights as other members of society. Within supportive relationships, the following factors need to be present for the relationships to be effective for the individual and the worker:

Humanistic approach

This optimistic approach to relationships arose out of counselling work. It is based on helping people to realise their potential by assisting them to explore their understanding of themselves, how they see themselves and their experience. The aim is to increase self-awareness to enable the person to apply their understanding into their everyday life and the challenges they encounter. This exploration is conducted in an accepting and non-judgemental atmosphere. It is designed to enable the person to identify their strengths and find their own answers, as they are more likely to change if they understand and determine their own goals. This approach to a supportive or counselling relationship enables individuals to focus on their capabilities and their creativity, personal growth and choice.

Helping and enabling

Health and social care work is often considered to be about helping people to do those things they are unable to do for themselves. While this remains true in part and indeed some individuals require considerable help, the emphasis on how that help is provided has changed. It is no longer accepted good practice to help an individual so much that they

> **remember**
>
> You can still help someone without doing everything for them. Take things at the individual's pace and encourage them to tell you how and when they want things done.

become dependent and 'helpless'. Too much help may cause a person to lose the ability or skills to undertake certain tasks for themselves, for example, they may lose the ability to wash and dress themselves because the worker does everything for them. On the other hand, the worker's role is not to stand by and watch while someone struggles with a task that is beyond their capability at that time. Judging the right amount of help an individual requires while supporting their independence is one of the skills that health and social care workers need to learn.

The emphasis in the supporting role today is that of enabling. Enabling refers to the ability to provide an individual with the resources, authority or opportunity to do something themselves. Examples of enabling are when the worker provides appropriate information to enable an individual to make informed decisions or provides an individual with learning disabilities appropriate training and practice to enable them to use public transport safely. This also includes ensuring the individual can communicate with others using their preferred method.

See page 3 in Unit 1 for more information about types of communication.

Empowering and giving choices

As well as enabling, health and social care workers seek to empower service users to exercise their rights and take control of their lives and the decisions about what happens to them. Empowerment means gaining more control over your life, often through being aware of and using personal as well as external resources and rights. It is also about overcoming obstacles in order to meet your needs and aspirations and having your voice heard in decision making. Empowerment is also about being able to challenge inequality and oppression in your life. Not only must the worker understanding an individual's rights, they must also work with the individual to enable them to understand those rights and how they may challenge and exercise those rights.

> **remember**
>
> Not everyone understands what 'choice' is. You may have to explain what choice means before individuals are able to make choices for themselves.

Part of the enabling and empowering relationship relates to giving the individual choices so they can make their own decisions about their lives. However, understanding choices is not always as simple as saying 'Would you like a hot or cold drink?' For some individuals, the concept or idea of choice may be difficult to understand and so a variety of ways to communicate choices and what they mean should to be considered if we are to offer real choice. Some choices are complex with each alternative option having an impact that requires some consideration. For example, the choice may be about staying at home or moving into supported accommodation. Each option has implications not just practical but also economic, emotional, **psychological** and social. Whatever capability an individual may have, they should always be offered choices. The challenge is for health and social care workers to interpret how the individual communicates their choice.

Maintaining privacy and confidentiality

Maintaining privacy is generally accepted as the foundation of good care practice. Maintaining privacy means ensuring the individual is free from unwanted attention, intrusion or observation by other people.

> **Professional Practice**
>
> Within health and social care settings privacy can be maintained by:
>
> ■ providing a private area for residents to meet their visitors
>
> ■ drawing curtains around a patient's bed when supporting them with personal care tasks
>
> ■ providing residents with a key to their room.

Taking time to ensure that an individual is not seen, heard or disturbed when they choose not to be, such as while attending to their personal care, while upset and crying or when behaving in a way that challenges others is an important part of the health and social care workers responsibility. Privacy also relates to personal information and so maintaining confidentiality is also essential.

Maintaining confidentiality means keeping an individual's personal matters private and not telling anyone else about them unless the individual has given their permission to disclose information to others. Confidentiality relates to all information whether spoken, written or held on electronic records and is subject to conditions of the Data Protection Act (2000).

An individual can consent to information being shared with others as long as it is informed consent, that is they know what information will be shared, with whom, when, where, how, the purpose as well as the potential consequences of not sharing information. An individual can give consent with limitations and specify what information can be shared and with whom. For example, they not may wish their family to know their diagnosis if unwell. Health and social care workers have a legal responsibility to maintain confidentiality, and guidance on their role is found in organisational policies and procedures.

See page 70 in Unit 2 for more information about the Data Protection Act (2000).

Advocacy

Advocacy is the process of representing the needs of individuals who would otherwise find it difficult to communicate their views to others and be listened to, as they are regarded by society as being unable either to hold views or to express them coherently. Individuals who need this type of support include children and young people, and adults with learning disabilities or mental health problems. An advocate might, for example, put forward the move to a more independent living environment for a person with mental health problems.

For advocacy to be successful and effective, an advocate needs to understand the individual's circumstances, values, beliefs, wishes and aspirations. Advocates need to be skilled at communicating without unduly influencing the individual so that they can represent the individual's views and not their own.

Advocacy is one way of ensuring an individual's rights are maintained when they are not able to speak out for themselves. Family members may not be the best advocates as they may represent their own views of what they want for the individual and not what the individual would choose for themselves.

remember
Independent advocates may be available to support individuals with specific needs, such as advocates for older people, adults with learning disabilities or mental health issues.

Promoting rights

Enabling, empowering, maintaining privacy and confidentiality and advocacy are all ways in which an individual's rights can be promoted. Health and social care workers need to firstly understand what rights people have and how these can be both promoted as well as infringed. Promoting something suggests taking an active role and so that means taking action to ensure this happens as well as taking action when it is not happening.

See page 57 in Unit 2 for more information about individual rights.

Non-judgemental support

Supportive relationships require those involved to accept one another as they are with both the good and not-so-good qualities. We are all unique with individual likes, dislikes, values and beliefs and this is a reason for celebration rather than condemnation. We live in a free society where people have a right to express themselves (as long as it is not discriminatory) in any way they wish to. If we wish this freedom for ourselves, we must be prepared to give others the same freedom and not make judgements that place the other person in an inferior position or belittle them. We may not like what someone does or says, but we must accept that it is their choice and they have a right to be themselves. We can be supportive by explaining why we may find something difficult or unacceptable but our explanation should contain no condemnation and we should not treat them less favourably because of it.

Relationships

Relationships of any kind teach us things about other people, their motivations, how we can adjust our approach to respond to different people with different needs, experiences, attitudes, behaviours, values, and so on. Each relationship is as unique as the individual we relate to. Relationships also teach us about ourselves. They can provide valuable insights to enable us to understand ourselves better. Through these interactions we gain an understanding of our values, beliefs, culture, motivations, strengths and weaknesses, as well as the impact our behaviour has on others. Self-awareness can come through our own reflection but also through the constructive feedback we get from others that tell us how they perceive us.

remember
Building relationships with others is a core activity in being a human being.

Promoting views, preferences and independence of individuals and key people

Supportive and positive relationships with others enrich our lives. Supportive relationships should enable a person to grow in confidence and feelings of self-worth. They will feel comfortable with themselves as a unique and valued individual. For this to happen, a person must feel secure enough to express themselves with the other person.

Within health and social care, the focus of the service user-worker relationship is promoting the independence, views and preferences of the individual being supported. Consideration also needs to be given to those people who are significant to the individual, such as family, friends, and the relationship should promote their opportunity to express their views, preferences and promote their independence. An essential part of this relationship is creating a sense of security.

To achieve this you need to be yourself with no pretence about being more skilled or knowledgeable than you really are. People will soon identify if you are not being genuine and will be less likely to trust you. You also need to demonstrate warmth or what Carl Rogers refers to as 'unconditional positive regard'. This is the ability to convey acceptance of another without question or judgement.

See page 284 in Unit 8 for more information about Carl Rogers.

Showing real interest in the individual, being responsive to them and attempting to place yourself in their situation in order to understand it better (empathy) are also important aspects of relationship building, and contribute to creating a sense of security and trust as a foundation for the relationship to grow from.

Supporting individuals with communication of their needs and preferences

See page 3 in Unit 1 for more information about communication needs and preferences.

Communication is a vital part of building and sustaining relationships. Being responsive to others is achieved through active listening. This is not just listening to what is being said but listening to voice tonality and observing the non-verbal signals being conveyed through the conversation. Interpreting these as a way of understanding the whole of the communication is really important as this information will give you an insight into the individual's emotional state and their needs and preferences. This will help you in determining your approach when asking questions, for example what type of questions they are likely to respond to (open, probing, closed). Summarising and reflecting back to the individual are also ways of demonstrating that you are being responsive to them in a supportive manner. You also need to be aware of your non-verbal (body language) as this will either be congruent (agree) with what you are saying and therefore reinforce it or will be in conflict which is likely to undermine your words and create feelings of mistrust.

Encouragement and approval can be conveyed through both verbal and non-verbal communication and are essential if you hope to demonstrate unconditional positive regard towards the individual.

Differences between family, friends and professionals

Family relationships

The first relationships we experience are with our parents or carers as a baby and child and are therefore instrumental in helping us to form ideas about the world and our place within it. These relationships should be supportive, caring, nurturing and protective. We know from research that if these are missing from an individual's early life this has a lifelong impact on their sense of identity, security and ability to form effective and long-term relationships with others. Family or primary care givers, such as foster parents, are our role models for personal relationships with others and we generally expect our family to support us through life's ups and downs, giving us unconditional love, although this is not always the case. The foundations for primary (parental) relationships are from our own experiences of being parented. If a person's role models are poor, for example due to parental **abuse**, neglect or failure to protect from abuse by others, this can impact on their confidence and ability to

Supporting and protecting adults

> **remember**
>
> There are different types of parental relationship: biological, adoptive or foster.

Fig 11.1 Different types of family

form those primary relationships with their own children. Family relationships can be very close where lives are intertwined and the bonds between members are not only of a shared inheritance and experiences but also of friendship and common interests and ideas. Research studies relating to identical twins have shown, however, that even a shared inheritance and upbringing does not ensure that experiences are interpreted identically as the relationships we have with one another are unique. Some would say that our family relationships are where we can experience our greatest joys as well as our greatest pain.

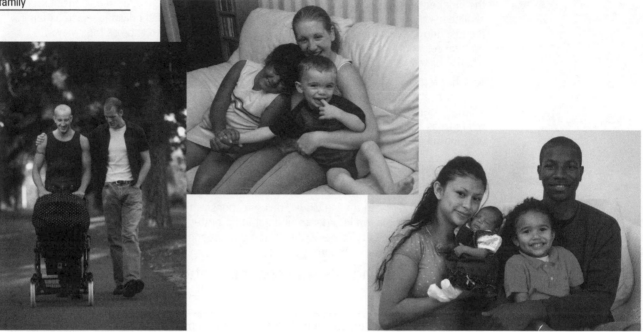

Family relationships often include an element of expectation and assumption in relation to how individuals within the family should behave towards one another. For example expectations may include loyalty to family members in any and every circumstance, a hierarchy of importance with deference to older, wiser, members of the family, an expectation that the needs of the family come first and that the needs and wishes of more senior members of the family will be met unquestioningly. Within families, alliances will be forged between different members to ensure their needs and interests are served. This can create all kinds of tensions that put pressure on those relationships. The consequence of this can be a breakdown in those relationships with members not communicating with one another and being excluded from the family sometimes for long periods of time. Family relationships are, in most cases, not chosen relationships and for some this creates a tension especially where the complexity of those relationships involves favouritism, rivalry and jealousy.

Some people find family relationships stifling, especially if their family impose expectations or limitations upon them that are different from their own. Often in these circumstances individuals feel closer to their friends.

Friendships

The main difference between family relationships and friendships is that friendships are chosen relationships. Our motivations for friendships are likely to be as varied as the people we are friends with. Friendships are often made a result of mutual interests. For example, we may have friends we went to school or college with, we work with or we play sport with. We may share a number of areas of common ground with some people and so meet up with them frequently as part of our life. Other friends we may have less contact with but still have things we share with them that form the basis of that friendship. We are friends with other people because we like them and the relationship with them in some way meets our emotional, intellectual or spiritual needs. We may be friends with someone because they meet our need for intellectual stimulation and, for example, we may spend our time with them discussing issues that affect our lives or we may argue with them but the relationship stimulates us to think and challenges us so that we learn more about our self and our views. Other friends may be fun to be with, so we like spending time with them because we relax, unwind and this brings out other aspects of our identity. Each friendship has a unique value to us and through that relationship we learn and grow as human beings.

> **remember**
>
> Friendships can be formed as a result of people growing up together, sharing school, college or university experience, through work, being parents and having common interests.

Fig 11.2 Friendship

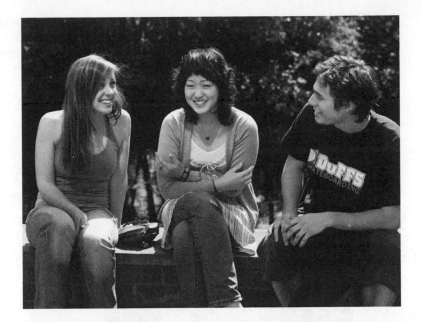

We negotiate friendships in a different way from family relationships. We informally establish the rules for our friendship. This may be, for example, how often you see one another, how you contact one another, what is shared and the status of that information (is it confidential or common knowledge?) and what each expects from the relationship. The last two points are often the most difficult as they are frequently unspoken and can lead to tensions if there is a mismatch in expectation.

Professional relationships

Professional relationships between the health and social care worker, other professionals and users of health and social care services should be clearly described to avoid ambiguity and to protect both the user and the worker from abuse. To achieve this, there must be clear guidance about roles and responsibilities as well as expectations and limits in terms of behaviour within the relationship. This type of relationship is generally described through a health and social care worker's job description, professional code of practice, organisational policies and procedures and legal responsibilities.

Fig 11.3 Job description

Position Description

Company:

Position Title:

Department:

Reports to:

Position Summary/Facts
(describe the overall purpose and objective of the position)

Does the position have supervisory responsibilities? No

Skills/Abilities
(categories and description of specfic skill/ability)

Position Prerequisites *(e.g. qualifications, experience)*

Major accountabilities
To work with publishing, brand management and sales to plan and implement marketing initiatives:

Authorised: (Position Holder)

Authorised: (Manager)

Authorised: (Director/Senior Manager)

Date:

In professional relationships, the areas of common ground are the work being undertaken and the focus of the relationship is to ensure the needs of the users of health and social care services are met in an enabling and respectful way. The worker's needs are of less importance and they should not seek to meet their own needs through professional relationships as it is at this point that the relationship changes to one that is exploitative and abusive.

Relationships between equals

In this type of relationship, there are mutual benefits to both people involved. The status of each person in the relationship is not contested (in question) as the gains from the relationship are equal on both sides. For example, in the relationships between care givers and care receivers, the care receiver works with the person giving care to ensure their needs and the best ways to support and meet those needs are understood. The care giver provides that support and their need for job satisfaction is achieved through meeting the care receiver's needs.

Fig 11.4 Maintaining a professional relationship

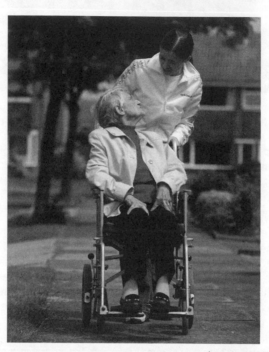

case study 11.1   Wendy and Ruby

Wendy works as a domiciliary care worker. For the past three years, she has been visiting Ruby, who is 86 years old. Wendy is having a lot of family problems which is causing her a lot of worry. When Wendy visits Ruby, she spends most of the time telling Ruby all about her problems and seems less interested in supporting Ruby. Wendy says that Ruby is the only person she can talk to. However, Ruby is beginning to find this distressing as it worries her but she feels unable to tell Wendy to stop as she does not want to upset her or appear unfriendly.

activity
GROUP WORK

1   Why is this relationship no longer professional?
2   Why do you think Wendy is behaving in this way?
3   How should Wendy behave within this relationship?

Power and subservience

Power or the ability to influence others is an aspect of any relationship and few relationships are totally equal. Power over the other person in a relationship can result due to one person's **status**. For example, in family relationships, this may be because one person is older (a parent), in professional relationships it may be because one person holds a position of authority or respect (a manager) or has a greater level of knowledge and as a result of this greater status (a doctor). Power has a tendency to have negative connotations as it can so easily be misused. However, having power within a relationship can be beneficial if it used to influence others in a positive way.

The misuse or abuse of power is a fundamental aspect of abusive relationships where one person exerts power over another to make them do things they do not wish to do and to behave in ways that are damaging to their identity and well-being. The relationship becomes a **subservient** one, and therefore abusive, when one person is exerting power over another person to the extent that the other person will follow the wishes or orders of the other without question or consideration of their own needs and well-being.

Patronising and belittling

Nowadays, we consider the attitudes displayed towards individuals with health and social care needs and in particular disabilities in the past to be **patronising**. In general, services were organised in a way that treated those receiving support as if they were less intelligent or knowledgeable than those providing support. Responsibility for decisions about their lives were taken away from service users, as it was felt they would be incapable of dealing with such responsibilities, or it would be too stressful for them. Things were 'done to' people as opposed to being 'done with' people.

Although such patronising attitudes are no longer at the heart of the health and social care services, sometimes, a worker may behave in a way that is belittling to a service user, making less of them in a way which is disrespectful and has a negative impact on the service user's identity. One example of such belittling behaviour is using language that is inappropriate to the individual's age by talking to a person with a disability or dementia using words and a tone of voice appropriate for talking to a child. When this happens, it suggests that one person considers themselves to be superior or more powerful than the other. Being patronising or belittling towards another person infringes that person's rights to independence of thought and action which is not acceptable in today's society.

Development of relationships

In order to establish, develop and sustain relationships, individuals must find some way of communicating with one another.

See page 3 in Unit 1 for more information about communication.

Through communication

Communication is the process of encoding, sending and decoding signals in order to exchange information and ideas between people. It lies at the very heart of relationships. When we communicate with others, only around 7 per cent of our message is communicated verbally. Thirty-eight per cent is communicated through tone of voice and 55 per cent of the message is conveyed through non-verbal communication or body language. As the saying goes 'our actions speak louder than words'. We also communicate through the written word, which can clarify things, although it can also complicate things if the words are misinterpreted.

See page 17 in Unit 1 for more information about the communication cycle.

Body language

We can tell a great deal by observing body. The way a person holds their body (their posture), the way they stand or sit, their position in relation to another person, the distance or closeness to the other person, the position of their hands, their head, the direction of their gaze all reveal more than the verbal conversation. For example, body language can reveal how at ease or anxious the person is in the situation, how interested or bored they are and if they are concentrating on what is being said. We pick up signals from body language subconsciously and use this to interpret the verbal communication. Often non-verbal communication reveals the intention behind the verbal communication. Body language can also reveal a persons' emotional state.

Facial expression

This is an important part of non-verbal communication. Facial expressions reveal a great deal about our emotions and can be a clear communication method. However, you need to be aware of the cultural differences in both facial expressions and body language to avoid misinterpretation. For some people with disabilities, their main form of communication is through facial expression and eye contact.

Touch

> **remember**
>
> Never assume it is okay to touch someone even on their hand or forearm. Always check first.

Communication through touch can convey emotions when words are inadequate. Touch can also be useful in certain situations, for example, if someone has a hearing impairment or when the background noise is too loud for verbal communication to be heard. However, touch needs careful consideration, as touch can convey messages to an individual which may be unwelcome, distressing or misinterpreted as a result of their past experiences, such as if they have experienced physical or sexual abuse. It is important that health and social care workers gain the individual's permission regarding touch and be clear about what is appropriate and inappropriate within their role and responsibility.

Trust

> **remember**
>
> Once trust is broken it is hard to re-establish a relationship and in many circumstances it may end a relationship.

If any relationship is to be sustained and develop, trust must be present. One of the main causes for relationships to falter or breakdown is the loss of trust, often due to one person not maintaining the confidentiality of the other. Part of building a relationship is getting to know someone and building up the trust that will sustain the relationship. People in the relationship need to have reasons to trust one another. Keeping your word, treating one another with respect, being able to rely on one another to be caring, honest, fair and truthful are all elements of trust. As a health and social care worker, building up trust is essential in a supportive relationship as many of the people you work with will be vulnerable and will need to be confident that they can trust and rely on you to not only support them but also protect them if the need arises.

Fig 11.5 Reading facial expressions

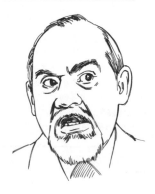 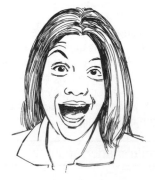 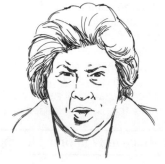 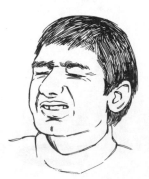

Reliability

Reliability, that is being consistent and doing what is expected of you, are essential elements of a supportive relationship. Relationships falter if one person is unreliable to the extent that the other person is never sure what their actions will be and so the element of trust is missing. Reliability in a supportive relationship is even more important especially when the service user needs support from the worker to enable them, for example, to undertake daily living activities. When trust and reliability are missing, the individual will feel unsupported and anxious as they are unable to predict what the other person will do. This creates a feeling of unease which may change their behaviour, for example they may become agitated or withdrawn.

Consistency of approach

Although we are all different and will have different approaches, it is important that when an individual is being supported by a number of different workers support is provided in a consistent way. The individual's care plan will provide information about their care and support and it is essential that workers follow this so that the individual gains confidence in the service and feels secure. Consistency is especially important when carrying out particular procedures or responding to individual needs, such as behaviour guidelines or an exercise programme. If the approach is inconsistent, the individual can become confused and lose trust and therefore confidence in those who do things differently. It can also create tensions between workers and individuals, for example if the individual seeks not to follow guidelines that they find difficult, saying that another worker said it was not important or did things differently. This inconsistency may have a negative impact on the individual's progress, for example slowing down the rehabilitation or behaviour management process.

Fairness

Being fair involves treating everyone in the same way and not showing favouritism or unequal advantage to one person. As a health and social care worker, this is important as in the supportive relationship the individual needs to have confidence you will not treat them in a way that will disadvantage them.

Managing your own feelings

From time to time, we all experience difficulties or problems in our relationships with others in working or in our personal lives. If we are struggling with a problem, it can become overwhelming to the extent that it is difficult to concentrate on anything else and it feels like it is taking over our life. If our focus and concentration is on other things, this will have an impact on how we relate to other people. A health and social care worker has a responsibility to concentrate on the needs of others in the workplace to ensure their needs are met and everyone is kept safe. When things are worrying us, we can become intolerant of the needs and concerns of others and this can lead to mistreating the other person, such as being curt in our responses or not taking time to respect or support them. Although it may be difficult, it is imperative to find ways of managing problems and concerns so that they do not damage relationships with service users or colleagues, such as seeking support from a manager or colleagues, for example through supervision.

Professional Practice

- Ensure you receive regular supervision with your manager.

- Use supervision to discuss areas of practice you are concerned about.

- Use supervision as a means to get constructive feedback to enable you to learn and develop your practice.

Individual rights

Promoting the rights of the individual is one of the health and social care worker's responsibilities and is one way to make those being supported feel less vulnerable. Being aware of an individual's rights and supporting them to understand these, and through that knowledge empowering them to exercise their rights, is a powerful way of reducing an individual's vulnerability to abuse by others.

See page 57 in Unit 2 for more information about individual rights.

Fig 11.6 Individual rights

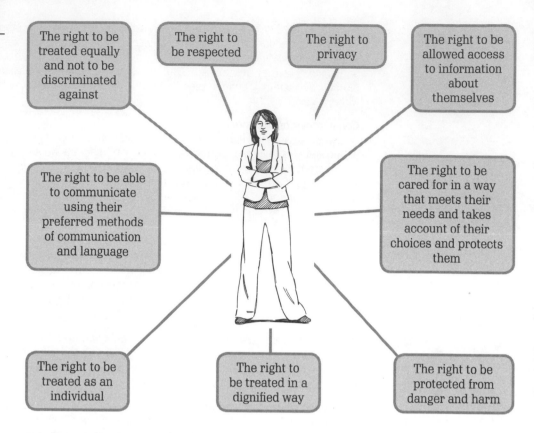

- The right to be treated equally and not to be discriminated against
- The right to be respected
- The right to privacy
- The right to be allowed access to information about themselves
- The right to be able to communicate using their preferred methods of communication and language
- The right to be cared for in a way that meets their needs and takes account of their choices and protects them
- The right to be treated as an individual
- The right to be treated in a dignified way
- The right to be protected from danger and harm

Diversity and difference

Individuals also have a right to be different without fear of intimidation, abuse or harm by others. Within society, people come from diverse backgrounds all of which are equally valuable in their contribution to society. People have a right to express their difference whether that is related to their nationality, belief, religion, culture, race, disability, gender or sexuality. Within health and social care settings, organisational policies are clear about acknowledging individual differences and celebrating the richness they bring to our life experience. However, when considering difference and individual rights, it is important to remember this extends to all expressions including an individual's behaviour, such as their eating and hygiene habits. We may not agree with these, however we have a responsibility to respect the individual and all their differences.

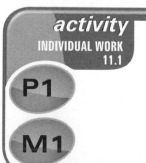

activity
INDIVIDUAL WORK
11.1

P1

M1

The relationship between a health and social care worker and a service user is described as a supportive relationship.

1   Using examples, explain how you as a health or social care worker can demonstrate that you respect the rights of the individuals you support.

2   With reference to these examples, explain how your supportive relationship with individuals who use care services improves their life experiences.

activity
GROUP WORK
11.2

D1

With reference to the examples used in activity 11.1, discuss the value to the individual of your supportive relationship with them in terms of their quality of life (that is, what they are able to do as a result of that relationship that they may not otherwise be able to do).

Types of abuse and indicators of abuse in health and social care contexts

Types of abuse

Abuse may be physical, psychological, sexual, financial, negligent, reckless behaviour which endangers self or others as well as self-harm. It also includes discrimination, bullying, and violent ill-treatment, speaking harshly, roughly or using harsh and vulgar comments to an individual. Abuse may be intentional or unintentional. It may be about doing something (an act of commission) or doing nothing (an act of omission). When a person abuses another person they violate their human and civil rights. Abuse may occur regularly and systematically or just once.

There are nine main types of abuse. These are:

- physical
- sexual
- psychological or emotional
- financial
- neglect
- institutional
- discriminatory
- self-harm
- domestic.

Physical abuse

Physical abuse is non-accidental injury or harm to the body. Physical abuse can include:

- hitting, slapping, shaking, punching, pulling or dragging a person
- handling a person in a rough manner without consideration of their well-being
- burning or scalding a person
- inappropriate restraint (not in accordance with agreed protocols)
- locking up or confining a person
- depriving a person of food or drink
- forcing a person to eat or drink
- misusing medication, such as not giving medication according to doctor's instructions, withholding medication, overdosing, infrequent medication review or giving medication intended for another person
- withholding aids for daily living, such as glasses, hearing aids or walking aids
- withholding care which causes physical discomfort, such as ignoring requests to go to the toilet, causing physical discomfort and or incontinence.

Physical abuse is often accompanied by other forms of abuse such as psychological and sexual.

Sexual abuse

This is involving any individual in sexual activities which they do not understand, have not given consent to or which violate the sexual taboos of family custom and practice. Sexual abuse can occur either through contact or non-contact.

Sexual abuse through contact can include:

- vaginal or anal rape
- buggery
- incest
- touching someone in a sexual manner
- forcing a person to touch another person in a sexual manner.

Sexual abuse through non-contact can include:

- forcing a person to watch pornography or adult entertainment without full understanding of what this may involve
- subjecting a person to indecent exposure, sexual innuendoes, harassment or inappropriate photography

remember

Sexual abuse can happen to adult men and women as well as children and young people.

- not giving a person a choice to have a care worker of the same gender to provide intimate personal care
- looking at a person's body inappropriately.

Psychological or emotional abuse

This type of abuse relates to any action that damages an individual's mental well-being. The effects of emotional abuse will reduce an individual's quality of life and their self-esteem to the extent that they will be less likely to achieve their full potential.

Emotional or psychological abuse can include:

- subjecting a person to threatening behaviour
- ignoring a person
- disregarding a person's opinions, life experience or personal history
- bullying or harassment
- forcing a person to live in fear or in a culture of intimidation, for example, always blaming them for things
- humiliating, ridiculing or teasing a person, for example, insulting them all the time
- blaming a person for something they are not able to control, such as being incontinent
- coercing, pressurising or manipulating a person into doing something against their will
- rejecting a person or intentionally withholding emotional support or affection from them
- treating someone inappropriately for their age or cultural background, such as using 'baby talk' to an adult with learning disabilities or dementia.

Financial abuse

This is the theft or misuse of an individual's money or personal possessions to advantage another person.

Financial abuse can include:

- stealing a person's money or belongings
- not giving a person access to their money or controlling their money and benefits
- spending a person's money without their consent
- removing, buying or selling a person's belongings without their knowledge or consent
- asking a person for money under false pretences, for example in payment for a service not provided
- altering the ownership of property without the person's knowledge or consent
- taking loans out in a person's name without their knowledge or consent
- asking a person to sign financial documents when they have been assessed as not having the mental capacity to consent
- borrowing a person's money or possessions.

Neglect

Neglect is the deliberate or unintentional failure to meet an individual's needs for care which results in a deterioration in their well-being. This can be either acts of omission (not doing something) or acts of commission (doing something on purpose).

Neglect can include:

- not responding to a person's care and health needs, such as their physical, emotional, social, cultural, intellectual and spiritual needs or preventing others from doing so
- withholding care, including medication or access to medical or care staff and services
- not providing the basic standards of care, such as meeting basic human needs, warmth, food, drink, safety
- preventing a person from seeing visitors or spending time with other people
- not undertaking appropriate risk assessments and allowing the person to self-harm or harm others
- not intervening when behaviour is dangerous to the person or to others.

Discriminatory abuse

This exists when the values, beliefs or culture within society or an organisation results in the misuse of power so that individuals who are different, or perceived as different, are denied the same opportunities as others in society. Discrimination may be on the basis of ethnicity, gender, age, disability, sexuality, health status or religion.

Discriminatory abuse also includes:

- excluding a person from opportunities in society
- explaining a person's opinions and behaviour in relation to their age or disability
- treating a person in an inappropriate way for their age or cultural background
- verbal abuse and inappropriate use of language
- harassment and slurs.

Institutional abuse

This is the mistreatment or abuse by a regime or the people within an institution. Everyone has a right to feel safe, be treated with respect and dignity. In situations of institutional abuse, the routines, systems and accepted behaviour ('how things are done around here') within the organisation are for the benefit and convenience of the staff and organisation and not for the individuals being supported.

Institutional abuse can include:

- inappropriate or poor standards of care
- misusing of medication, such as sedating a person to make life easier for staff
- using restraint inappropriately
- denying a person access to visitors or phone calls
- restricting access to toilet, bathing facilities or a comfortable place to rest
- restricting access to appropriate medical or social care
- lack of privacy or dignity (including failing to provide access to appropriate privacy)
- being inflexible in terms of bedtime and mealtimes, choice of food
- lack of adequate procedures to ensure clear roles and responsibilities of all staff and management
- the existence of controlling relationships between staff and individuals in their care
- repeated acts of poor professional practice.

Self-harm

An individual who has experienced harm or abuse may have such low self esteem and motivation that they self-neglect or self-harm. They may feel that if they are less attractive, the abuse (especially sexual abuse) may stop. Sometimes the act of self-harming, such as cutting their arms, releases them from the mental pain they are experiencing. If they have experienced abuse, this often results in feelings of self-loathing or worthlessness.

Self-harm can include:

- self-inflicted injuries, for example, to the arms or abdomen
- misuse of drugs (prescribed and illegal)
- misuse of alcohol
- inappropriate behaviour which increases their vulnerability, such as sexually precocious behaviour, taking undue risks with their safety
- overeating or starving themselves, for example, bulimia or anorexia
- self-neglect in terms of personal hygiene

Domestic violence or abuse

Domestic violence is any incident of threatening behaviour violence or abuse between adults who are or have been in a relationship together, or between family members, regardless of gender or sexuality. Home Office statistics identify the following facts about domestic violence:

- It accounts for 16% of all violent crime and has more repeat victims than any other crime.
- It claims the lives of two women each week and 30 men per year.

- It will affect one in four women and one in six men in their lifetime.
- It is the biggest cause of morbidity worldwide in women aged 19 to 44, greater than war, cancer and motor vehicle accidents.

Source www.homeoffice.gov.uk

Domestic violence is rarely a one-off incident and is a pattern of controlling and aggressive behaviours. It can be physical, sexual or psychological. Financial abuse and social isolation are also common features of the controlling behaviour. The abuse comes from the abuser's desire for power and control over another person. Domestic abuse has no boundaries and can happen to anyone regardless of social class, age, race, disability, gender or sexuality and can occur from the beginning of a relationship or after years of being together.

Contrary to many people's perception of domestic violence, men can also be subjected to it from their female or male partner. For men, seeking help can be especially difficult because of society's expectations of the male role and the lack of facilities to support men. Children are affected by domestic violence in both the short and long term.

Domestic violence is usually a combination of different types of abuse as the violence, physical, sexual or both are accompanied by psychological abuse. This takes the form of constant criticism, belittling, humiliation with the abused person being told how worthless they are and how the abuse is their fault ('you make me do it'). The abuser is likely to lose their temper over trivial things and threaten the person with more violence or their life being worse if they tell anyone about the abuse. The abuser may control the person to the extent of wanting to know exactly where they are at all times or restricting how often they go out or forbidding it altogether. The person being abused is likely to be in a state of anxiety most of the time as they live in fear of 'doing something wrong' without knowledge of what that 'wrong' is most of the time so are unable to prevent the abuse by avoidance tactics. They are likely to spend their time trying to appease the abuser acting in a subservient manner in an attempt to avoid inflaming the abuser's temper and the inevitable violence that results.

case study 11.2 — Karen's job

Karen has recently started work as a support worker for four people with mental health needs who live in a small group home. This is her first job in health and social care. She really enjoys the work but is concerned about some of the things she is being asked to do. She feels that lots of the 'routines' are designed to suit staff needs rather than those of individual users, for example meals are quite sparse and no alternatives are offered. Food is locked away and users are not allowed in the kitchen due to health and safety, even though all are capable of making themselves drinks and snacks. Karen is also concerned about the way other staff talk about the service users as she feels their language is derogatory and discriminatory. More worrying is the fact that one or two users are repeatedly given medication and quite forcefully restrained when they get 'aggressive'. This 'aggressive' behaviour seems to occur when staff ignore repeated requests by the users for help with something.

activity
GROUP WORK

1 What type of abuse is this?
2 What action do you think Karen should take?
3 What dilemmas do you think Karen faces in taking action?

Indicators of abuse and self-harm
Inappropriate injuries and bruising

When a person falls or hurts themselves, the bruising that results is normally on the outer areas of the body. Bruising to the more protected areas of the body, such as the inner thighs, abdomen, breasts, inner surface of the arms are less likely to result accidentally. Bruising should also be consistent with the individual's account of what happened and if it is not then this should be a cause for concern and further action.

remember

Don't make assumption or jump to conclusions. If you suspect abuse, follow procedures and never make decisions on your own.

Another sign of potential abuse is the presence of multiple or minor bruising of different ages. Bruising results from the release of blood from the fine blood vessels (capillaries) into the tissues under the skin. As the red blood cells break down, they release their pigments (colours) hence the changes in colour from red, blue, yellow and brown, gradually fading as the blood is reabsorbed into the tissues. The colour of the bruise can therefore tell you if the injury is recent or not. People who are repeatedly physically abused are likely to have bruises of different colours as well as bruises on top of older bruises. The bruising may also be oddly shaped, especially if the individual has been hit with something, such as a belt buckle, ring, or implement of some kind. Bruising usually occurs as a result of an injury, but be aware that bruising can sometimes happen spontaneously and indicate an allergic reaction, or more serious disease.

Marks of slaps, fingertips, scratches, bites, pinches or kicks are also indicators of injuries that are not accidental.

Burns and scalds

Again, if these are in places that are unusual, such as on the back, side or bottom or are distinctive in shape or size, for example cigarette burns or electric fire burns, these may also indicate that the person has been abused. Another indicator may be the number of burns the individual has or the presence of previous burns that have healed, suggesting that the injuries have been inflicted over a period of time. Again, inconsistencies in the individual's account of their injuries and the actual site of the injuries should raise suspicion.

Malnourishment

Indications of malnutrition include the person looking thinner than average for their age and height. They may show signs of hunger and thirst. Their skin often shows signs of dehydration in that it has lost its elasticity and does not return to its original position when a section of skin is pinched between the thumb and first finger. The person may also have poor skin condition with sores and minor ailments. Dehydration causes sunken eyes and dry lips. The individual's hair and nails will also be in poor condition. Malnourishment may cause women who are not menopausal, taking oral contraceptives or pregnant to stop menstruating.

Low self-esteem

Having self-esteem means having confidence in your own value or worth as in individual that you have something to give to others and are worthy of receiving in return. Individuals who value and respect themselves have positive self-esteem and a positive idea of who they are through an understanding of how others see them (self-concept). Self-esteem is influenced by how other people make us feel. If other people give us warmth and love regardless of our personality or capabilities, we can have good self-esteem. However, if an individual has received little warmth, love, affection of praise and encouragement in their life they are likely to have low self-esteem. One of the consequences of being abused is low self-esteem, as often the abuser makes the abused person feel worthless, useless and unlovable. Abusers often accompany physical or sexual abuse with psychological abuse by telling the person the abuse is their fault. The guilt this creates as well as the intimidation and humiliation all add to the individual's feelings of low self-esteem and worthlessness. Low self-esteem shows itself in a lack of confidence and a reluctance to try things or be involved with other people.

Emotional withdrawal

Changes in an individual's normal behaviour is often a sign that they are being abused or have been abused. For example, this could be someone who was previously outgoing and friendly becoming passive, with no spontaneous smiles and not wanting to see, speak or be with other people, in effect withdrawing both physically and emotionally from relationships with others. Changes in appearance, such as not changing their clothes, washing or putting on make-up can also an indicator that the person is being abused. They may show signs of being depressed or their actions may indicate avoidance of certain situations especially if they involve the person who is abusing them. They may also seem to be undecided or uninterested in things going on around them and decisions being made about them. Alternatively, they may be uncharacteristically tearful or fearful. When an individual becomes withdrawn, they place themselves in an even more vulnerable position than before as they can become isolated and ignored by others and considered 'unfriendly' 'difficult', and so on, all of which makes it harder for them to speak out about what is happening to them. These changes to behaviour would need to be investigated further to determine the underlying cause.

Neglect and other risk factors

Individuals who have been subjected to abuse often neglect themselves, self-harm or engage in behaviour that puts them at risk. The individual may be reluctant to seek medical help if they are ill, or refuse treatment when advised. Some people may become so self-neglecting that they place no value on their life and so are not concerned about the detrimental effect their behaviour is having on their well-being.

activity
INDIVIDUAL WORK
11.3

P2

P3

1   Describe the different forms of abuse a vulnerable adult may experience.
2   What are the signs and symptoms that may be present which would indicate they are being abused?

Potential for abuse within health and social care contexts

Contexts

The context of something is the set of circumstances which surround or lead to it, including the setting and the people involved. There are a number of different settings in which health and social care workers may be working and supporting individuals.

Home

More individuals are supported within their home environment by a range of health and social care services than ever before. Home is where most people would choose to remain when they have health or social care needs that require support from others. Individuals may be supported at home by family or friends as well as health and social care service providers, such as domiciliary care or district nursing services. The home environment does, however, present a number of potential opportunities for abuse not only of the individual being supported but also of those providing that support.

If an individual is living alone and receiving service to support their needs, they have a level of vulnerability. Individuals at home are more at risk from abuse by strangers than if they were living in supported accommodation. They are at risk from people calling at the door and gaining access through force or intimidation, who either steal from them or charge exorbitant rates for minor repairs.

They are also at risk from physical and sexual abuse as there is no one there to stop the perpetrator (person who commits the abuse).

If the individual lives alone and has health and social care needs, in particular physical or mental needs, they are also at risk from self-neglect or neglect by others, including services if insufficient or inappropriate support is provided to adequately support them and monitor their well-being.

Home may be the individual's choice. However, it may not be the carer's choice especially if they also have support needs. The stress and physical demands of caring for someone 24/7 is known to have a detrimental effect on a carer's health and well-being. Most informal carers are family members and it is generally the emotional bond of that relationship that leads them to take on the caring role. However, this may be severely tested through the physical tiredness of constantly broken sleep, a lack of understanding of the individual's condition, needs and how to meet these (made worse if there are changes in personality as a result of illness), the lack of freedom and constant state of alertness that often comes with the role of caring for another person. Both the informal carer and the cared for are at risk of abuse by each other.

Informal carers and service users in their own homes may also present a risk of abuse for the health and social care worker. Workers may be intimidated into doing more for the individual than agreed, for example by being threatened that the individual will make a complaint or accuse them of malpractice. The potential for the health and social care worker to abuse the service user is also greater within the individual's home. Within this environment, there is little or no supervision or close monitoring of the worker's activities and so the opportunity to abuse without detection is present. This potential is greater still if the individual lives alone, has no close friends or relatives and little or no contact with other people.

Fig 11.7 Bogus callers

89 YEAR OLD MAN 'TRICKED' OUT OF HIS LIFE SAVINGS

On Tuesday a 89 year old man had his life savings stolen after two men posing as water supply engineers tricked their way into the man's house telling him they needed to urgently turn off the water supply.

While one of the men distracted the 89 year man the other stole the man's cheque book, Bank cards and savings books. The man did not realise anything had been stolen until he sat down to pay his bills on Thursday and first found his cheque book missing. When he contacted his Bank and the building society to let them

know they informed him that all the money in his accounts had been withdrawn on Tuesday.

This is the latest in a series of 'distraction' burglaries in the area and police have again issued warnings about bogus callers.

The police were able to get a good description of the two men and have released e-fit pictures and Detective Inspector Ian Justice leading the investigation urged anyone who with information to contact them as soon as possible. They can either contact their local station or Crimestoppers on 0800 555 111

Community

There are a number of initiatives to safeguard individuals from abuse within their community. Two examples are Neighbourhood Watch schemes and the more recent National Community Safety Plan (NCSP) as part of the Crime Reduction government initiative. The NCSP seeks to involve citizens in identifying community safety priorities for their neighbourhoods and working with agencies to tackle these effectively. There is increasing concern about antisocial behaviour especially the intimidation of others by small groups or individuals. There is a need to improve the design of common spaces, such as residential housing estates and shopping areas, so that there are fewer places where individuals are isolated and concerned for their safety. The past five years have seen an increased use of close circuit television (CCTV) surveillance in public areas to increase public confidence in the safety of their community and to apprehend those committing offences.

In the community, we are potentially at risk from abuse by others. That can take the form of verbal abuse, such as swearing or using discriminatory language, physical abuse, such as being physically attacked or murdered, psychological abuse, such as being humiliated, intimidated, bullied or threatened, financial abuse, such as being robbed, or sexual abuse, such as being sexually assaulted or raped. There is a common misconception that most people are abused by strangers. The reality is that by far the majority of abuse is committed by people known to the individual. We need to be aware of the behaviour of others and ensure we think through our plans when in the community to avoid placing ourselves in danger. For example, being out late at night with no means of transport home or walking in unlit, unpopulated areas. One sensible precaution is to ensure that someone knows where you are if you are going out and the approximate time you will be back, when, for example, you go on a visit to see a service user.

Service users can be particularly vulnerable when in the community if they look or behaviour differently to the accepted norms in society. They are vulnerable to all forms of abuse and may be targeted by groups or individuals as they anticipate they will put up less resistance and not be considered reliable witnesses if a crime is committed against them due to their frailty, vulnerability or perceived lack of capacity.

Residential care

Residential settings provide the potential for abuse to occur for a number of reasons. Firstly, the fact that a number of individuals share the same living space can lead to tensions and conflicts. If the living environment is not managed effectively this can lead to tensions rising to the point where there is a loss of control, patience and tolerance of others and abuse occurs.

Trying to balance the needs and wishes of a diverse group of individuals who have generally not chosen to share their living space with one another is one of the difficult but important aspects of providing residential care.

Seaview Residential Care Home

A group of residents all share the same lounge area at the Seaview Residential Care Home. A new resident, Harry, has memory loss and is constantly calling for help. The other residents find this very wearing and have asked staff to move Harry so they can have some peace and quiet. Staff just shrug their shoulders and say there is nothing they can do to make him stop and Harry does it all the time.

One afternoon, Harry is particularly agitated and has been calling out for the past hour. Staff have come once and told him to be quiet and gone away again. After another hour of this, one of the other residents, Bill, gets up and slaps Harry around the face and tells him to stop or 'he'll get more where that came from'.

activity
GROUP WORK

1 What type of abuse is this?
2 Who is being abused?
3 What could have been done to minimise the potential for abuse?

Meeting the needs of a group of individuals can lead to compromise and, although activities, such as mealtimes, may be flexible some of the time, most residential care settings have some routines in place. Routines in themselves are not abusive. It is only when they are rigid and inflexible that they can become so, such as if someone is ill and they are still made to get up for meals or they are offered no alternative if they do not want to eat what is on the menu.

Within residential care settings, individuals can be isolated from other people who may notice changes in their behaviour and this increases their vulnerability. The nature of the one-to-one work involved in supporting personal care activities can also lead to the potential for abuse.

Institutional care

When we think of institutional care, we tend to think of the large psychiatric long-stay hospitals that were a part of health care provision in the middle of the last century. There individuals were segregated from society not just because of psychiatric problems, but for a wide range of reasons, such as being an unmarried mother as a result of being raped. These large psychiatric long-stay hospitals were dismantled as a result of a number of revelations and inquiries that uncovered systematic and widespread abuse of patients. Individuals were relocated to smaller homes, but many found it difficult to adjust to caring environments after years of living in a brutal and dehumanising regime. Institutionalisation is often considered as only happening when individuals live for long periods of time in large institutions. However, individuals can also become institutionalised within a short period of time or in a small home, as it is the nature of the experience that creates the effect of institutionalisation. One of the main features of institutionalisation is the change to the individual's self-concept as it is taken over by the institution. The ability to think for themselves and make choices appears to dissipate, as the individual's interaction with others and the world around them leads them to lose their sense of self as an autonomous individual. Individuals lose their concept of themselves as an 'I', and think only as a 'we', since they never do anything on their own.

The regime within institutional care leads to the breaking down of self or the 'mortification of self'. This happens in a variety of ways, such as:

- not treating people as individuals to the extent where they may not be addressed by name
- making everyone wear the same regimented clothing
- not allowing people to have individual possessions
- giving no choice in aspects of personal appearance, for example giving everyone the same hair cut
- making people undertake activities that are punitive rather than beneficial to their well-being
- humiliating people in front of others, for example telling everyone that an individual is incontinent in a derisory manner

- lack of privacy including open access of personal details and information, censorship or withholding of letters
- regularly subjecting people to abuse and ill-treatment (acts of omission and commission).

The level of control over individuals' lives is almost complete and this makes it more difficult to speak out about what is happening from either inside or outside the institution. By its very nature, an institution is closed from public scrutiny and those who work within it often feel their behaviour is justified as the individuals are viewed by many as a burden on society and have been placed in the institution to separate them from society.

Although the large long-stay hospitals are gone the potential for institutional care remains. Even today, many individuals who live in care homes have little contact with the outside world, few opportunities for going out and often minimal access to activities to occupy their time and energy. In some homes, staff still behave in an authoritarian manner towards residents and the fact that they wear uniforms (particularly in homes for older people) sets them apart as being in a superior position. A contributory factor is working with a medical model of care, where the focus is on the individual's disease, condition or ill health and, therefore, what they are unable to do as opposed to all they can do. This leads staff to take a task-orientated approach where care is seen merely as a series of tasks (for example, baths, meals, medication round) to be got through, often in the shortest possible time, so they can spend time talking with colleagues rather than residents. There is little consideration of the individual and their quality of life and recognition of the fact that having a bath may be one of the few times in the week that a resident receives one-to-one attention and feels as if they are an individual. All of these things can create a situation of institutional care where the needs of the staff or the smooth running of the home assume greater importance than the needs of the individual.

Institutional abuse is not a thing of the past. In July 2006, the Healthcare Commission and the Commission for Social Care Inspection (CSCI) produced a report which revealed the widespread institutional abuse taking place at Budock Hospital near Falmouth in Cornwall. Budock Hospital was a treatment centre for people with learning disabilities. The report highlighted the use of excessive, illegal physical restraint and the overuse of medication as part of the intuitional abuse that had been taking place there since 2001. They found staff had received extensive training in restraint but little other training. The environment was stark with no curtains in the rooms. There was nothing for people to do to and the activities cupboard was empty apart from one Beano annual. Staff were more interested in talking to one another than caring for patients. Inspectors found evidence of staff hitting, pushing and dragging patients, withholding food and giving people cold showers as well as regular financial abuse. It was also found that Cornwall NHS Trust who ran the hospital had failed to act to stop the abuse in spite of several internal inquiries. As a result of the report, Budock Hospital closed in December 2006 and CSCI was asked to inspect every service for people with a learning disability in England and Wales more rigorously to avoid this happening in the future.

Relationships involving power

Where there are inequalities in power in a relationship, there is the potential for the misuse of that power. Power or the ability to influence others can be used to positive effect, such as encouraging someone to try something new, or to negative effect, such as persuading them to do something against their will or better judgement. Situations where power can be abused are where one person is in a more senior position, has more authority or status than the other person, such as a manager and worker, a parent and a child or a professional and a service user. Evidence from inquires such as Beech House (1996) and Budock Hospital (2006) confirmed that power had played a part in institutional abuse continuing, as managers were either directly involved, colluded with the abusers or intimidated staff into colluding and not reporting what was happening. Patients in these settings were not only abused by the staff whose job it was to care for them, they were also abused by the organisational processes that enabled senior staff to avoid taking action when concerns were raised.

 See page 68 in Unit 2 for more information about the Beech House inquiry.

The health and social care worker or informal carer may be in a position of power if the individual they support has limited abilities, for example if they are physically disabled, have dementia, have learning disabilities, are unable to speak or have other communication differences. Service users, to some extent, rely on the worker or carer to do those things they are not able to do for themselves and to protect them from harm or abuse. If there is no mechanism for those relationships to be monitored to ensure power is not misused, the potential for abuse to happen increases. Relationships are complex and in particular those between partners and marital relationships. A dependency on an emotional level may lead to differences in power, which may lead to the relationship becoming abusive, thus increasing the power differential as the damaging effects of abuse attack the self-esteem of the abused person to the extent they become subservient in the relationship.

Caring relationships

The potential for abuse within informal caring relationships can come from a variety of stresses within this situation. The role reversal that often occurs in caring relationships within families, such as husband caring for wife or child caring for parent, can create tensions in the relationships and the carer can become bitter and resentful which can lead to punitive actions as they feel they have been made to take on this role out of a sense of duty rather than choice. They have had to give up a considerable amount of freedom to care for the other person too which can also make the relationship strained. If the individual being cared for is also resentful at being in a position where they have lost their status in the family and are now dependent on another person, they too can become abusive to the carer (formal or informal). Caring relationships often include the performance of intimate tasks and this can lead to misinterpretation of intentions and abusive actions.

Potential

There are a number of factors that may contribute to the potential for abuse to occur.

Bullying within care services

Bullying does not just happen in the playground. It can happen within any group of people and care services are sadly no exception. Bullying refers to the intimidation or mistreatment of a person who is seen as weaker or more vulnerable by another or others. Bullying usually takes place when someone exerts power over another person in order to get them to do something they do not really want to do. Bullying is often accompanied by physical violence or psychological abuse or both. The bully is likely to threaten the individual in order to get what they want. The threat may be to withhold something, for example, something the individual needs such as medication, food or support, as well as to actually harm the individual. Bullying, like other forms of abuse, usually takes place where the person cannot be overheard or seen and this isolation adds to the individual's fear, making them more likely to give in to the bully's demands. Bullying may also take the form of persistent pressure to in effect wear the individual down so they feel they have no option but to agree to something they do not want.

Invasions of privacy

Most people take for granted their privacy and the freedom to decide how much of their lives they wish to share with others. Living in any group environment or needing other people to support you to meet your needs places an individual in a position where privacy can be hard to achieve and decisions about how much they wish to share with others even harder. However, it is the health and social care worker's responsibility to maintain an individual's privacy.

Within care settings, the individual's privacy could be invaded by:

- people not knocking on their door before entering the individual's room or home
- not being able to be in a private place when they see visitors or when they are distressed
- having no key to their room
- having nowhere lockable and safe to keep private and personal possessions
- the bathroom or toilet door being left unlocked or open when the individual is undertaking personal care activities
- being left exposed when personal care or clinical procedures are being undertaken
- workers going in and out of the bathroom while an individual is in the bath
- records not being stored in locked cabinets
- information being shared with others without the individual's informed consent
- personal matters being discussed in public areas where they can be overheard by others
- individual's private matters being discussed by others in inappropriate settings, such as in open areas of the care setting or outside the care setting.

remember

All organisations will have a whistleblowing policy in place to enable workers to raise concerns about practice with the workplace.

Abuse by carers

Carers, whether they are formal paid carers or informal unpaid carers, are in a position of power when supporting individuals merely by the nature of providing that support. The opportunities for misusing that power are many, as they are often working alone on a one-to-one basis with individuals they support and therefore unseen by others. Carers are also in a position of trust and this brings with it opportunities to be involved in the individual's life to a greater extent than other types of relationship may afford. This relationship creates the potential for abuse to occur and research has shown that carers are capable of subjecting the individual to any type of abuse.

Many factors may contribute to carers abusing the individuals in their care, such as:

- care workers having unclear role boundaries between personal and professional relationships
- increased dependency of the vulnerable individual
- when informal carers are in situations where there is more than one dependent person within the family or social network
- when informal carers are in situations where there are several generations of the same family living together and where this is creating conflicts of personal interests and loyalties
- for informal carers, where there is a reversal of role or significant change in the relationship between them and the individual
- for informal carers, where there is a history of abuse in the family, including domestic violence
- if carers are experiencing significant levels of stress
- where the demands of caring for the individual means that the informal carer is isolated from practical and emotional support from others
- where there is a lack of understanding about the individual's condition and care needs which results in inappropriate care
- where there is dependency on the vulnerable individual to meet their needs, such as emotional or sexual needs
- where the vulnerable individual displays challenging behaviour which the carer finds intolerable or stressful
- if there is a history of the carer being abused or being a perpetrator of abuse
- if the carer feels exploited, resentful, angry or guilty
- if the carer has financial difficulties
- if the carer is ill or disabled
- if the carer is experiencing significant and long-term stress.

It is important to remember that only a small number of carers abuse those they care for. However, one abuser is one too many and some would say that it is a failure of the health and social care system that abuse continues to happen. Informal carers are entitled to an assessment of their needs and services to support them continue caring if they wish to do so under the Carers (Recognition & Services) Act (1995) and the Carers and Disabled Children's Act (2000). Accessing support services can make a significant difference to an informal carer's ability to support the individual as well as reducing the risk of unintentional abuse that can result from exhaustion, frustration, stress, lack of skills or understanding.

System abuse

Sometimes the arrangements for health and social care support are inadequate to meet the needs of those individuals who require support. An insecure or overcrowded environment is likely to be a stressful environment. This increases the likelihood of harm or abuse occurring as people struggle to adequately manage individuals' needs. If individuals are living a long distance away from family and friends, they can become isolated and this makes it more difficult for them to communicate their concerns to others. Also the more isolated the individual is from people who know them the harder it is to recognise the subtle changes that may occur as a result of harm or abuse. Poor management and high staff turnover are also likely to mean that tensions created by a diverse group of individuals living together are not managed and this increases the chances of harm and abuse going unnoticed.

When staffing levels are low, training to equip staff to meet the needs of individuals appropriately is not a priority and so inappropriate and inadequate standards of care can result through lack of knowledge and skills. The failure to provide services that meet the prevailing standards of good care practice is also an abuse as it fails to recognise and meet the individual's human rights.

The presence of abusive behaviours, actions, practices and punitive regimes in a health and social care setting that are not challenged and become accepted practice is institutional abuse and is also a failure of the system to protect those it seeks to support.

Inappropriate placement of individuals is an abuse of the individual and occurs when there are inadequate provision of the right type to meet the individual's needs. For example, placing an individual with acute mental health needs resulting in erratic and aggressive behaviour in a residential care home for people who are frail and have no mental health needs is abusive to both the individual, as their needs cannot be adequately met, and also to the other users, as the individual's behaviour can be frightening and intimidating. Failing to assess an individual's needs adequately or to provide appropriate and timely packages of care to meet those needs can also be viewed as an abuse by the system. For example, the inappropriate placement of individuals or discharging an individual from hospital without contacting other agencies to arrange support for them when they return home.

Individuals within health and social care settings can also abuse the system by continuing to claim the need for services they no longer require or by misusing the services that are provided. Threats and intimidation have been used by some individuals to get services they are no longer entitled to but feel they have a right to, for example, by threatening to sue or go to the national press. The requirement for minimum staffing levels, qualifications, appropriate and adequate training and regular supervision as described in the Care Standards Act (2000) are all intended to minimise the risk of abuse.

Abuse by service users

The power in relationships is not always where you think it is, and in some relationships the power lies with the person requiring support and not with those providing it. Anger and resentment of their situation can lead an individual to project their feelings onto those supporting them and this is often displayed as abusive behaviour. However, understanding the reason does not excuse it and whatever the reason the individual should be supported to examine their behaviour and understand the impact that it has on others and that is not acceptable to continue.

Such abuse may be physical, causing injury to the carer or to other users. Sometimes the abuse is sexual, through inappropriate and unwanted touching or subjecting the carer to actions they feel uncomfortable about, such as washing the user's intimate areas when they are capable of doing this for themselves. Sometimes the abuse is verbal, through swearing, insults, using racist or sexist language, sexual innuendo or through humiliation. Service users can be intimidating to those who support them, for example, by saying they will tell others that the carer abused them. Abuse of another person is not acceptable whoever the perpetrator is and no carer is expected to accept abuse as part of their caring role.

Informal caring relationships are likely to be complex and understanding the past as well as the present is always important in these situations if a resolution to abuse is to be found. The carer may be reluctant to tell others for fear of people believing the user and not them.

In formal paid caring roles, the carer may be led to believe that it is 'all part of the job' and the individual 'can't help it' or that it is a failure on their part to manage the situation better.

Service user to service user abuse can also take place and again it can take any form. In particular, physical, psychological, financial, discriminatory and sexual abuse can occur. Where individuals live together, if there are not systems in place to maintain user's privacy, they may be subjected to abuse, such as other users stealing their possessions or invading their privacy. Unclear guidelines for staff regarding relationships between service users and inadequate support for those who wish to form personal relationships, increase the potential for one service user to coerce another into sexual activities they are not able to or do not fully consent to. In this circumstance, carers are often uncertain about intervening as they do not wish to infringe user's rights and so do nothing to check if the relationship is an informed and fully consenting one.

Abuse of carers

Within health and social care settings, carers may be abused by service users, by other carers as well as by the system. This abuse can be physical, psychological, sexual or discriminatory.

In particular, the potential for carers to be abused because of unacceptable levels of stress exists when:

remember

Organisations supporting adults with learning disabilities should have a relationships policy in place to clarify the worker's role and responsibility in safeguarding adults while maintaining the users' rights.

- they are inadequately trained for the job they are required to do
- they are poorly supervised or receive insufficient management support
- they are unsure of the boundaries between personal and professional relationships
- staffing levels are inadequate to meet the needs of the individuals being supported
- they are encouraged to work within rigid routines
- they are poorly paid (this also increases the service user's vulnerability to financial abuse)
- they work long hours.

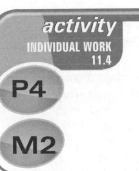

remember

Being abused by others is not in a health and social care worker's job description and is therefore not 'part of the job'. Abuse should always be reported and recorded.

In addition, if carers work within a closed system with little contact with others and are isolated from professional discussions and ideas, this can add to their feelings of vulnerability as they have no way of checking that what they are doing meets acceptable standards or if the expectations of them as a carer are reasonable. In situations of institutional abuse, this was found to be a significant factor in enabling the abuse to continue over a long period of time. All of these can make the carer feel powerless to influence practice and afraid to report their concerns.

Informal carers are also at risk from abuse, not only from the individual they support but also by the system. Carers who are left to care for an individual without adequate information, advice or support or beyond the time they have clearly stated they are able to do so could be considered as being abused by the health and social care services that have a responsibility to meet their needs as well as those of the individual being cared for. A lack of understanding of those in health and social care about the impact caring can have on the carer, their health and their relationship with the cared for can lead to a lack of resources being made available to adequately support individuals. Health and social care workers can intimidate the carer into continuing to care for an individual at home by using the emotional bond between the carer and the cared for and the guilt the carer would feel at not caring, thereby putting pressure on the carer to carry on even though this is having a detrimental effect on their health and well-being. Not providing information and advice about available support options is another abuse as it infringes the person's rights to make informed decisions.

activity

INDIVIDUAL WORK 11.4

P4

M2

1   Identify four health and social care settings and for each one describe what circumstances create the potential for abuse to occur.
2   Analyse the reasons why this potential exists in these four settings.

Predisposing factors

 Link

See page 51 in Unit 2 for more information about vulnerability to abuse.

Fig 11.8 Individuals vulnerable to abuse

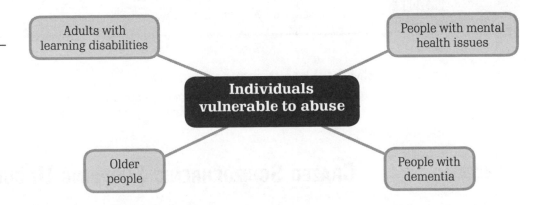

Adults with learning disabilities

People with mental health issues

Individuals vulnerable to abuse

Older people

People with dementia

One thing that people with health and social care needs have in common is their vulnerability to abuse. Many people in society may discriminate against them and, in so doing, do not consider and treat them as equals with equal rights and responsibilities. They may be viewed as having needs that may make self-expression difficult or they not be taken seriously.

Learning disabilities

Adults with learning disabilities are particularly vulnerable if they use other communication methods, such as using eye movement, touch, pictures or Makaton, rather than speech as not everyone will be able to communicate with them therefore increasing their isolation. They may be perceived as being less able to understand or express what is happening to them. They may be easier to coerce into doing something they are uncomfortable with as they may not fully understand the implications of their consent. In reality, the difficulties they may have with complex, higher thinking processes such as abstract thought and analysis are as much as consequence of their exclusion from or lack of access to education as their intellectual ability. The individual's vulnerability is increased by the fact that they may not be considered to have the capacity to consent and so it is a matter of one person's word against another. Reports, such as MENCAP's report Behind Closed Doors (2001), have shown that the likelihood is that the abuser will be believed rather than the person with learning disabilities if any investigation takes place. Often no criminal charges are brought in cases of abuse because the individual is deemed unreliable and there is little chance of them being believed in a court of law. This could be viewed as abuse by the system.

Link

See page 21 in Unit 1 for more information about alternative communication methods.

MENCAP	www.mencap.org.uk
Ann Croft Trust	www.anncrafttrust.org

---

case study 11.4   **Luke and Pete**

Luke is 26 years old and has learning disabilities. He lives at home with his parents and works part-time at the local supermarket. He used to like working there and was always keen to get up on the days he worked. Recently, however, he has refused to get up or said he feels unwell. He refuses to talk to his parents about it and so his mother phoned his support worker, Pete, to arrange an earlier visit. Luke tells Pete that the other young people at the supermarket have been calling him 'stupid' and other nasty names, making fun of him, teasing him and getting him into trouble. He was told off by the manager in front of other people for putting the wrong things on the shelf and when he tried to explain it was not his fault, the manager wouldn't listen and told him if he was not up to the job perhaps he should leave.

activity
GROUP WORK

1   What type of abuse has Luck experienced?
2   What action do you think Pete should take?

Mental health issues

People with mental health issues are often portrayed in the media as being dangerous, unpredictable in their behaviour, irrational and to be avoided.

Fig 11.9 Public perception of schizophrenia

CRAZED SCHIZOPHRENIC SHOPPING UNSUPERVISED

The fact that one in four people are likely to experience some form of mental health issue appears not be heard above the voices of alarm that discriminate against this group of people. There is a lack of understanding about mental health issues and the diversity of illness. Society has for a very long time constructed this group of people as being a threat to others and less worthy of our compassion as those with physical illness and disease. All of this makes them vulnerable to abuse from others through exclusion, intimidation and actual physical violence as people are fearful of their difference.

Age

See page 60 in Unit 2 for more information about discrimination against older people.

Youth is celebrated in our society and older people can be discriminated against. One of the consequences of negative attitudes towards older people is their vulnerability to abuse by others who do not value them as individuals or their contribution to society. Twenty-two per cent of all people abused are aged between 80 and 84, with over half of all elder abuse committed against people aged 70 and over. It is not just frail older people or women who are abused either, although women are more likely to be abused than men.

One type of abuse on the increase with abusers targeting older people is fraud. Older people are often intimidating into sending money to fraudsters who persistently telephone them either asking for donations to charities (which often do not exist) or with promises of financial investments to enable them to leave money to their children. Leaving an inheritance is something that many older people would like to be able to do for their families, to the extent that they often live frugally themselves, and so this financial opportunity seems particularly attractive to them. Once they have sent money, however, they are then telephoned persistently often several times a day with calls become more frightening and intimidating until they sends more money. In addition, many older people respond to unsolicited junk mail, telling them they have, for example, won a prize which they can claim if they send a certain sum to cover administration and postage, not realising that it is in fact a fraudulent activity as there is no competition and no prize just someone stealing their money. Local trading standards officers and the police often warn people about these illegal activities, but many older people are too embarrassed to admit they have been taken advantage of and it is only when they have lost all their savings, get into debt or someone close to them finds unpaid bills that what has been happening comes to light.

Many older people do not speak out about the abuse they are experiencing as they feel embarrassed or ashamed that they have in some way allowed it to happen to them. Others feel trapped by their dependence on their relatives or carers or fear that if they do say anything this will make the abuse worse or they may be made to leave their own home and 'put into a home or hospital' and that loss would to their mind be worse that what they are experiencing. Many also believe that nothing can be done and mistrust that anyone would believe them and so say nothing.

Counsel + Care	www.counselandcare.org.uk
Help the AGED	www.helptheaged.org.uk
Action on elder abuse	www.elderabuse.org.uk

Dementia

Many people believe that only older people have dementia. In fact, according to the Alzheimer's Society dementia currently affects over 750,000 people in the UK and approximately 18,000 of this number are under 65 (2006 statistics). Dementia is a progressive disease that affects the brain and the individual's short-term memory, speech and comprehension creating, among other symptoms, confusion. Impairment of the ability to remember things that have just happened or you have just been told makes the individual particularly vulnerable as other people can assure the individual they did or did not do something and they have no recollection of it at all to establish what really happened. Other people can therefore abuse them and then deny any wrong doing and due to the dementia the individual is unable to dispute the abuser's denial. Even though people with dementia have moments of insight and clarity, they are more often confused and unable to remember recent events. Therefore, if they do speak out about the abuse, the reliability of their account will still be in doubt. This situation is compounded if the abuser is in a caring role or has some status.

As the dementia progresses, the individual becomes unable to recognise people familiar to them, such as their partner, which can cause great distress to both but even more so if their partner also acts as their carer and every time they support them with intimate personal care tasks the individual accuses them of assault or rape. An abusing carer may feel even more protected in these circumstances, as the individual's accusations can be dismissed as part of the dementia and not a reality.

In addition to short-term memory loss, problems with speech and understanding isolate the individual with dementia even more and this increases their vulnerability. People with dementia can be confused about the time of day and abusers can use this and poor memory to treat individuals in ways that others would consider unacceptable. For example, in cases of institutional abuse routines have included getting residents up very early and making them sit for two or more hours before giving them their breakfast or getting them ready for bed in the middle of the afternoon.

Alzheimer's Society   www.alzheimers.org.uk

Previous history of being abused

If individuals have been abused in the past then they are particularly vulnerable to being abused again. This may be because the reasons for their vulnerability remain, for example they may have limited communication, or due to the negative impact that the experience of being abused has on the individual's self esteem and responses to others. Because they lack a sense of self-worth they may be more inclined to please others to gain acceptance and affection. This subservient role may lead to them being taken advantage of and abused by others. The experience of abuse may have been so damaging that as a result the individual self-harms or has little or no regard for their own well-being. This again increases their vulnerability to further abuse. They may have no experience of supportive non-abusive relationships and without help and support may be unable to break with patterns of learned behaviour which leads them to form relationships with abusive partners. Low self-esteem is another contributory factor in repeating patterns of learned behaviour. If the individual's past history is known to others, this can make them more vulnerable as the potential abuser may identify this as an opportunity to manipulate the situation to hide their actions. For example, the abuser may discredit the individual's accusations claiming that as they had been abused in the past they see everything as abuse. It will also highlight their vulnerability to a potential abuser.

Working strategies to minimise abuse

Working practices, strategies and adult protection policies and procedures as well as legislation are all intended to minimise the potential for abuse.

Strategies

Protection of Vulnerable Adults Scheme (POVA)

Unfortunately someone who abuses a vulnerable individual is likely to do so many times before they are caught, especially if they leave their employment before the abuse is discovered or they are dismissed. Since July 2004, it has been a statutory requirement for employers and the Commission for Social Care Inspection (CSCI) to report people considered unsuitable to work with **vulnerable adults** (people over 18 years of age) for inclusion on the POVA list. The POVA scheme is run by the Department of Health and covers England and Wales. People are included on the POVA list if they have abused or harmed a vulnerable adult in their care or placed that individual at risk of harm.

POVA applies to:

- registered service providers of care homes
- domiciliary care agencies
- adult placement schemes
- employment agencies or businesses that supply care workers to the above providers.

The POVA guidance included changes to the requirements for the Criminal Records Bureau (CRB) disclosures. People are unable to start working with any of the above service providers until a full CRB disclosure has been completed. Following guidance from the Department of Health in May 2006, changes to this requirement have been made that allow people to start work in exceptional circumstances subject to safeguards including a POVAFirst check.

The circumstance when a POVAFirst check can be carried out is when there is a real danger that if the worker is not able to start staffing levels will fall below statutory requirements. POVAFirst applications are monitored by CSCI to ensure compliance. The POVA scheme is another line of defence in protecting vulnerable adults from potential abuse as it is in addition to the pre-employment checks, such as the interview process, qualifications, references and CRB disclosure.

Research into the first 100 POVA referrals by King's College London and the Social Care Workforce Research Unit published in July 2005 identified the following facts:

- Most referrals from care homes involved physical, psychological and verbal abuse.

- Financial abuse was the main reason for referrals by domiciliary care providers.

- Male staff were more likely to be referred for physical abuse whereas female staff were more likely to be referred for financial abuse.

- The majority (70%) of those people referred were dismissed from their jobs.

- 40% of the referrals involved the police and resulted in convictions (in 20% of referrals the police investigations or criminal proceedings were ongoing when the research took place).

Care Homes Regulation

The Care Standards Act (2000), introduced the National Minimum Standards (NMS) for the delivery of care in a number of settings. Registered care homes for older people, younger adults and adult placements and domiciliary care services are all required to meet NMS, which describe the quality of care considered to be the minimum that individuals should be receive within these settings. The standards relate to all aspects of daily life and include protection from abuse. The standards relating to protection of the individual from harm and abuse are Standard 18 for older people, Standard 23 for younger adults and adult placements and Standard 14 for domiciliary care. All state the expectations and responsibilities within this area of care provision. This includes the requirement for providers to have robust policies and procedures in place that are underpinned by effective working practices that protect vulnerable adults.

National Service Framework

The government introduced National Service Framework standards (NSF) in April 1998 as a rolling programme of long-term strategies with the aim of improving specific areas of care. Each standard has a set of measurable goals and timescales within which these are to be achieved. There are NSF standards for older people, children and people with mental health issues as well as for specific diseases, such as coronary heart disease, cancer, long-term conditions, renal conditions, chronic obstructive pulmonary disease (COPD) and diabetes.

For older people, Standard 1, rooting out age discrimination, and Standard 2, person-centred care, both emphasise the treatment of people with dignity and respect and as individuals. Both of these standards relate to protecting the individual from abuse. The NSF standards are described as outcomes, or expectations of service provision quality, and so these can be used to measure and regulate service provision thereby acting as a protection for the users of those services.

Multi-agency working

Lessons learnt from child abuse cases included the vital role that multi-agency working has in protecting vulnerable adults from abuse. Multi-agency working across statutory and non-statutory health and social care agencies as well as the police is the foundation of all adult protection polices and procedures. All organisations that come into contact with vulnerable adults need to be aware of circumstances that may potentially increase that vulnerability and cooperate with one another to minimise the risk. In addition, when there is a suspicion of abuse, all agencies must adopt the same strategies for managing the situation and investigating the allegations and dealing with the outcome. Consistency in approach is a vital strategy in safeguarding adults from abuse.

Working in partnership with service users

Health and social care agencies working together is only a part of the overall strategy to protect vulnerable adults from abuse. Enabling service users to recognise abuse and knowing how to alert others to this is another important strategy. It is important that health and social care workers act as good role models in terms of worker-user relationships as this helps the service user to recognise when the relationship is abusive. In addition, it is important for workers to enable service users to know how to protect themselves, such as building positive self-esteem through knowing their rights and knowing how to complain. Many organisations also operate a key worker system where the service user has one particular worker they relate to and who takes an individual interest in the user's well-being. Because of the relationship, the key worker is often the person to pick up early signs that indicate all is not well with the service user. Any interventions implemented to protect the service user should be discussed with them so they can make informed decisions and agree to those interventions.

Strategies between professionals and within organisations

Inter-agency working is also important, especially when the service user is accessing a number of different services. Effective communication between professionals and organisations is vital to ensure the service user is protected. Communicating information about changes, significant events and actions ensures that all those involved with supporting the service user are monitoring their well-being. For example, a day care provider should be made aware of any behaviour strategies and contract that have been agreed between the service user and residential care provider so there is continuity of practice. A lack of communication can lead to inconsistency as well as misinformation and accusation, none of which are in the service user's best interest. In situations where the service user is identified as vulnerable, there should be interagency agreements regarding monitoring and review as well as what action to take if the situation changes or escalates.

Decision-making processes and forums

Local authority social service departments are responsible for taking the lead in adult protection and, to that end, may have set up an adult protection forum. If not, then the local policy and procedures will describe the decision making process in situations where suspected or actual abuse require investigation. A case conference is a key element of any investigation and would be made up of all those involved with the service user. You will need to look at the local policy and procedures when you are on placement to find out how decisions are made in your area.

Organisational policies and training

Organisational policies and procedures will be based on the multi-agency adult protection policies in your area. Organisational policies and procedures will contain information about signs and symptoms of harm and abuse and what actions to take in specific circumstances. Part of the policy will include the requirement for all staff working with vulnerable adults to receive training about abuse and POVA to enable them to recognise and report any factors that they consider may be dangerous, harmful or abusive to individuals and what action to take in accordance with those policies and procedures. Training should include information about your organisation's whistleblowing policy and how to report incidents or suspicions of abuse when those suspected are in positions of authority within the organisation.

Working practices

Policies and procedures alone will not protect vulnerable adults; this can only happen when these are integrated into working practice.

Needs assessment

The starting point when supporting individuals is to identify and understand their needs and circumstances. A detailed needs assessment which identifies areas of strength as well as areas that require support will help health and social care workers to plan appropriate levels of intervention. Abuse can occur when individual needs are not adequately identified or met either intentionally or unintentionally. The individual should have a holistic assessment of needs which explores all the relevant areas of their life and the impact that their circumstances, for example illness or disability, has on their day-to-day life, potential and quality of life. A needs assessment should identify an individual's vulnerability and should inform the next stage of the care process, that is, care planning.

Care planning cycle

The effectiveness of care planning depends on the effectiveness of assessment. If needs are clearly identified, agreeing actions and interventions to meet the individual's needs will be easier. The care planning cycle could be described as a journey. You start the journey by identifying where the individual is (their needs). The next part is to identify where they are going (the goal or outcome). The care plan is the map that tells the individual and worker the route to follow to reach where they are going (the steps along the way that need to be undertaken to get to the goal or outcome). The care plan details the different tasks that will be undertaken to meet the individual's needs and take them a step closer to achieving their goal. For some, the goals may be limited due their circumstances, for example if they have a life-limiting disease. For others, the care plan may involve gaining new skills to achieve greater independence, such as life skills for person with learning disability or mental health issues. If the individual has needs related to protecting them from potential or actual abuse by others or themselves, the strategies agreed by all involved should be recorded in the care plan and communicated to everyone supporting the individual. This should ensure consistency of practice and also be a mechanism for monitoring their well-being.

Person-centred practices

Person-centred approaches were first used in supporting older people with dementia. A person-centred approach is one where the individual is valued and respected and where their best interests are placed at the centre or core of everything that happens to that individual, such as assessment, care planning and interventions. In relation to supporting and protecting adults, this means considering the situation from their viewpoint and ensuring they are involved in decision making and supported to voice their views and concerns. If they are unable to do this, consideration of an advocate to act on their behalf and in their best interest needs to be explored. In adult protection cases, there are often dilemmas about removing the individual from a risk situation or leaving them with close support and monitoring as this may be their wish. If a person-centred approach is used, the individual must be empowered to state their wishes and make informed choices about the risk and how these should be managed.

Oral and written communications

Communication both with service users and others involved in their care and support is essential if the potential for harm and abuse is to be minimised. Systems for communicating information about individuals must be confidential. However, those who have a responsibility to support individuals must have adequate access to appropriate information. Most organisations will have information-sharing agreements or protocols in place to ensure people are clear about what information can be shared and with whom. The misuse of information is abusive as it removes an individual's rights. There may be a variety of recording systems within the workplace and workers must ensure that each is used appropriately. Written information can provide vital evidence in situations where abuse is systematic. All health and social care records are legal documents and as such information recorded must be factual, accurate, legible, signed and dated. Care must be taken when communicating information verbally to ensure it remains confidential, for example, that it is not overheard by others. Written records must be kept in a secure location and accessible only by those who need to know or who the individual has consented to information being shared with.

Use of IT in sharing information between professionals

Most health and social care workplaces use computers to store service user records and it is important to have procedures in place to ensure these records remain confidential and meet the requirements of the Data Protection Act (2000). The use of passwords, secure email and agreed information-sharing protocols are all ways in which sensitive information can be protected. In situations where abuse is suspected or alleged, information about the situation is highly sensitive as the individuals involved have a right to privacy and the breach of confidentiality may place them in further danger from others (this is true of the accused as well as the abused person, as the accused may be subjected to abuse or harm by others). Agreements about what information is to be shared and with whom must be with the individual's informed consent. They have a right to place limitations on this.

See page 71 in Unit 2 for more information about the Data Protection Act (2000).

Anti-oppressive practice

In relation to supporting and protecting adults from abuse, it is important that information is not withheld from those who have a right to that information. In addition, it is important that all allegations of abuse are fully investigated if possible by an independent party. All investigations must be carried out in a way that respects the rights of those involved and is non-judgemental. Within British law, people are innocent until proven guilty and it is important therefore that workers and others do not jump to conclusions or make assumptions about an individual's guilt or the truth of an allegation without the correct procedures being followed to establish the facts and truth of the situation. Adult protection procedures are in place to ensure that people are not treated in an oppressive manner as this in itself is abusive.

Anti-discriminatory practice

Recognising abuse, reporting it and acting to protect the individual in a non-judgemental, respectful and confidential manner are all ways in which anti-discriminatory practice should be demonstrated. Anti-discriminatory practice is demonstrated when workers follow procedures and do not make judgments or attribute blame without gathering all the facts first. All those involved in an adult abuse situation have rights and maintaining those rights does not in any way condone the action of the abuser.

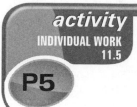

activity
INDIVIDUAL WORK
11.5

P5

Use examples to describe the different working practices and strategies that can be used to minimise abuse within health and social care settings.

Procedures for protection

Organisational policies and procedures

Every health and social care organisation will have policies and procedures related to protecting adults from abuse. These should have been made clear to each worker as part of their induction and they should be kept informed if these change. Within these, there should be information about who to report concerns to. This could include a named person, such as the manager as well as the commissioning or inspection authority, such as CSCI.

See page 76 in Unit 2 for more information about organisational policies and procedures.

Fig 11.10 Policy and procedure documents

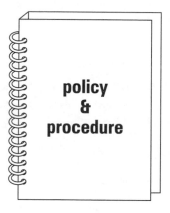

policy
&
procedure

Organisational policies and procedures will also contain information regarding confidentiality and information-sharing agreements and the rights of the service user in situations of suspected or actual abuse. This should also include information about advocacy services that could support the service user and how to contact them. The main part of the document will relate to the actions that workers need to take if they suspect or witness abuse. Although polices and procedures will vary some general principles apply. These include:

- The worker must ensure that any action they take does not place the individual or others in further danger of harm or abuse.
- The worker must never confront the suspected perpetrator. This may place the individual raising the concern at risk.
- The worker must know who to report any suspicions or disclosures of danger, harm or abuse to and the time scales for this.
- The worker's report and records must maintain confidentiality as far as their responsibility and authority allows. If their report is verbal, they must ensure that this takes place somewhere where they will not be overheard.

- The worker must not discuss the situation with other members of staff.
- Reports and records must be factual and not contain subjective opinion unless this is clearly stated as such.

Actions to take in the event of disclosure

Health and social care workers may become aware of potential or actual harm and abuse through a **disclosure**. This could be made by the individual, the perpetrator (abuser) or another person.

In the event of disclosure:

- do remain calm and try not to show shock, disbelief or anger
- do listen very carefully to what is being said and respect their wishes
- do show concern by acknowledging, if appropriate, your regret about what has happened
- do reassure the person by telling them they have done the right thing in telling someone and that you take what they are saying seriously
- if the person disclosing is the individual who has been harmed or abused, do reassure them it is not their fault
- do be honest about your responsibility to act upon the information disclosed
- do reassure the individual that information will not be shared with other individuals supported within the service
- do tell the individual what you are going to do and who you are reporting the disclosed information to
- do explain that the person you report to will then talk to them about the next steps
- do, if appropriate, take urgent action to protect the individual from any immediate danger
- do be aware, if it is a recent incident, you need to preserve any material evidence that may be required for an investigation
- do not interrupt or ask questions to gain more details
- do not promise a level of confidentiality you do not have the authority to maintain as this will mislead the individual
- do not be judgemental
- do not break confidentiality between the person disclosing, yourself and your manager
- if a person other that the alleged perpetrator and victim discloses, do not alert the alleged perpetrator or victim..

It is vital that workers do not make assumptions about what has happened and report exactly what was disclosed without opinion. Effective action at this point is crucial for both the alleged abuser and the individual who may be being abused. It is important that procedures are followed correctly throughout so that a proper investigation can be conducted if appropriate. Failure to do so may jeopardise the objectivity of the investigation. This may mean the alleged perpetrator can continue abusing or if the allegation is unfounded, leave suspicion lingering.

Recording and reporting requirements

These will be clearly documented in the procedures and it is imperative that workers adhere to the guidelines if adults are to be adequately protected. Patterns of behaviour are often only identified through examination of service user records. Records kept at the time of an allegation or incident will be vital evidence in the event of a criminal prosecution. The procedures may include the need to complete specific documents, such as an incident report and this would be copied to senior managers as well as to the commissioning or regulatory authority as part of the multi-agency procedures.

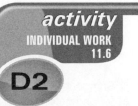

activity

INDIVIDUAL WORK 11.6

D2

Explain the role of multi-agency working in minimising the risks of abuse in health and social care settings and provide reasons why this is an effective strategy.

Legislation

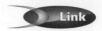

See Unit 28, in BTEC National Health and Social Care Book 2, for more information about legislation.

There are a number of pieces of legislation that contain information about legal responsibilities in relation to the support and protection of adults from abuse.

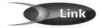

See page 71 in Unit 2 for more information about the Data Protection Act (1998). See pages 68–69 in Unit 2 for more information about Bournewood.

Policies and procedures

Protection of Vulnerable Adults Scheme (POVA) and Practical Guide for Placement of Adult Carers

POVA is an important strategy in protecting vulnerable adults.

Refer back to page 372 to remind yourself about POVA.

All employers must ensure that all staff have an understanding of what constitutes abuse, the local policy and procedures and their role in these. Employers must ensure they know who the local social services adult protection coordinator is and must refer to them in situations where abuse is suspected or alleged before they take any action.

Criminal Records Bureau and enhanced disclosure

The role of the Criminal Records Bureau (CRB) is to reduce the risk of abuse by ensuring that those who are unsuitable are not able to work with children and vulnerable adults. A CRB disclosure is made under the Police Act (1997) and it contains information held by the police and government departments. It is used by employers and voluntary organisations to make safer recruitment decisions. A standard CRB disclosure gives details about criminal convictions, cautions, reprimands and warnings held on the Police National Computer (PNC). The enhanced CRB disclosure includes looking at the PNC database records, local police records and the three government lists of those banned from working with children or vulnerable adults. A standard CRB disclosure check may be considered to be sufficient when a health and social care worker is employed, but many organisations will require an enhanced CRB check. This is in part due to the changing nature of health and social care work where many workers work one-to-one with individuals and outside the confines of a care or nursing home environment.

Local and national guidelines for staff and volunteers

Health and social care workers need to be aware of local guidance regarding CRB and POVA checks in relation to themselves and to volunteers. This may vary depending on the service user group and the type of service provision. The national guidance is outlined in the POVA and CRB regulations. The national guidance is that volunteers who work with vulnerable adults may also be subject to CRB disclosure checks. The guidance states that those people who regularly care for, train, supervise or are in sole charge of vulnerable adults must have an enhanced CRB check. This would include for example, teachers, scout or guide leaders and activity club leaders. According to the CRB, the decision of whether or not to require CRB disclosure checks of volunteers should be based on:

- a thorough risk assessment of the role performed by the volunteer and the extent to which this brings them into contact with children and vulnerable adults
- whether the person's voluntary work is carried out in someone else's premises where it is a requirement that CRB checks are done in order to comply with statutory regulations, such as a school or care home

If a volunteer needs a CRB check this will be done free of charge by the CRB as long as they meet their volunteer definition criteria.

In October 2005, the Association of Directors of Social Services (ADSS) produced Safeguarding Adults, a national framework of standards of good practice and outcomes in adult protection work. The intention in setting the 11 sets of standards is to achieve consistency and reliability of service provision and response to suspicions and allegations of

Legislation relating to abuse

Legislation	Section
European Convention on Human Rights and Fundamental Freedoms (1950)	This states fundamental civil and political rights and freedoms of individuals.
Sexual Offences Act (1976, updated in 2003)	This includes sections relating to consent, and definitions of different types of sexual offence. SOA (2003) is gender-neutral although some offences remain gender specific. It includes sections relating to the capacity to consent of individuals with mental health needs or a learning disability. The act was updated by 2004 amendments.
Mental Health Act (1993) & Codes of Practice	The Act outlines the arrangements for the compulsory detention of people with mental health needs for assessment or treatment. Section 7 relates to the guardianship of individuals with mental health needs in the interests of their welfare or for the protection of others.
Nursing & Residential Care Homes Regulations (1984)	These Regulations provided guidelines about standards of care prior to the Care Standards Act (2000). They were repealed with the introduction of the Care Standards Act.
NHS & Community Care Act (1990)	Section 47 relates to rights of individuals to have an assessment of their needs. Section 48 relates to the inspection of nursing and care homes.
Disability Discrimination Act 1995	This establishes rights for people with disabilities to be treated fairly and without discrimination and to be afforded the same opportunities as others.
Human Rights Act (1998)	This establishes the following fundamental human rights: ■ The right to life ■ Freedom from torture, inhuman and degrading treatment ■ Freedom from forced labour or slavery ■ The right to liberty and to a fair trial ■ Freedom from facing retrospective crimes or penalties ■ The right to privacy ■ Freedom of conscience ■ Freedom of expression ■ Freedom of assembly ■ The right to marriage and family ■ Freedom from discrimination
Data Protection Act (1998)	Individuals have a right to access information about them that is held by organisations.
Special Educational Needs Act (2000)	This extends the Disability Discrimination Act (1995) to cover every aspect of education. It re-emphasises the rights of children and adults to be educated within mainstream education at all levels with appropriate provisions being made to enable this to occur.
Care Standards Act (2000) (No Secrets and Speaking up for Justice)	This introduced new registration, regulation and inspection processes and extended these to all care services. No Secrets also included the need to minimise the risk of abuse through rigorous recruitment practices. Both led to the introduction of the POVA register.
Race Relations (Amendment) Act (2000)	This strengthens earlier legislation and extends to all public bodies who now have a duty to eliminate unlawful racial discrimination as well as enhancing the powers of the Commission for Racial Equality.
Care Homes for Older People NMS – Care Homes Regulations (2003)	Standard 18 relates to the protection of service users from abuse.
Mental Health Bill (2006)	This provides more safeguards than the Mental Health Act (1993) in relation to detention and more independent checks, rights to appeal and the appointment of a representative to look at an individual's rights (the 'Bournewood provisions').

abuse. In addition, Safeguarding Adults recognises the need to include all adults who may be eligible to receive community care services within policies and to enable those users who choose to manage their own care through using Direct Payments or In Control funding to access support of their own choosing. As a result of the changes in how health and social care services are accessed by users, the wider term 'safeguarding adults' is beginning to replace the terms 'vulnerable adults' or 'adult protection'.

Fig 11.11 POVA flowchart

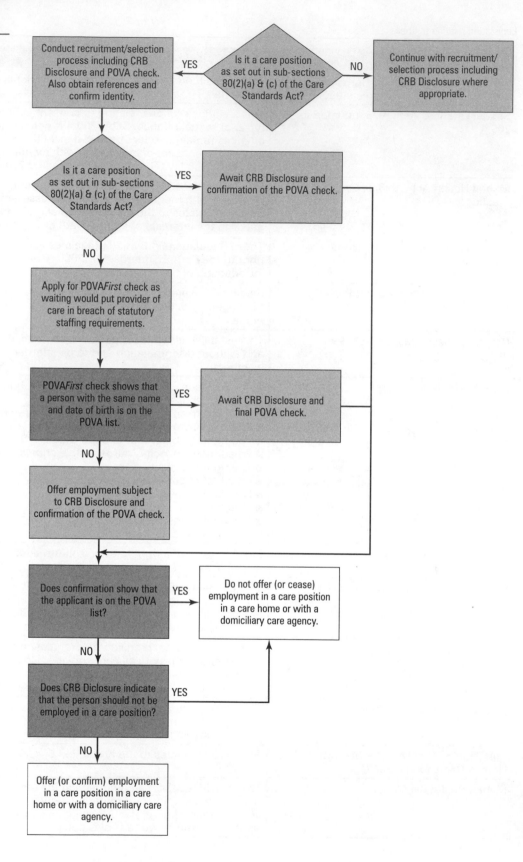

Fig 11.12 NMC Code of
Professional Conduct

Fig 11.13 GSCC Code of
Practice

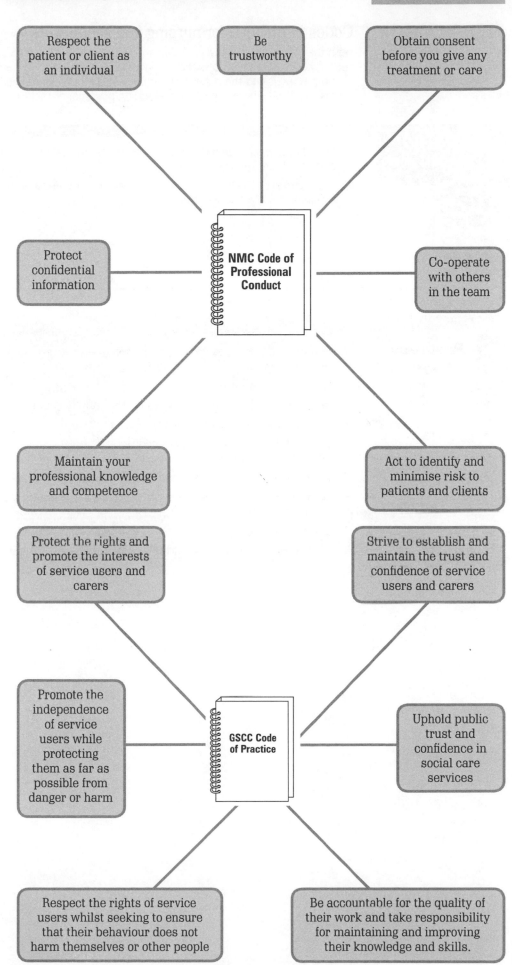

Respect the patient or client as an individual

Be trustworthy

Obtain consent before you give any treatment or care

Protect confidential information

NMC Code of Professional Conduct

Co-operate with others in the team

Maintain your professional knowledge and competence

Act to identify and minimise risk to patients and clients

Protect the rights and promote the interests of service users and carers

Strive to establish and maintain the trust and confidence of service users and carers

Promote the independence of service users while protecting them as far as possible from danger or harm

GSCC Code of Practice

Uphold public trust and confidence in social care services

Respect the rights of service users whilst seeking to ensure that their behaviour does not harm themselves or other people

Be accountable for the quality of their work and take responsibility for maintaining and improving their knowledge and skills.

Codes of practice for nursing and social work

Both the Nursing and Midwifery Council (NMC) and the General Social Care Council (GSCC) set out codes of practice for people working in health and social care. Clarifying expectation for both workers and the public is an important step in safeguarding adults. In addition to the professional code there is guidance regarding practitioner-client relationships.

activity
INDIVIDUAL WORK
11.7

P6

M3

1 Identify the legislation, polices and procedures that safeguard adults receiving health and social care services.

2 Use examples to help you explain how these contribute to protecting vulnerable adults within health and social care settings.

Progress Check

1 Explain, using examples, how you would maintain a service user's confidentiality.

2 Compare the relationship between a health and social care worker and a service user and that between two friends.

3 What is adult abuse?

4 What are the different types of abuse that adults could experience?

5 Explain, using examples, where abuse can occur.

6 What signs would indicate that institutional abuse may be present within a health or social care setting?

7 Which groups of people are particularly vulnerable to abuse?

8 What national strategies are in place to safeguard adults receiving health and social care?

9 Explain how effective needs assessment can protect individuals from abuse.

10 Explain what action you would take if you suspected or witnessed abuse.

Glossary

abuse
to cause physical, emotional or sexual harm to an individual or to fail or neglect to protect them from harm

accurate record
a factual written record made of an event

active listening
the process of communicating with a person without being distracted or talking over them

adoption
the legal basis for assumption of parental responsibility

advocacy
the process of representing the needs of an individual

anatomy
the science of the physical structure, especially the internal structure, and the relationship between structures of the human body

autoimmune disorder
a disorder by which a person's immune system attacks their body's own tissues

caecum
the first part of the colon which is a dilated part of the intestine, blind at one end and continuous with the ascending colon

capitalism
an economic system with private ownership of organisations that produce, distribute and sell good and services. It is a system of free competitive markets driven by profit

care order
an order made by the courts placing the child in the care of the local authority

care value base
the fundamental rights that people should expect when receiving care and on which professionals in health and social care should base their practice

carer
a person who looks after a relative or friend who needs support because of age, physical or learning disability or illness, including mental illness

cataract
a condition in which the lens of the eye becomes opaque, resulting in blurred vision

centile (percentile)
each of the 100 groups into which a population can be divided according to, e.g. height or weight

child protection register
a list of children who are deemed by the local authority to be at risk of harm

children's centre
a point of access to integrated services for children under five and their families

chromosome
a rod-shaped structure in a cell nucleus carrying the genetic material that determines sex and other characteristics an organism inherits from its parents

client
a person receiving care, also known as a service user or patient depending on the care setting or service

cochlea
the inner ear

cognitive
concerned with thinking

communication cycle
the pattern of interaction that occurs when giving or receiving information from a person that includes encoding and decoding words and symbols

condition
to train or accustom to behaving in a certain way

confidentiality
the act of ensuring that information is seen strictly by those who have a right or need to see it

cultural and social norms
the traditions and customs that govern a culture or society

cyanosis
a bluish discolouration of the skin due to poor circulation or insufficient oxygen in the blood

dermatitis
a skin condition that can make skin dry and sore. It is not contagious but is usually a reaction to something that has come in contact with the skin

differentiation
the process by which stem cells specialise

disclosure
a secret fact that is made known, often about current or past abuse

DNA
(deoxyribonucleic acid) the substance carrying an organism's genetic information. It is a nucleic acid molecule in the form of a twisted double strand (double helix) that is the major component of chromosomes and carries genetic information

E. coli
(*Escherichia coli*) bacteria that causes diarrhoea, vomiting, kidney damage and kidney failure

Early Years Foundation Stage
part of the National Curriculum for the education of children aged three until the end of their reception year

elective mutism
a condition in which an individual chooses not to speak

empower
to give someone who may be disadvantaged, e.g. through age, a learning disability or non-verbal communication, control of their life and opportunities to meet their needs and aspirations

empowerment
the process of gaining more control over your life by becoming aware of and using personal and external resources and overcoming obstacles in order to meet your needs and aspirations, having your voice heard in decision-making and being able to challenge inequality and oppression in your life

enhance
to improve

enzyme
a powerful protein which controls chemical reactions

faeces
waste product eliminated from the body. It is made up of water, inorganic salts, bacteria and decomposed bacteria, dead alimentary canal cells, indigestible food (e.g. vegetable fibres that cannot be broken down), digested food not absorbed, bile salts and pigments and mucus

formal communication
information passed following professional terms and guidelines

foster care
local people who provide a safe and caring environment for children and young people in their own homes

gaseous exchange
the exchange of gas that takes place at a respiratory surface

gene
the basic unit of heredity capable of transmitting characteristics from one generation to the next. It contains a specific sequence of DNA and RNA that occupies a fixed position on a chromosome

group communication
information passed among several people together

hair cell
a cell in the cochlea that is sensitive to sound waves

hazard
something which has the potential to cause harm

health care setting
a place where health care treatment is carried out, e.g. hospital, health care centre, dental surgery

hegemony
a controlling or dominating influence by one person or group over others

hoist
a piece of mechanical equipment usually with a body sling to transfer immobile individuals

holophrase
a one-word expression which conveys several meanings by changing sound and using gestures, used in the early stage of language development before telegraphic speech

homeostasis
a state of constant equilibrium within the body's internal environment

ideology
a meaningful system of social beliefs, ideas and values that are closely organised to form the basis of a social, economic or political philosophy

informal communication
information passed in a friendly or familiar manner

inhibit
to hinder, restrain or prevent an action occurring

interaction
communication between one or more people that involves a response and feedback which can be verbal or non-verbal or both

interpersonal skills
communication skills between people, e.g. using body language, verbal and non-verbal skills, awareness, empathy and understanding to maintain communication

invasive procedure
a medical intervention that enters the body, e.g inserting a urinary catheter

Irlen syndrome
(also known as scotopic sensitivity syndrome) a visual perceptual problem affecting the way the brain encodes and decodes visual information

jargon
the language used by a particular group, profession or culture, often in the form of an abbreviated short form for specific terms, phrases and words

keratin
a fibrous protein that is the main structural part of nails and hair

key people
significant people who provide and give care to service users, clients, patients, e.g. doctors, nurses, carers

kinship
a family or blood relationship, or a sharing of characteristics or origins

learning difficulty
a significant impairment in the ability to learn

lethargy
tiredness or fatigue

macrophage
a type of white blood cell whose function is to 'eat' or engulf bacteria or cell debris and by so doing destroy it or limit its ability to damage tissues

meconium
the sticky green substance secreted from a baby's bowels while in the uterus

medicalisation
the way in which medicine has increased its power within society. This includes the use of medical technology and the professional power of doctors to make decisions about social and ethical problems

menstrual cycle
a regular, approximately four-weekly cycle of changes that prepare the body for pregnancy

metaphor
something which is symbolic of something else

microscopic
extremely small and not visible to the eye. It can only be seen using a microscope

molecule
the smallest part of a substance that can exist independently, consisting of one or two atoms held together by chemical forces

Glossary

monogamous
having a relationship with one sexual partner during a period of time

mutation
a change in structure

neurotransmitter
a chemical that crosses the gap between neurones, allowing the electrical impulse to travel to the next neurone

non-verbal communication
ways of passing information that are not spoken, e.g. body language, gestures, written, typed media

numeracy
the knowledge of number and number operations

one-to-one
communicating with one other person only

oppression
harsh or unfair domination over another

organelle
a specialised structure within a cell, e.g. nucleus, mitochondria

organism
a living thing

ovulation
the release of an egg cell from an ovary

palate
the roof of the mouth, separating the cavities of the mouth and nose

palliative
pain relieving but not providing a cure

pathogen
a microorganism that can cause disease

patronise
to treat somebody as if he or she were less intelligent or knowledgeable than yourself

peer pressure
the influences that people of the same status or age have on each other

perception
the ability to become aware of something through the senses

person-centered approach
planning for care that places the service user at the centre of the process

phonemes
the units of sounds produced to make words, e.g. b-e-d (buh-eh-duh) equals bed

physiology
the science of body functioning

play therapy
structured play activities to help children who have suffered abuse

pluralism
the existence or tolerance in society of a number of different groups, such as ethnic or cultural groups, religious believers, political groups

polygamy
the practice of having more than one spouse at the same time. This is illegal in the UK and many other countries

predispose
to make someone liable or inclined to a specific attitude, action or condition

probability
the extent to which something is most probable or certain

procedure
an instruction to follow in a certain situation

proxemics
the study of social distance rules and personal body space used in interactions between people

psychological
to do with the mind and emotions

psychology
the study of the mind and emotions

reflex responses
actions performed without thinking in response to a stimulus, e.g. stimulation of a part of the body

reinforcement
the action of strengthening or supporting something (such as conditioning)

reminiscence
the act of remembering past experiences, e.g. childhood, people, places

residential child care
short, medium and long term placements for children and young people

respite care
a period of rest, or a break from caring for another person which enables the carer to recover from the physical and emotional demands of caring for someone who requires significant levels of support

ribosome
a cluster of proteins and RNA

risk
the possibility that something might be dangerous or harmful

RNA
(ribonucleic acid) a nucleic acid containing the sugar ribose found in all living cells and essential for the production of proteins according to the instructions carried by genes

self-image
a person's own view of themselves

service users
People that health and social care services help. They include patients and social care clients and their friends, families and carers.

semantics
the meaning of words and phrases

shivering
a series of involuntary muscular contraction and relaxation cycles creating movements that are usually small and repeated as a response to feeling cold. It is a short-term response by the body to raise the metabolic rate

short-term memory
the part of the memory that is available for short periods of time, e.g. the memory of a telephone number in the time it takes to dial the number

significant others
people who play an important role in one's life

slip sheet
a piece of nylon material used to slide a patient, usually on a bed, rather than lift them onto their side or into a sitting position

social care setting
a place where social care is carried out, e.g. day care centre, family centre, social service centre

social exclusion
being kept out of mainstream society due to poverty, poor housing, unemployment

socialisation
the process by which human behaviour is shaped through experience and being in different social situations. Through the socialisation individuals learn the values, beliefs, formal and informal rules or norms of the society in which they live

socio-economic disadvantage
a poorer quality of life due to unemployment, poverty, isolation

sociology
the study of the structure and functioning of human society

squint
a deviation in the direction of the gaze of one eye

statement
to produce a Statement of Special Educational Need, a legal document outlining a child's special educational needs and the provision to meet those needs

status
Position compared with others, e.g. sister, manager, chief inspector

stem cell
an unspecialised cell that gives rise to a specific specialised cell, such as a blood cell or nerve cell

stereotype
to view people as part of a particular group, based on perceived outward signs or characteristics

stigma
a sign of social unacceptability creating a sense of shame or disgrace

stigmatised
regarded as socially unacceptable or undesirable

stimulus
(plural, stimuli) something that encourages activity or interest

subservient
too eager to follow the wishes or orders of others

substance abuse
dependency on alcohol, drugs or illegal substances

syntax
the way words are put together to give meaning

synthesis
the process of combining different substances, elements together to create a new whole

telegraphic speech
two-word phrases, e.g. 'drink now', the next stage of language development after holophrases

terminal illness
a deteriorating condition that will lead to untimely death

therapeutic
having a beneficial effect on the body or mind

voluntary arrangement
an agreement entered into willingly, whereby parents allow their child to be cared for by the local authority

vulnerable adult
an individual who is in need of the care services by reason of mental or other disability, age or illness, and who is, or may be, unable to take care of themselves or protect themselves against significant harm or exploitation

vulva
the external opening of the vagina

Welfare Checklist
a reference point for the courts when considering any question relating to a child's upbringing

young offender
a person under the age of 18 years who is found guilty of criminal activity

Bibliography and suggested further reading

General

Books

T. Bruce & C. Meggitt, *Child Care and Education* (Hodder Arnold, 2006)

P. Crawford and P. Bonham, *Communication in Clinical Settings* (Nelson Thornes, 2007)

C. Hogg & K. Holland, *Cultural Awareness in Nursing and Healthcare* (Hodder Arnold, 2003)

J. Miller, *Care Practice for S/NVQ 3* (Hodder Arnold, 2003)

B. Myers and L. Shaw, *The Social Sciences* (Nelson Thornes, 2004)

Y. Nolan, *S/NVQ Level 3 Health and Social Care Candidate Handbook* (Heinemann, 2005)

Y. Nolan, *S/NVQ Level 3 Health and Social Care Candidate Book Option Plus* (Heinemann, 2006)

J. Richards, *Complete A–Z Health and Social Care Handbook* (Hodder Arnold, 2003)

B. Stretch, *Core Themes in Health and Social Care* (Heinemann, 2007)

B. Stretch and M Whitehouse, *BTEC National Health and Social Care Book 1* (Heinemann, 2007)

H. Thomson, C. Meggitt, S. Aslangul & V. O'Brien, *Further Studies for Health* (Hodder Arnold, 2002)

H. Thomson, C. Meggitt, S. Aslangul & V. O'Brien, *Further Studies for Social Care* (Hodder Arnold, 2002)

M. Walsh, P. Stephens, M. Billingham, M. Crittenden, A. Thomson & D. Thomson, *Health and Social Care A2* (Collins, 2006)

Journals

Care and Health
Community Care
Health Service Journal
Nursing Times

Websites

www.basw.co.uk
  British Association of Social Workers
www.bbc.co.uk
  BBC
www.bmjjournal.com
  British Medical Journal
www.careknowledge.com
  Care Knowledge
www.community-care.co.uk
  Community Care
www.dh.gov.uk
  Department of Health
www.dss.gov.uk
  Department of Social Security
www.eoc.org.uk
  Equal Opportunities Commission
www.guardian.co.uk
  Guardian newspaper
www.hse.gov.uk
  Health and Safety Executive

www.imagesofdisability.gov.uk
  Images of Disability (Department of Work and Pensions initiative)
www.lsc.gov.uk
  Learning and Skills Council
www.ncb.co.uk
  National Children's Bureau
www.nursingtimes.net
  Nursing Times
www.onlineclassroom.tv
  online learning resource
www.parliament.uk
  UK Parliament
www.rightsnet.org.uk
  welfare rights for advice workers
ww.scie.org.uk
  Social Care Institute for Excellence
www.scils.co.uk
  Social Care Information and Learning Service
www.skillsforcareanddevelopment.org.uk
  Sector Skills Council for Care and Development
www.skillsforhealth.org.uk
  Sector Skills Council for Health
www.statistics.gov.uk
  Government statistics resource
www.who.int
  World Health Organization

Unit 1

Books

R.B. Adler, L.B. Rosenfeld, R.F. Proctor *Interplay: The Process of Interpersonal Communication* (Oxford University Press, 2003)

E.T. Hall, *The Hidden Dimension.* (Anchor Books Edition, 1990)

C. Petersen, S.F. Maier, M.E.P. Seligman, *Learned Helplessness: A Theory for the Age of Personal Control* (Oxford University Press, 1995)

Unit 2

Books

P. Clements & J. Jones, *The Diversity Training Handbook: A Practical Guide to Understanding and Changing Attitudes* (Kogan Page, 2002)

H. Malik, *A Practical Guide to Equal Opportunities* (Nelson Thornes, 2003)

N. Moonie, *Diversity and Rights in Care* (Heinemann, 2004)

N. Roper, N. Logan, & A. Tierney, *Using a Model for Nursing* (Churchill Livingstone, 1983)

E. Thomas, *What about Me? An Equal Opportunities Support Pack* (HLB Associates, 2003)

Websites

www.bcodp.org.uk
  British Council for Disabled People

www.kingsfund.org.uk
    The King's Fund
www.rnib.org.uk
    Royal National Institute of the Blind
www.rnid.org.uk
    Royal National Institute for Deaf People

Other

Department of Health, *Change Your Mindset* (DoH, 2003)
an activity pack for youth groups about discrimination and mental
    health, available from www.mindout.net

Unit 3

Books

G. A. Owen, *HACCP Works* (Highfield Publications, 2005)
R. Sprenger *The Foundation HACCP Handbook* (Highfield Publications)
R. Sprenger and I. Fisher, *The Essentials of Health and Safety (Carers)*
    (Highfield Publications)

Leaflets

Five steps to risk assessment (HSE Publications)
Health and Safety Law: What you should know (HSE Publications)

Websites

www.bohs.org
    British Occupational Hygiene Society
www.ccwales.org.uk
    Care Council for Wales
www.foodstandards.gov.uk
    Food Standards Agency
www.hsebooks.co.uk
    Health and Safety Executive Books
www.lshtm.ac.uk
    London School of Hygiene and Tropical Medicine
www.niscc.info
    Northern Ireland Social Care Council

Unit 4

Books

E. Cumming & W. E. Henry, *Growing Old* (Basic Books, 1961)
E. Kübler-Ross, *On Death & Dying* (Macmillan, 1969)
B. W. Lemon, V. L Bengston, J. A. Peterson, *An exploration of the
    activity theory of ageing* (Journal of Gerontology, 27 (4), 1972)
J. Lindon, *Understanding Child Development* (Hodder Arnold, 2005)
C. Meggitt, *Child Development: An Illustrated Guide* (Heinemann, 2006)
P. Minett, *Child Care and Development* (Hodder Arnold, 2005)
J. Richards, *Caring for People: A Lifespan Approach* (Nelson Thornes,
    1999)

Journals

Child Care, Health and Development

Unit 5

Books

J. Clancy & A. McVicar, *Physiology and Anatomy: A Homeostatic
    Approach* (Hodder Arnold, 2002)

B. Myers, *The Natural Sciences* (Nelson Thornes, 2004)
L. Shaw, *Anatomy and Physiology* (Nelson Thornes, 2004)
J. Ward, R. W. Clark and R. Linden, *Physiology at a Glance* (Blackwell
    Publishing, 2005)

Journals

Biological Science
New Scientist

Websites

www.bbc.co.uk/science/humanbody
    BBC resource pages on the human body and mind

Unit 6

Books

J. Bell, *Doing your Research Project* (Open University Press, 2005).
Department for Education and Skills, *Skills for Life, Teacher's Reference
    Pack, Social Care* (DfES)
G. Gibbs, *Learning by Doing. A Guide to Teaching and Learning Methods*
    (Further Education Unit, Oxford Polytechnic, 1988)
P. Honey & A. Mumford, *The Manual of Learning Styles* (Peter Honey,
    1992, 1986).
M. Jasper, *Beginning Reflective Practice* (Nelson Thornes, 2003)
D. A. Kolb, *Learning Style Inventory: Technical Manual* (McBer and
    Company, 1976).
P. Race, *Making Learning Happen* (Paul Chapman, Publishing, 2005)
D. Schön, *The Reflective Practitioner: How Professionals Think in Action*
    (Basic Books, 1983)

Websites

www.csci.org.uk
    Commission for Social Care Inspection

Unit 7

Books

P. Aspinall & B. Jacobson, *Ethnic Disparities in Health and Health Care:
    A Focused Review of the Evidence and Selected Examples of Good
    Practice* (London Health Observatory, 2004)
A. Barry & C. Yuill, *Understanding Health, a Sociological Introduction*
    (Saga Publications, 2005)
M. Blaxter, *Health and Lifestyles* (Routledge, 1990)
K. Brown, *Introductory Sociology for AS Level* (Polity Pres, 2002)
E. Durkheim, *The Division of Labor in Society*, translated by George
    Simpson (The Free Press, 1947)
S. Earle, *Sociology for Nurses* (Polity Press, 2003)
E. Goffman, *Asylums* (Penguin, 1968)
I. Illich, *Limits to Medicine* (Calder and Boyars, 1976)
M. Marmot, *Social Determinants of Health* (Oxford University Press,
    2005)
K. Marx, *Capital: An Abridged Edition* (Oxford University Press, 1999)
K. Marx & F. Engels, *The Communist Manifesto* (Penguin, 1981)
G. H. Mead, *Mind, Self and Society* (University of Chicago Press, 1934
    & 1962)
G. Murdock, *Social Structure* (Macmillan, 1949)
J. Naidoo & J. Wills, *Health Studies* (Palgrave, 2001)
S. Nettleton, *The Sociology of Health and Illness* (Polity Press, 2006)
D. Pilgrim, *Mental Health and Illness* (Palgrave Macmillan, 2002)
M. Senior & B. Viveash, *Health and Illness* (Palgrave, 1998)

G. Davey Smith, *Health Inequalities: Life Course Approaches* (The Policy Press, 2003)

K. Tudor, *Mental Health Promotion: Paradigms and Practice* (Routledge, 1996).

M. Whitehead, P. Townsend & N. Davidson, *Inequalities in Health: The Black Report and The Health Divide* (Penguin, 1992)

R. Wilkson, *The Impact of Inequality: How to Make Sick Societies Healthier* (Routledge, 2005)

Journals

Politics Review
Sociology Review

Articles

H. Graham, 'Women's Smoking and Family Health' *Social Science and Medicine*, 25 (1987), 47–56

Websites

www.adviceguide.org.uk
  Citizens Advice Bureau
www.intute.ac.uk/socialsciences
  Free social sciences resource

Unit 8

Books

A. Bandura, *Social Learning Theory* (Prentice-Hall, 1977)

C. Brain, *Advanced Subsidiary Psychology Approaches and Methods* (Nelson Thornes, 2007)

M. Donaldson, *Children's Minds* (Fontana, 1984)

E. Erikson, *Childhood and Society* (Vintage, 1950)

S. Freud, *Collected Papers* (Vol 11) (Hogarth, 1914)

A. Gesell, F. L. Ilg & L. B. Ames, *Infant and Child in the Culture of Today* (Harper Collins, 1974)

A. Gesell, F. L. Ilg & L. B. Ames, *The Child from Five to Ten* (Harper Collins, 1977)

S. W. Kelly, S. Griffiths & U. Frith, *Evidence for Implicit Sequence Learning in Dyslexia* (John Wiley & Sons, 2002)

C. Rogers, *Client-Centred Therapy: Its Current Practice, Implications and Theory* (Constable, 1951)

C. Rogers, *On Becoming a Person: A Therapist's View of Psychotherapy* (Constable, 1961).

J. Russell, *Introduction to Psychology for Health Carers* (Nelson Thornes, 2005)

M. Sheridan, M. Frost & A. Sharma, *From Birth to Five Years: Children's Developmental Progress* (4th Ed) (Routledge, 1997)

B. F. Skinner, *About Behaviorism* (Vintage, 1976)

B. Tizard & M. Hughes, *Young Children Learning* (2nd Ed) (Blackwell 2003)

J. Watson, *Behaviorism* (Norton, 1930)

Unit 10

Books

J. Barker, *The Child in Mind: a Child Protection Handbook* (Routledge, 2004)

C. Beckett, *Child Protection: an Introduction* (Sage, 2003)

H. Ferguson, *Protecting Children in Time: Child Abuse, Child Protection and the Consequences of Modernity* (Palgrave Macmillan, 2004)

J. Fowler, *A Practitioner's Tool for Child Protection and the Assessment of Parents* (Jessica Kingsley, 2002)

R. Gardener, *Supporting Families: Child Protection in the Community* (Wiley, 2005)

C. Hobart & J. Frankel, *Good Practice in Child Protection* (Stanley Thornes Publishers)

C. Karp & T. Butler, *Treatment Strategies for Abused Children* (Sage, 1996)

V. Makins *The Invisible Children: Nipping Failure in the Bud* (David Fulton, 1997)

P. Tassoni, *BTEC National Early Years* (2nd Ed) (Heinemann, 2006)

P. Trevethick, *Social Work Skills* (Open University Press, 2000)

Websites

www.baaf.org.uk
  British Association of Adoption and Fostering
www.childpolicy.org.uk
  Four Nations Child Policy Network
www.dfes.gov.uk/rsgateway
  National statistics bulletin
www.dhsspsni.gov.uk/publications/2003
  Children Order statistics
www.everychildmatters.gov.uk
www.jrf.org.uk
  Joseph Rowntree Foundation
www.lgdu-wales.gov.uk/eng/project
  Social Services statistics Wales
www.nspcc.org.uk
  National Society for the Prevention of Cruelty to Children
www.savethechildren.org.uk
  Save the Children

Reports

People like us; The Report of the Review of Safeguards for Children Living Away From Home (The Stationery Office, 1997)

A Better Education for Children in Care (Social Exclusion Unit, Office of the Deputy Prime Minister, September, 2003)

Unit 11

Books

J. Hendrick, *Law and Ethics* (Nelson Thornes, 2004)

Index